NATIVE AMERICAN HERBALIST'S BIBLE

13 in 1. Ancient Herbal Remedies & Medicinal Plants to Heal Naturally and Improve Your Wellness. A Modern Herbal Dispensatory to Build Your Apothecary Table

Ashley Ahoka

Copyright ©2025 by Ashley Ahoka. All rights reserved.
Native American Herbalist's Bible

All rights reserved

*Copyright ©2025 by **Ashley Ahoka**. All rights reserved.*

This document is geared towards providing exact and reliable information in regard to the topic and issue covered.

From a Declaration of Principles which was accepted and approved equally by a Committee of the American Bar Association and a Committee of Publishers and Associations.

In no way is it legal to reproduce, duplicate, or transmit any part of this document in either electronic means or in printed format. All rights reserved.

The information provided herein is stated to be truthful and consistent, in that any liability, in terms of inattention or otherwise, by any usage or abuse of any policies, processes, or directions contained within is the solitary and utter responsibility of the recipient reader. Under no circumstances will any legal responsibility or blame be held against the publisher for any reparation, damages, or monetary loss due to the information herein, either directly or indirectly.

Respective authors own all copyrights not held by the publisher.

The information herein is offered for informational purposes solely and is universal as so. The presentation of the information is without contract or any type of guarantee assurance.

The trademarks that are used are without any consent, and the publication of the trademark is without permission or backing by the trademark owner. All trademarks and brands within this book are for clarifying purposes only and are owned by the owners themselves, not affiliated with this document.

*All rights reserved by **Ashley Ahoka***

Table of Contents

BOOK 1: NATIVE AMERICAN HEALING HERBS 21

INTRODUCTION 22

NATIVE AMERICAN HEALING HERBS OVERVIEW 23

    HISTORY OF NATIVE AMERICAN HERBALISM 23

    FUNDAMENTALS OF NATIVE AMERICAN HERBALISM 25

NATIVE AMERICAN HERBS 27

HERBAL REMEDIES BENEFITS 31

NATIVE AMERICAN MEDICINE TODAY 32

    NATIVE AMERICAN HERBALISM IN MODERN TIMES 32

CONCLUSION 34

BOOK 2: NATIVE AMERICAN SPIRITUALITY 35

INTRODUCTION 36

THE ROLE OF RELIGION AND SPIRITUALITY 38

    SPIRITUALITY AND CONNECTION 38

    HEALING AND KINDNESS 40

    SPIRITUALITY AND RELIGION 41

    NATIVE AMERICAN RELATIONSHIP WITH NATURE 42

NATIVE AMERICAN HEALERS 43

DREAM CATCHERS AMONG NATIVE AMERICANS 46

NATIVE AMERICAN TRADITIONAL HEALING RITUALS AND CEREMONIALS 47

    POW WOW 48

    MUSIC: DANCE, DRUM, FLUTE 48

    SMUDGING 49

    STORY-TELLING 49

    INIPI/SWEAT LODGE 49

THE DANCES 51

OTHER CEREMONIES 55

    PAINTING THE BODY OF A NATIVE AMERICAN 55

  Pipes of Peace for Native Americans 55

  Totems and Animal Medicine in Native American Culture 57

CONCLUSION 59

BOOK 3: HERBALISM ENCYCLOPEDIA VOL. 1 62

INTRODUCTION 63

THE TWELVE CATEGORIES OF HERBS 64

NATIVE AMERICAN HERBS 68

  Agave 68

  Alder 68

  Alfalfa 69

  Aloe Vera 70

  Angelica 70

  Arsemart 71

  Amaranth 72

  American Licorice 72

  American Mistletoe 73

  American Raspberry 74

  Arnica 74

  Arrowwood 75

  Ashwagandha 76

  Aspen 76

  Balsam Fir 77

  Balsam Poplar 78

  Balsam Root 78

  Black Alder 79

  Blueberry 79

  Black Locust 80

  Black Walnut 81

  Blazing Star 81

  Boneset 82

  Borage 82

  Buckthorn 83

  Buffaloberry 84

  Burdocks 85

- California Poppy ... 85
- Catnip ... 86
- Cattail ... 86
- Chamomile ... 87
- Corn ... 88
- Candle Bush ... 88
- Cat's Claw ... 89
- Chaga ... 90
- Chaparral ... 90
- Chicory ... 91
- Cow Parsnip ... 91
- Cranberry ... 92
- Dandelion ... 92
- Devil's Club ... 93
- Echinacea ... 93
- Elderberry ... 94
- Evening Primrose ... 95
- False Unicorn ... 95
- Fendlerbush ... 96
- Feverfew ... 96
- Geranium ... 97
- Ginseng ... 97
- Hawthorn ... 98

HERBAL ALPHABETIC INDEX ... 99

CONCLUSION ... 100

BOOK 4: HERBALISM ENCYCLOPEDIA VOL. 2 ... 101

INTRODUCTION ... 102

TIPS FOR USING NATIVE AMERICAN HERBS SAFELY ... 104

NATIVE AMERICAN HERBS ... 106

- Honeysuckle ... 106
- Hops ... 106
- Horsetail ... 107
- Hyssop ... 107

Ironwood	108
Juniper	108
Lady's Slipper	109
Larch	109
Lemon Balm	110
Licorice (Wild American)	111
Mayapple	111
Milkweed	112
Mullein	112
Mexican Yew	113
Mint	114
Nettle	114
Oak	115
Oregon Grape	115
Oshà	116
Partridge Berry	117
Pasque Flower	117
Passionflower	118
Plantain	119
Prickly Pear	119
Queen of Meadow	120
Red Clover	120
Sagebrush	121
Sassafras	122
Saint John's Wort	122
Sarsaparilla	123
Saw Palmetto	124
Skullcap	124
Skunk Cabbage	125
Slippery Elm	125
Sumac	126
Tobacco	127
Toothwort	127
Turtlehead	128
Usnea	128

Valerian	129
Verbena	130
Water Birch	130
Watercress	131
Wild Yam	131
Willow	132
Witch Hazel	132
Yarrow	133
Yellow Dock	133
Yew	134
Yucca	135

HERBAL ALPHABETIC INDEX ... 136

CONCLUSION ... 137

BOOK 5: HERBAL APOTHECARY ... 138

INTRODUCTION ... 139

ALLERGIES ... 141

How to Know If You Are Allergic To Plants ... 141
Always Try Small Quantities First ... 142
Be Aware of the Herbs' Potential Side Effects ... 143

REMEDIES TO TREAT THE MOST COMMON ILLNESSES AND PAINS (80-100 RECIPES) ... 144

Digestive System ... 144
- *Bloating* ... 144
- *Constipation* ... 145
- *Heartburn* ... 146
- *Indigestion* ... 147

Cardiovascular System ... 148
- *Anemia* ... 148
- *Bruise* ... 150

Respiratory System ... 151
- *Asthma* ... 151
- *Bronchitis* ... 152
- *Cough and Cold* ... 153

Nervous System ... 155

- *Headache* *155*
- *Insomnia* *157*
- *Stress* *158*

EXCRETORY SYSTEM *159*
- *Uremia* *159*
- *Kidney Stones* *159*
- *Oedema* *160*

SKELETAL SYSTEM *160*
- *Abscess* *160*
- *Backache* *161*

MUSCULAR SYSTEM *162*
- *Sprains and Strains* *162*

ENDOCRINE SYSTEM *163*
- *Body Odor* *163*
- *Chapped Lips* *163*
- *Menopause* *164*
- *Irregular Menstrual Cycle* *164*

IMMUNE SYSTEM *165*
- *Cold Sores* *165*
- *Fever* *165*
- *Gingivitis* *167*
- *Hangover* *169*
- *Immune System Boosters* *171*

INTEGUMENTARY SYSTEM *172*
- *Acne* *172*
- *Allergies* *173*
- *Athlete's Foot* *174*
- *Bee Sting* *175*
- *Burns* *176*
- *Rashes* *177*

LYMPHATIC SYSTEM *178*
- *Fibrocystic Breasts* *178*
- *Swelling* *179*

REPRODUCTIVE SYSTEM *179*
- *Erectile Dysfunction* *179*
- *Menstrual Cramps* *179*

RECIPES ALPHABETIC INDEX 183

CONCLUSION 184

BOOK 6: HERBAL DISPENSATORY VOL. 1 185

INTRODUCTION 186

GETTING STARTED 187

START YOUR HOME APOTHECARY 188

    ESSENTIAL TOOLS 188

    APOTHECARY SUPPLIES FOR THE HOME 190

    PREPARATIONS OF NATIVE AMERICAN HERBS 191

    HERBAL PREPARATIONS 191

HOW TO GET HERBS 194

    BUYING HERBS 194

        Purchasing Herbs from the Grocery Store 194

        Purchasing Herbs from a Nursery 194

        Purchasing Herbs from the Farmers Market 194

        Wild/Foraged Herbs 195

        Buying Herbs Online 195

    GROWING HERBS IN OUR GARDEN 195

        Herbs Grown from Seeds 195

        Herbs Propagated Through Cuttings 196

        Herb Division for Propagation 196

    WILD CRAFTING 197

        Benefits Of Wild Crafting 197

        Tips for Wild Crafting Herbs 197

SAFETY TIPS AND ABUSE OF HERBS 200

    SAFETY TIPS WHEN USING NATIVE AMERICAN HERBS 200

    ABUSE OF NATIVE AMERICAN HERBS 203

CONCLUSION 205

BOOK 7: HERBAL DISPENSATORY VOL. 2 206

INTRODUCTION 207

PREPARATIONS OF REMEDIES USING FRESH HERBS 208

    EQUIPMENT NEEDED 208

HARVESTING: STEP BY STEP GUIDE 209

DRYING: STEP BY STEP GUIDE 210

METHODS TO DRY HERBS 210

REMEDIES PREPARATION USING DRIED HERBS 212

EQUIPMENT NEEDED 212

QUALITY CONTROL ISSUES WHEN BUYING DRIED HERBS 213

CAPSULES 213

TABLETS 213

NUT BUTTER BALLS 214

REMEDIES PREPARATIONS MAKING EXTRACTION 216

WATER-BASED EXTRACTIONS 216

Infusions 216

Decoctions 216

Syrups 217

ALCOHOL EXTRACTIONS 217

Tinctures 218

Dried Herbs Tinctures (Macerations) 218

Fresh Plant Tinctures (Macerations) 218

GLYCERIN EXTRACTS (GLYCERITES) 219

How Glycerites Are Made 219

Seales Simmer 219

EXTRACTING IN VINEGAR 219

TOPICAL PREPARATIONS 221

WHAT IS A TOPICAL PREPARATION? 221

OIL-BASED HERBAL PREPARATION 221

LOCAL APPLICATIONS 222

OTHER APPLICATIONS 222

HOW TO STORE HERBS AND KEEP THEM SAFE 224

DIFFERENT METHODS OF STORAGE 225

Drying 225

Freezing 226

Extracting or Tincturing 226

Infusions of Herbs 226

Canning 226

Herbal Butter 227

CONCLUSION 228

BOOK 8: HERBAL REMEDIES FOR CHILDREN 229

INTRODUCTION 230

15 HERBS PERFECT FOR YOUR CHILDREN'S HEALTH 233

HERBAL REMEDIES FOR CHILDREN OF 0-2 MONTHS 240

GRIPE WATER 240

HOMEMADE POWDER FOR THE SOFT SKIN OF NEWBORN 240

YARROW RECIPE FOR BABIES 240

HERBAL REMEDIES FOR CHILDREN OF 2-12 MONTHS 240

CREAMSICLE BATH 241

HERBAL BATH 241

REMEDY FOR TEETHING 241

BABY POWDER 241

HERBAL REMEDIES FOR CHILDREN OF 12 MONTHS-5 YEARS 242

ROSY ROLL-ON 242

LEG ROLLER 242

YOGA GROUND INHALER 242

PALMAROSA CALMING AROMA 242

HERBAL REMEDIES FOR CHILDREN OF 5 YEARS TO 12 YEARS 243

CARROT PUREE 243

APPLE NUTMEG 243

PEAR-NUTMEG PUREE 243

COLIC 243

EAR ACHES 244

FEVERS 244

LEMON BATH 244

BABY LOTION 244

CONCLUSION 245

BOOK 9: EVERYDAY HERBAL REMEDIES 246

INTRODUCTION 247
BEST COMMON DIY HERBAL TEA RECIPES 248
Juniper Tea 248
Mint Tea 248
Honey Drink 249
Apricot Tea 249
Sassafras Tea 249
Medicinal Pine Needle Tea 249
Burdock Root Tea 250
Lung Tea 250
Hawthorn Tea 250
Buck Brush Tea 251

DIY PERSONAL CARE HERBAL RECIPES 252
Yucca Shampoo 252
Wild Rose Toner 253
Honey Face Mask 254
Aloe Vera and Almond Oil Face Mask 254
Coffee and Turmeric Face Mask 255

DIY HERBAL REMEDIES FOR PETS 256
Treatment for Fleas 256
Flea Treatment with a Body Bath 256
Diarrhea 256
Catnip and Sienna Tea for Diarrhea in Pets 256
Animal Injuries 256
Hyssop Poultice for Pet Injuries 256
Coughing in Animals 256
Elecampane Root Tea for Cough in Dogs and Cats 257

HOME HERBAL RECIPES 258
Mold Production on The Ceiling 258
Garlic and Thyme Compress to Prevent Mold Growth on Walls and Ceilings 258
Keeping Lizards Away 258
Keeping Lizards Away from Your Home with Black Pepper and Coffee Balls 258
Mosquitoes in the House 258

- *Lavender and Lemongrass Candles for Mosquito Repellent in the Home* 258
- KILLING BUGS 259
  - *Bug Spray with Witch Hazel, Peppermint, Spearmint, Lavender, and Lemongrass* 259

CONCLUSION 260

BOOK 10: ESSENTIAL OILS 261

INTRODUCTION 262

ESSENTIAL OILS. THE HISTORY 263

INTRODUCING ESSENTIAL OILS THERAPY 267
- HOW DO ESSENTIAL OILS WORK? 267
- WHAT ARE ESSENTIAL OILS USED FOR? 267
- AROMATHERAPY AND FLOWER ESSENCES 268
- ESSENTIAL OIL SAFETY 269
- AROMATHERAPY ESSENTIAL OIL SAFETY TIPS 270
- SOME SAFETY TIPS TO NOTE BEFORE BUYING ESSENTIAL OILS 271

HOW TO PREPARE ESSENTIAL OILS DIY 274
- STILL OR STEAM DISTILLATION METHOD OF EXTRACTING ESSENTIAL OILS 274
- ALTERNATIVE METHODS OF EXTRACTING ESSENTIAL OILS 275
- THE PROCESS OF BLENDING DIFFERENT ESSENTIAL OILS 276
  - *Formulating the Blend* 276
  - *Diluting the Essential Oil Blends* 277
  - *Finish the Essential Oil Blend* 278

ESSENTIAL OILS BENEFITS 280
- HEALING 280
- PAIN RELIEF 280
- REDUCING INFLAMMATION 280
- ANTISEPTIC 280
- STRESS RELIEF 280

USING ESSENTIAL OILS 282
- DILUTING OILS 282
- TOPICAL USE 282
- DIFFUSION 283
- INHALATION 283

- INTERNAL USE 283

7 MUST-KNOW ESSENTIAL OILS REMEDIES 285

- ANTI-ALLERGEN ESSENTIAL OIL 285
- ESSENTIAL OIL FOR ARTHRITIS 285
- BODY PAIN RELIEF OIL 286
- MINTY OIL FOR SWELLING 286
- ESSENTIAL OIL FOR MENSTRUAL PAIN 286
- ESSENTIAL OIL FOR HEADACHE 287
- ESSENTIAL OIL FOR COUGHS 287

CONCLUSION 288

BOOK 11: HERB GARDENING FOR BEGINNERS 290

INTRODUCTION 291

SIMPLY HERBS 292

ANNUAL, BIENNIAL, AND PERENNIAL HERBS 293

HOW TO PLANT IN YOUR GARDEN 294

- ESSENTIAL TOOLS 295
- STEP-BY-STEP GUIDE 297
  - *Choosing Your Herbs* 297
  - *Garden Size* 298
  - *Finding the Best Location for Your Plants* 298
  - *Designing Your Garden* 298
  - *Fertilizers* 299
  - *Determining If You Need a Greenhouse* 299

HOW TO PLANT HERBS IN A CONTAINER 300

- WHAT DO I NEED FOR CONTAINER HERB GARDENING? 301
- WHAT ABOUT THE SOIL? 302
- THE SEEDS AND THE PLANTS 303

HARVESTING 304

- HOW TO HARVEST 304
- WAYS TO HARVEST HERBS 304
- HOW MUCH TO HARVEST AND WHEN TO HARVEST 305
- TOOLS NEEDED 306

METHODS IN HARVESTING HERBS 307

7 HERBS TO GROW AT HOME 308

ROSEMARY 308

BASIL 308

GINGER 308

GARLIC 308

THYME 309

PEPPERMINT 309

OREGANO 309

BENEFITS OF SELF-CULTIVATION OF MEDICINAL PLANTS 310

CONCLUSION 312

BOOK 12: FORAGING WILD EDIBLE PLANTS 314

INTRODUCTION 315

FORAGING 316

WHAT IS A FORAGER? 317

WHAT ARE WILD EDIBLES? 318

THE FUNDAMENTALS OF FORAGING 320

ETHICAL FORAGING 320

SAFE FORAGE 320

BEGINNER FORAGERS' GUIDE TO BASIC RULES 320

FORAGING TIPS 321

TOOLS FOR FORAGING 322

Picking Tools 322

Knives 322

Storage Containers 322

First Aid Kits 322

Water and Rags 322

Illustrated Books 323

Sun Protection 323

Magnifying Glass 323

Proper Clothing 323

Snacks 323

WILD EDIBLES 324

BEST WILD EDIBLES AND HOW TO GATHER THEM IN WINTER 324
- *Big Leaf Maple* 324
- *Bittercress* 324
- *Crab Apples* 324
- *Peppergrass* 325
- *Siberian Miner's Lettuce* 325

BEST WILD EDIBLES AND HOW TO GATHER THEM IN SPRING 326
- *Asparagus* 326
- *Blue Camas* 326
- *Catnip* 326
- *Common Plantain* 327
- *Mustard* 327
- *Sheep Sorrel* 327
- *Wild Ginger* 327
- *Wild Strawberry* 328
- *Yarrow* 328

BEST WILD EDIBLES AND HOW TO GATHER THEM IN AUTUMN 329
- *Arrowhead* 329
- *Black Hawthorn* 329
- *Bog Cranberry* 329
- *Evergreen Huckleberry* 329
- *Hazelnut* 330
- *Jerusalem Artichoke* 330
- *Juniper* 330
- *Oregon Grape* 330
- *Silverweed* 331
- *Springbank Clover* 331
- *Milk Thistle* 331
- *Wild Licorice* 331

BEST WILD EDIBLES AND HOW TO GATHER THEM IN SUMMER 332
- *Chokecherry* 332
- *Cloudberry* 332
- *Coastal Black Gooseberry* 332
- *Oval Leaf Blueberry* 332
- *Pearly Everlasting* 333

Pipsissewa 333

Red Currant 333

Salmonberry 333

Yerba Buena 334

CONCLUSION 335

BOOK 13: ROSEMARY BASIL AND THYME BEST RECIPES 336

INTRODUCTION 337

ROSEMARY 337

BASIL 337

THYME 338

10 ROSEMARY RECIPES 339

BEST RECIPES AS A MEDICINE 339

Rosemary Oil 339

Rosemary Tincture 339

Rosemary Tea 339

Rosemary Salve 339

Orange Rosemary Salt Scrub 340

BEST RECIPES FOR THE HOME 340

Rosemary Shampoo Bar 340

Rosemary Pest Deterrent 340

Rosemary Tooth Paste 340

Rosemary Conditioner 341

Rosemary Toner 341

10 BASIL RECIPES 342

BEST RECIPES AS A MEDICINE 342

Fresh Basil Steam For Congestion 342

Basil Essential Oil 342

Basil and Honey Tea For Digestion 342

Simple Basil Tea For Cough 342

Basil Vinegar For Warm Bath 342

BEST RECIPES FOR THE HOME 343

Basil Hair Oil 343

Basil Perfume 343

Basil Based Insect Repellent 343

- *Unclogging Steam Bath* *344*
- *Basil Salt* *344*

10 THYME RECIPES **346**

BEST RECIPES AS A MEDICINE 346

- *Thyme Essential Oil* *346*
- *Thyme, Ginger, Garlic, and Mint Tea for Tonsillitis* *346*
- *Thyme Tea* *346*
- *Honey Thyme Cough Syrup* *346*
- *Thyme Tincture* *346*

BEST RECIPES FOR THE HOME 347

- *Thyme Based Repellent for Mosquitoes* *347*
- *Thyme Based Mouthwash* *347*
- *Thyme Disinfectant* *347*
- *Homemade Thyme Insect Repellant* *348*
- *Frozen Thyme Cubes* *348*

CONCLUSION **349**

BOOK 1: NATIVE AMERICAN HEALING HERBS

Introduction

Native American medicine is a broad field with many varied techniques and practices. Some of these medicines and practices have been passed down within families for generations, while others are shared openly with the community. Indigenous people in North America may not have had formalized methods of diagnosis or treatment, but they did have an extensive knowledge of medicinal plants that could be found nearby or gathered from local markets. For example, the Cherokee people use black walnut hulls to treat cystitis; white oak bark to make a sweat tea for colds; and burdock root for inflammation.

Native American herbalism has been adopted into the practices of modern Western herbalism in different ways. Some of these plant medicines were discovered by European settlers and then adopted by whites. Others were adopted into Western culture with formal medical practices, such as the use of Red Clover (traditionally used for respiratory ailments) with regular honey treatments for TB. Modern herbalists also learn about the historical uses of various medicinal plants from Native Americans, including dandelion (bitter tonic), milkweed (diuretic), wood sorrel (astringent), and elderberry (digestive).

Much like the plants themselves, Native American practitioners are varied in their approach to healing. Some Native American medicine men and women use prayers to ask the Great Spirit to heal those in their care. Others seek to let the body heal itself by avoiding medical treatment or using minimal medicines. Some, like Black Elk (an Oglala Sioux healer), combine these two approaches.

Diseases believed to be caused by witchcraft can be treated using traditional Native American medicines, such as burning juniper smoke (to clear poison from the air) or giving tobacco water (to eliminate bad medicine). Still other ailments are treated through sweat lodges, massage, and music. Sweat lodges are used for a number of reasons: as a social gathering place; as an aid in healing; or as part of spiritual purification ceremonies. Massage helps circulation of blood and lymph, relieves musculoskeletal tension, and improves the immune system. Music is used as a way to help medicine penetrate deeper or work more quickly. Other forms of treatment include medicated steam baths, which are used for muscle pain or respiratory problems; hot rocks that are placed on the body to stimulate it; or medicinal teas that can be drunk to improve health.

Some plants have a long history of use in Western herbalism prior to their discovery by Native Americans. Such is the case with Echinacea (purple coneflower), which has been used since at least 1776 in Europe for its supposed ability to cure colds. However, Native Americans had been using the herb for years prior to that. The Sioux believed it could be used to treat snakebites and even smallpox.

Many Western herbalists praise the healing properties of plants used by Native Americans, but they are quick to add that these plants also can be toxic. For example, both lobelia and ephedra have powerful effects on heart rate and blood pressure, which can make them extremely dangerous if not properly used.

Native American Healing Herbs Overview

History of Native American Herbalism

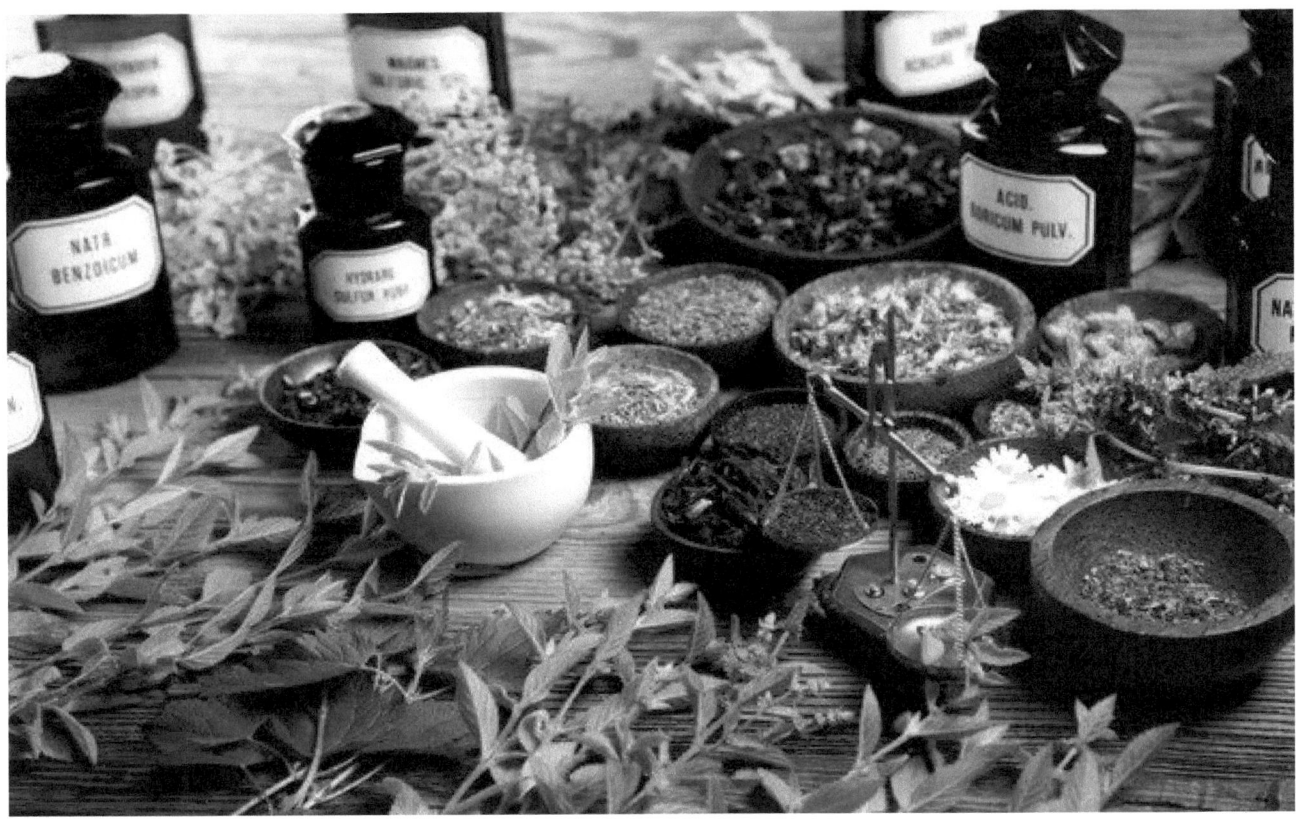

With over 2000 indigenous tribes in North America, it should come as no surprise that there is a rich history behind Native American herbalism. Each tribe has contributed its own touch to healing practices, which vary from tribe to tribe and region to region. The natives live off of the land and even today, many Natives retain a rich history and closeness to their ancestral ways.

There is no one standard of healing that all tribes follow. However, most shared a belief that the physical health of an individual was directly related to their spiritual strength and health. Health was a perfect combination of physical, spiritual, and mental wellness. When that harmony was achieved and maintained, then sickness would be kept at bay.

When someone would get ill, it was believed that it was directly related to thoughts and actions, which would have consequences. By restoring harmony of body, mind, and spirit, health could be restored as well. In healing the body, mind, and spirit, often the indigenous people turned to herbal remedies. Medicinal plants and herbs were a way of assuaging the physical pains and ailments while also creating harmony with the spirit.

The practices have been developed and passed down orally, like much of Native American history. However, their methods were effective. As European settlers arrived in what is now the United States, they were shocked to find that many of the illnesses and injuries that would be deemed fatal by their standards were healed with the Native American medicinal practices. However, many of the diseases that were unique to the settlers spread like wildfire, killing thousands of Native Americans as measles, smallpox, and the like were introduced for the first time.

Prior to 1900, Native Americans relied on their medicine people, trained in their medicinal ways, to heal and care for injuries and illnesses of their people. However, slowly over the 20th century, hospitals and clinics were opened and modern medicine was introduced. Especially for "white-man" diseases, the diseases brought from Europe that the natives had no cure for, were treated in these clinics.

However, despite the shift toward modern medicine, a swing toward the traditional and a deep-seated need to reconnect with ancestry has encouraged the revival and popularization of many Native American practices. Natives and non-natives alike have taken an interest in natural treatments for ailments that may usually be treated with medication. Due to a concern with toxicity and side effects associated with medications, more and more are interested in holistic, herbal treatments that many times are quite effective.

Many times, herbal remedies are perfectly effective at treating all sorts of ailments. There is little reason to medicate when herbal treatments can cure many illnesses, ailments, and diseases with fewer side effects. The world around us has provided us with several natural options that bring us closer to nature.

Native American medicine was essential for the indigenous tribes prior to the arrival of European settlers, and it remains essential for them today. Life all around us is interconnected, and looking at Native American solutions for many ailments that we cannot yet treat with modern medicine is telling. If imbalances in mind, body, and spirit cause ailments, it is no wonder so much of the modern world is suffering. It is time to turn back to a more natural and holistic solution.

The simple focus on the health and wellbeing of the body, mind, and spirit in all aspects of life is what brings health and healing to the Native people. The healthy native diets, spiritual ceremonies, and reverence for nature all combine and contribute to the healing seen today.

One example to consider is diabetes. Though common elsewhere, less than a century ago, it was rarely diagnosed in Native American peoples. Today, however, as the American lifestyle is adopted, it has become more common. As the healthy, wellness-centralized mindset and traditions are abandoned, health is lost.

Fundamentals of Native American Herbalism

Herbalism itself is the process of drawing from herbs. The word "herb" can be a bit confusing for those only familiar with it in terms of cooking. Herbs are not just tiny shrubs that grow on the ground like parsley or basil; they are any plants or plant parts used for either culinary or therapeutic value. In many traditions, herbalism also acknowledges and uses fungi, mineral, and animal substances. For example, as you read, you will see several references to using honey in conjunction with herbs in order to create syrups or to sweeten teas. Honey, though an animal product, has its own medicinal values that make it an important part of herbalism, especially in regards to herbal medicine.

Herbal medicine is the practice of using plants to support health and wellness. Though sometimes believed to be nonsense today by those who believe there is no place for the solutions of yesteryear in today's modern society, naturopathic solutions to issues are becoming much more compelling and popular. More and more often, people are interested in turning their attention to natural solutions rather than taking pills at exorbitant prices.

Herbal medicine itself has been practiced as far back as humanity, with the first written history dating back over 5000 years. Many populations today still draw from herbal medicine to heal, and even in developed nations, many turn to it. According to the National Institutes of Health, over 50% of adults in the United States take some sort of herbal supplement on a regular basis. You may even be taking them now without realizing it.

In the United States, much of the traditional herbal medicines used are rooted in Native American traditions. Native American traditional healing works as a whole medical system. In other words, it functions as a medical system that employs several holistic treatments for several acute and chronic conditions. Each tribe has their own beliefs and practices, but there are several beliefs that are shared between them, and those are traditions that work to keep several aspects of themselves healthy.

Native Americans emphasize a holistic approach that aims to create a harmony of mind, body, and spirit. Many practices from many different tribes aim to integrate these together. Take, for example, the tradition of running to greet the dawn each morning. Not only does this help to connect the individuals to their heritage, their beliefs, and their spirituality, it also helps to keep the body healthy.

The healing systems are passed down through legends and stories, used to teach positive behaviors. They pass on their diets, their ceremonies, and the use of plants to promote further health. Part of this comes from a major fundamental of Native American tradition: symbolic healing and ceremonial gatherings. Native American ceremonies emphasize a togetherness; they bring together the patient, the family, and the community in hopes of healing the individual. Surrounding the ill or wounded with family can certainly have a good effect; we know that positivity and support are beneficial to people and help them to recover.

By implementing ceremonial gatherings and practicing prayer, song, dance, and music, the family and other loved ones get to contribute healing energy. Their presence and positivity help alleviate stress, which also helps the ill to heal and recover.

Because Native American healing ceremonies implement four constructs of spirituality (Creator, Mother Earth, Great Father), environment (nature and balance), self (inner peace, thoughts, and values), and community (family, clan, and tribe), all four must be present.

Symbolism is present in just about every culture in the world, and the Native American healing ceremonies are no different. While there are many different tribes out there, and this is certainly not a blanket statement, several tribes have their own traditional and Christian symbols that they use during these ceremonies. By restoring spiritual health, physical health can return as well.

One of the most common symbols in Native American cultures is the Medicine Wheel. This may look like a circle at a glance, but there is more to it than that. It has a high degree of symbolism and has been used as a sacred symbol in many tribes in the Plains. It represents the universe and the knowledge within it. It is also a sign of healing.

The Medicine Wheel has four key components: The circle, the lines, the feather, and the four directions. The circle is the outer boundary of the Medicine Wheel. It may be referred to as the Sun Dance Circle or the Sacred Hoop. This circle is indicative of the circle of life; it shows the pattern that we all go through of life and death. It shows the path of the sun and of the moon as well. It also is related to the family home, shaped like a traditional *tipi*. This outer boundary of Earth is the foundation of the Medicine Wheel.

Next comes the lines. There are two lines, one vertical and one horizontal. These represent the sacred paths of the sun and of man. They cross in the center, which is another indication of the Earth, in this case, of the center of the Earth.

Sometimes, there is a feather included within the Medicine Wheel. This is a sign of the Great Spirit's power over everything. The attachment of an eagle feather is used to mark accomplishment and ceremony.

Finally, there are the four directions on the Medicine Wheel. These are often included in color; each of the four segments created by the lines can be colored differently. Each of these colors represents one of the cardinal directions and the seasons. North is represented with red, East is represented by yellow, South is represented by white, and West is represented by black. Likewise, the four directions can represent the four elements, fire, water, earth, and air. It can also represent the four stages of life: Birth, childhood, adulthood, and elder.

Native American Herbs

Native Americans are highly remembered and popular for the medicinal plant knowledge that they possess. There has been a rumor that they were the first to start the use of herbs and plants for healing health conditions after watching the animals consume different types of plants when they get sick. Therefore, in order to protect all of these plants from over-harvesting, men started to pick every third plant that they found.

The Native Americans come with a spiritual view of life, and for being healthy, the person is destined to have a sense of purpose. Apart from that, the person should be harmonious, righteous, and should follow a balanced path in life. They had the belief that some of the illnesses were accountable as life lessons that the person needed in order to learn and understand that they should not interfere.

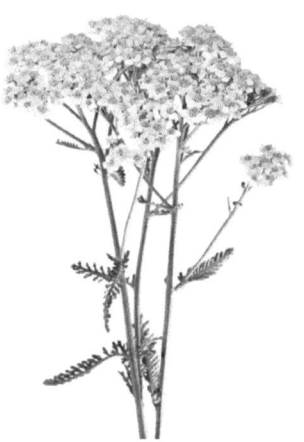

Most of the modern medicines and remedies are based upon the Native American knowledge of different herbs and plants, which they used for thousands of years in the past. Here are some of the versatile plants that the Native Americans used in their everyday lives for healing purposes and their significance:

Yarrow (Achillea Millefolium)

A fragrant and flowering plant has been in use since the Ancient Greece period. It served the purpose of stopping excessive bleeding conditions. It is said that the famous Greek hero Achilles used it over his wounds. Therefore, it has been given the name as that of his! The pioneers and aboriginal people used to apply it on open cuts and wounds in the form of a poultice. It was made from the leaves for clotting the blood and preventing its flow.

This plant was also used in the form of fresh Yarrow juice with a water blend for recovering from upset stomach problems. It is said that the Native Americans claimed it to have cured the intestinal disorders as well. Moreover, a tea made out of these leaves or stems will possibly act as a form of an astringent.

Sumac

This plant has been highly preferable for several medicinal remedies since the era of Native Americans. But, it is only one amongst the other few plants that are ideal for healing and treating eye problems. A sumac decoction was once known to be used for gargling to relieve sore throats or to heal diarrhea problems. The berries and leaves of these plants were also combined in the tea to reduce fever symptoms. It is also made in a poultice form for soothing poison ivy rash.

Blackberry

The famous Cherokee used this plant to treat upset stomach conditions. The Native Americans used blackberry for making tea to cure swollen tissues, swollen joints, and diarrhea conditions. The roots of the blackberry plant were used to make an all-natural cough syrup for healing sore throats. The roots of today are mixed with maple syrup and honey for adding taste to the tea.

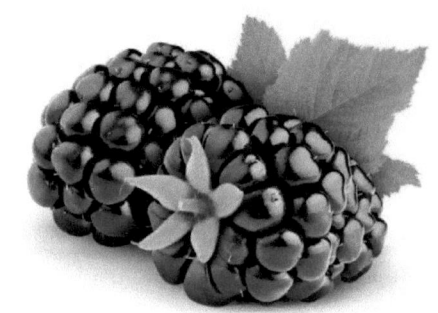

It is also an effective remedy for soothing bleeding gums by just chewing its leaves. It is also stated as an optimal remedy for strengthening the overall immune system of the body.

Rosemary

The Rosemary plant was considered sacred by the Native American tribes. They preferred to use it mostly as an analgesic for getting rid of sore joints. This herb is accountable for improving memory power, relieving muscle pain, spasms, and other such conditions. As per the records and tests, it is also stated that this plant helps in improving the circulatory and nervous systems. As a whole, it also treats digestion problems and strengthens the immune system.

Mint

All digestion problems during the era of Native Americans needed a form of beverage to soothe the symptoms. Therefore, they used mint to make tea. The Cherokee made use of it for healing purposes. They also made salve from its leaves to sooth rashes and itching skin conditions.

Red Clover

Native Americans used this plant for treating respiratory and inflammation conditions. Some recent and modern studies have elaborated that the red clover also has properties of preventing heart disease by lowering cholesterol and improving blood circulation within the body.

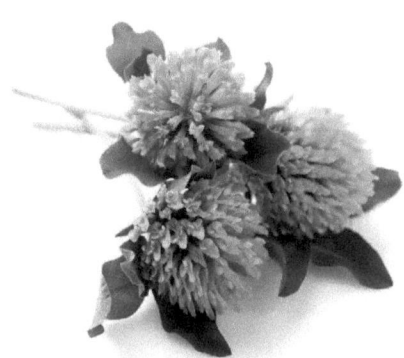

Cattail

This is one of the most famous and popular survival plants that the indigenous population or the Native Americans used as food. Apart from that, it was also used as a preventative medicine. As it is easily digestible, recovery potential from illnesses was high. Cattail is today popularly known as the supermarket of the swamp, as you can use it in multiple dishes to add taste.

Hummingbird Blossom or Buck Brush

The Native Americans preferred this plant for treating all types of throat and mouth conditions such as fibroid tumors, inflammation, and cysts. They used it in the form of a poultice for treating sores, wounds, and burns. With further research today, it also has been found to have diuretic properties that stimulate the functions of the kidney. Its roots can be used for attaining this kidney stimulation property.

All the early pioneers used this plant as an ideal substitute for black tea. Some of the recent and detailed studies have found that the humming blossom is effective in treating lymphatic blockages and blood pressure conditions.

Wild Ginger

The healers of the Native American era made use of this plant for treating ear infections and earache. They also used to make mild tea out of its rootstock to stimulate the digestion system and relieve bloating. It is also ideal for treating nausea and bronchial infections.

Prickly Pear Cactus

This is yet another popular plant that was used both as food and medicine for the Native Americans. They used it in the form of a poultice made out of mature cactus pads. The poultice was then used as an antiseptic for treating burns, boils, and wounds. The tea was also made for treating complex urinary tract infection problems. According to current research, this plant is ideal for strengthen body immunity.

The research shows further that this cactus plant can also help in lowering cholesterol levels and prevents serious chronic conditions such as diet-oriented cardiovascular disease and diabetes.

Ashwagandha

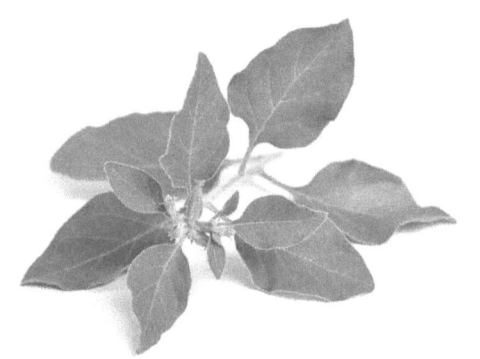

This is a powerful plant that was used by the Native Americans for its unusual medicinal properties. Today, people are well aware of the potential of Ashwagandha. It treats muscle weakness and tension as well as bone weakness. Apart from that, it can also prevent memory loss, teeth weakening, and rheumatism and is also used as a sedative.

The sedative properties of this plant impact an overall rejuvenating effect on the body to improve its vitality. The root bark and leaves can be used as an antibiotic. It can also be made into a poultice to help ease pain and swelling. Modern research and historical records show that this plant has toxic properties in it.

There is a saying, "Knowledge will help you survive when you have no one to help you out." The Native Americans made this practical by using surrounding herbs to make medicines for their survival. They did their research and tests without the help of the technological advancements we have today! And their discoveries are today helping medical scientists and pharmaceutical companies to prepare healing medications and remedies.

The world is no doubt grateful for the contributions made by the Native Americans in the field of healthcare and medicines. Today, some of these herbs are made in the form of capsules, syrups, powders and other forms of medicines. They are still serving the purpose for which they were discovered. In addition, with modern technology and increased manpower, sourcing these plants is now easy and more people across the globe can benefit from them.

Herbal Remedies Benefits

Herbal medicine is the use of plants for curing and even preventing illnesses. Many Native Americans made use of herbal medicine for healthy living. Even today and with the emergence of modern science, more than half of the world still uses herbal medicine because it works. Here are some of the numerous benefits of herbal medicine:

Affordability: modern medicine has been great for the overall health of humanity. However, things are getting more expensive, and getting medical care is more complicated and difficult for many people and this is where herbal medicine comes in.

It is just as effective as modern medicine and much cheaper. An added benefit of herbal medicine is that, properly used, it has no side effects.

Available in different forms: many people find it difficult to take any form of medicine – whether herbal or drugs. And then there are those who will take it in one form and not in another. Herbal medicines can be found in different herbal shops, pharmacies, and even on the internet, and this means you get your medicine close to you in whatever form. However, it is advisable to purchase herbs from the right source.

Efficacy of treatment: many of the herbal medicines have gone through numerous trials which has helped confirm their efficacy.

Immune-boosting properties: herbal medicine helps to strengthen and improve body immunity in a way that it does not interfere with the person's psychological processes; rather, it supports the body and helps keep those processes going. Every aspect of the body is boosted to the point that the body suddenly gets a lift and can function at its fullest.

Native America is one of the birthplaces of herbal medicine where the Native Americans' relationship with nature was so strong that they clearly understand the benefits of certain herbal medicines. This connection has been shared to many parts of the world today where it is being used by many more people.

Native American Medicine Today

Every culture has its distinct form of medicine, which they use to treat illnesses and injuries. In Native American culture, plants are there to be used as an important part of their lifestyle and spirituality. There is a reason that Native Americans were one of the first cultures to discover herbalism; it has been passed down through generations from ancient times when human beings were only just beginning to adapt to their harsh environment.

Traditional Native Americans practiced herbalism between 1300 and 1850 CE. They did not have hospitals would instead the herbs and plants surrounding them to cure sicknesses or treat injuries. Around 1500, many of them began to convert to European-style medicine, a more scientific form of medicine some of which had side effects because of harmful the chemicals they contained.

Native Americans were one of the first peoples in North America to discover herbalism as a form of medicine and they have continued to use traditional medicines for several generations.

Native American Herbalism in Modern Times

Native American herbalists have brought their knowledge of herbs and plants into modern medicine in the modern era. For example, they are currently using herbs to treat allergies and wounds. They have found out that some herbs work better on certain types of wounds than others and therefore rely on their knowledge of herbs to heal people instead of using harmful or potentially harmful chemicals.

The Herbal Medicines Act of 1990 has allowed Native American herbalists to practice modern medicine freely; it allows them to obtain herbs from areas with native herbs, such as the reservation lands and protected lands. It also allows the medical use of herbs found on reservation lands but does not allow Native American herbalists to go outside of their reservations to collect herbs. This is a big change from previous times when herbalists could collect plants anywhere as long as they respected their environment and did not harm plant life. These changes have helped many more people learn about and study herbalism and is a large part of what has created more interest in herbalism worldwide.

Native Americans used herbs to help them heal because they were among the first cultures to discover herbalism. They would gather the plants in a specific area and have an entire set of medicines. If someone became sick with a fever, they would try to pick a plant that would stop the fever quickly and then use it as medicine for the illness.

There are a few ways that Native Americans are using herbs in their lives today including restoring balance, treating illness, and promoting good health. They do this for example by educating those who wish to become holistic healthcare providers or herbalists on these plants and their uses. Another way is in the food they eat together with wild plants which allows them to treat their bodies naturally and also get the nutrients they need. One of the most common ways is the use of herbs for medical purposes. The

Native Americans have learned through their ancestors how to make and mix medicines from the plants around them to take care of illnesses and wounds.

Native American herbalists are not just using knowledge passed down through generations to practice herbalism; they also use scientific evidence to support what their ancestors have told them about handling their bodies. For example, herbalists have found that certain plants are used for specific ailments. When they treat these ailments themselves, they first try to find the root of the problem before treating it with herbs.

One example of how Native Americans are using scientific evidence to support their herbalism would be in the case of allergies. In many cases, allergies can be cured with the help of herbs, but there is also need to find the root cause of the allergy before trying out different treatments using herbs. In such a case, the herbalists rely on science and scientific methods to support their herbalism.

Today, many people are trying to use Native American herbs because they want to try something different when sick or because they have some knowledge about the herbs and their uses. Native American herbalism has been a part of many cultures, so it is not surprising that people today want to incorporate these medicines into their lives.

Conclusion

Plants and natural resources shape the foundation and contribute primarily to some industrial drug formulations developed today. In fact, about 25 percent of prescription medications globally are produced from plants. In addition, medicines are sometimes used in health treatment rather than in medications.

Herbal therapy is a favorite therapeutic form for others. Herbs are used as an adjunct treatment to traditional pharmaceuticals, among others. In several emerging societies, moreover, conventional medicine, to which herbal medicine is a central component, is the only accessible health care method.

Those using herbal remedies should be confident, irrespective of the cause, that the items they are purchasing are healthy and contain what they are meant to contain, whether it be a single herb or a certain quantity of a single herbal ingredient. Science-based details on dose, contraindications, and effectiveness should also be provided to customers. Global harmonization of laws is required to accomplish this in order to direct the responsible development and selling of herbal medicines. If there is ample clinical proof of an herb's usefulness, a law may allow it to be used properly to encourage its utilization such that those benefits may be appreciated for the protection of public health and for the diagnosis of illnesses.

You've reached the end of this book, but not the end of your journey to using herbal medicine. I hope you have enjoyed what you have learned so far. As you start to practice and use herbal remedies, take some time to reflect on how well they work for you. A great way of doing this is by keeping a journal with the remedy that you used, the recipe you followed, and whether it worked or not. You can also include any side affects you had or any allergic reactions, so you know which remedies are not for you. To maintain the safety and effectiveness of your herbal remedies, it is important to store them correctly. For infusions, you can store them in a covered jar in the fridge for 24 hours.

Finally, one must be thankful to the Native Americans for their role in providing us with these natural remedies using herbs and plants. We must also always remember that nature is always kind to us, so we should be comfortable while using these herbs.

BOOK 2: NATIVE AMERICAN SPIRITUALITY

Introduction

Traditional Native American healing is a broad medical practice that incorporates a range of therapeutic methods used by indigenous healers to treat a wide variety of acute and chronic illnesses, as well as to promote health and wellness.

Although tribal differences exist, there are also common wellness values and interventions, such as a health promotion foundation that promotes bio-psycho-social-spiritual methods and rituals.

Herbal treatments, coercive therapies, rituals, and prayer are also used to avoid and cure sickness in a variety of ways.

Thousands of years ago, this continent was populated by millions of Native peoples, who relied on orthodox herbal medicine to maintain their health and well-being. Local foods, seasonal and harvest rituals, and curing with indigenous plants have all been used to encourage longevity by living in harmony with nature.

The younger generations of indigenous peoples are leaving behind these rituals, which provide a profound link to the earth, resulting in a rise in illnesses and poor health.

Though ceremonies play a significant role in the lives of traditional Native Americans, their therapeutic importance is often overlooked by allopathic health professionals. Native American rituals include the patient, his or her relatives, and the community in the healing process.

Ceremonial gatherings can last days or weeks, and the more the participants, the more relaxing the effect. The patient's family and friends use poetry, prayer, music, and dance to help the patient recover.

Individuals from diverse religious and cultural backgrounds use symbols from their respective faiths and cultural traditions to address health concerns.

Native American healing ceremonies allow extensive use of idols, deities, and ritualistic objects associated with cultural and Christian worship. By re-establishing the requisite equilibrium for wellbeing, these symbols activate bio-psycho-social-spiritual healing responses.

Whether associated with rituals or with religious services, the symbolism may be integrated into the recovery process to create a positive healing synergy.

Today's Native Americans also use a combination of conventional and allopathic medicine to maintain health and vitality where allopathic medications are combined with indigenous herbal medicines and rituals. As a result, spiritual therapies play a critical role in the health and restoration of Native American culture.

Native American healing practices have been recorded in the United States since colonization. However, cultural enumeration has complicated the identification of Native American medicinal practices as fore runners of folk medicine and other natural remedies that have had a profound influence on western medicine.

Understanding Native American healing practices requires an understanding of Native American cultural value structures relating to health and nutrition, as well as the numerous forces that assist practitioners in strengthening the mind, body, spirit, and natural environment.

The Role of Religion and Spirituality

Native Americans focused mainly on natural curing techniques rather than on unnatural or man-made healing procedures. Healing activities adopted by Native Americans illustrated their cultural development. These traditional healing activities and methods were considered odd in the European world despite the fact that they had profound importance in Native American culture.

In actual fact, Native Americans are always acclaimed for medicinal plant knowledge as they were first to recognize the importance of plants or herbs in healing various diseases. They on their part had learnt about these healing herbs by observing ill animals who, when they were taken for grazing, and ate those plants, started healing; they started testing numerous herbs to cure the sick among them. Those that proved effective were recommended for specific disease; Native Americans' healing traditions were not all uniform as different tribes selected different herbs, roots and therefore acquired differing but equally valuable knowledge. Almost 2000 plus tribes resided in North America then and almost every tribe had a slightly different healing technique and criteria.

Native Americans contended that there is a strong connection between nature and people's health. They believed that it was important to have emotional and physical well-being while maintaining harmony with nature. Whereas today, technological inventions have strengthened their roots, concepts of Native American healing techniques are not given much importance because human beings have started relying more on knowledge and the use of different technologies. Nowadays, people have become more logical, so they like logical treatment rather than depending on unknown or baseless ancient healing techniques despite being quite helpful and effective.

Spirituality and Connection

The spirituality has been an integral part of Native American culture for centuries. For many of them, religion was not a realm separated from daily life but rather part and parcel of it. This section will look at the various aspects of this spirituality and how it affects them.

Native American spirituality has been influenced by and borrows from many religions. Among these are Buddhism, Taoism, Shintoism, Christianity, Hinduism, and Islam as well as the traditions and beliefs of its tribes and cultures. It therefore includes many complex elements which are reflected in their spiritual practices and individual expressions; most revolve around participating in ceremonies or rituals to mark rites of passage or spiritual growth.

Examples of these include the pow wow (a gathering where singers perform dances that tell a story), sweat lodge (a cleansing ritual based on American Indian traditions with participants purifying themselves through prayer), purification ceremony (an initiation ceremony performed at puberty), and vision quest.

The spirituality of Native Americans is one that many people do not associate with the mainstream. They have unique traditions, beliefs, and spiritual practices that may be foreign to those outside their community. Given this connection to their cultures, it is not surprising that the Native American perspective on spirituality would be very personal. All of this and the associated identity can be found woven into their culture and religion.

The spirituality of the Native American tribes may be similar to Christian spirituality in that it has both beliefs and practices. The Native American sees no separation between life and religion. They have a deep connection to their spiritual ways, influenced by their culture and their perspectives on life.

Connected within this is an essential concept of self-identity. Spirituality is reflected in everything from their art, music, and even social structures right down to how they behave toward one another. Through this exciting mix of interconnectivity with their culture and the resulting identity, they can live connected with all things; spiritually, physically, mentally, emotionally, and intellectually.

The spiritual beliefs of Native Americans are based on their traditions and folklore. It is the basis for their faith in animism, the idea that everything is possessed of a spirit; thus, it becomes necessary to honor these spirits to avoid angering them. It can often be seen through rituals; such as the pow wow, sweat lodge, purification ceremony, vision quest, or the Ghost Dance, which are all ceremonies or rituals that Native Americans have adopted to help ensure good health, prosperity in living conditions and abundance for future generations.

As mentioned earlier, a number of religions have influenced the spirituality and beliefs of Native Americans. One such religion is Buddhism whose adherents believe that through meditation, one can achieve Nirvana and transcend suffering, either through self-realization or by reaching enlightenment (the state of complete awareness).

The Native American shaman utilizes the idea of a higher power, which corresponds to the same concept in Buddhism. This higher power is believed to give them what they need for their personal spiritual growth, for example, healing abilities, visions, or psychic powers. The Native American shaman uses this in hopes of guiding his people to a better life.

The spirituality of the Native Americans relies on a set of individual beliefs and a connection to the land. It is seen in many ways, from those that hold ceremonies or rituals, such as sweat lodges or vision quests, to those that seek guidance from their spirit guides. While these are certain core beliefs, there is also a wide variety of unique traditions and practices connected with each tribe. These may have evolved via cultural adaptation over time; others may be associated with that particular tribe's location and history.

Many Native Americans see their spirituality as a calling or how they can serve their community. As such, it is something that is both personal and communal; this results in everything from their art to their music being filled with Spirit. It has been noted that spirituality is found in all facets of Native American life. It allows people to live their lives believing and acting, following what they know to be correct according to the beliefs and traditions of their tribe. Because of this connection between spirituality and culture, life is lived with an entire focus on these beliefs, bringing them into every aspect of day-to-day living.

With this focus on everything connected and how the spirituality of Native Americans arises from their culture, it is easy to see that there is a sizeable impacting factor between the two. It is especially true concerning identity. Thus, it is not surprising that spirituality remains one of the most defining aspects of Native American life today.

The spirituality that flows through every facet of Native American culture may be unique and complex, but it makes up an integral part of their being. With their core beliefs in animism, connection to the land is also found throughout their spirituality. Many Native Americans believe that there is a spiritual presence in all things, which shows up in everything from their traditions to everyday living.

Despite the different religions that have influenced the spirituality of Native Americans, they share many similarities. For example, one common belief is Animism. The spirits are believed to also influence the world around them. Paganism—this can be seen as similar to Animism since it is based on a belief in multiple natural forces. However, Karma typically describes how people determine their fate based on how they have treated others in the past or present. It is something that isn't apparent while following this critical value.

The beliefs of Native Americans are also connected to the land that they live on. It is evident in their connection with the spirit of this land and in their traditional ways of living off of it. It includes things such as hunting, gathering, and farming. The entire way they live and interact with their environment is done with a deep understanding of its spiritual value. Doing this makes it possible for Native Americans to live in the manner they feel is right.

Many different views have been placed on spirituality over the past few centuries. Even though some have tried to change or even eliminate this belief system, it still influences earth-based traditions throughout the world today, particularly within Native American culture.

Healing and Kindness

Traditionally, Native Americans had extreme love for the motherland earth. They express their love through humility and humbleness in their relationship with nature. The standard of success and happiness among Indians was not about how rich they were or how much strength they owned. Instead, the standard of success and happiness was that those who gave away more money and donations were considered happier and prosperous. They were of the view that to become rich; one has to give away more money.

Kindness was deeply rooted in their traditions; for example, if Native Americans would celebrate anyone's birthday, instead of expecting any gifts from his guests and neighbors, he gives away gifts to his guests to honor his birthday and honor his guests attending the event for his sake.

According to Native Americans, a person is afflicted by disease or illness only when he adopts immoral behavior called soul loss. To them, soul loss is when a person loses his beliefs and depicts selfishness, cheating, evilness, disrespect and dishonesty in his actions. As all these actions of that person go against nature, henceforth, nature would avenge for all the displeasing inflicted on it by anyone. A person's health will deteriorate until their soul returns to his body; otherwise, it would lead to a catastrophe and even death.

Although all these beliefs seem odd to human beings living in today's world, there is some reality to these beliefs, evident from the number of events, research, and inventions. According to recent research by scientists, it has been revealed that those who hold grudges and whose minds are always overwhelmed by negative thoughts are more prone to mental and cardiac diseases. These aggressive-minded people undergo more heart attacks than those who always maintain a positive attitude and remain calm and serene. Medical Scientists are now contending that those who undergo soul loss live unsatisfied lives, leading to a cellular breakdown. It is important to remain satisfied and humble and stay connected with our faith and nature to live a serene and healthy life.

Spirituality and Religion

Native Americans have their ways of prayer based on different beliefs that were quite distinct from that of the traditional Christian way of prayer and their belief in a single God. When they invaded Native American territory, Europeans called these Native Americans pagans; however, they found their supposition wrong with time. When Europeans came in close contact with Native Americans traditions, they realized that they did not believe in a single God but in the spirits of animals and plants. In their traditions, they proposed gifts to these spirits and asked the spirits of these plants and animals for their help in healing those who were sick, and those who were suffering at the hands of life or any other physical danger.

Usually, they pray in the form of a ceremony while collectively dancing and chanting songs in favor of these animals and plant spirits to appease them and, in some cases, to attribute them for their services towards their believers. Native American prayers were not brief, but they were quite long and more specific. In their prayers, even a single vowel had specific and different meanings. A doctor named Mehl-Madrona reported that a number of patients got cured through Native American spiritual traditional belief, which he had witnessed personally. He saw a woman getting cured of cancer, a child suffering from gallbladder disease got cured too, and likewise, a man got cured of liver cirrhosis.

All these cures were a miracle. As a doctor, Mehl-Madrona tried to rationalize the healing techniques of Native American medicine. Still, he had always warned other people to refrain from adopting such a procedure for the cure. He says that to get healed, you must first develop a firm belief that you will get cured. It has been noted that whenever a healing ceremony for any patient is staged, every relative of a healing person was expected to be present in the ceremony because they thought that more the member of the ceremony would be to pray for the healer, more will be the strength of prayers and the relation between nature and men would get stronger, henceforth improving the rate of healing of Native American doctor. He said that all of us naturally possess the ability inside ourselves to heal.

Native American Relationship with Nature

Native Americans find themselves very close to nature. They have built a connection with nature because they believe that it has the remedy for all the diseases and for balance mind, body and soul in harmony with each other. With nature, only then a person and a society can stay healthier and happy. In this regard, they discovered many medicinal plants and have used them to prevent and treat several diseases. They have made natural remedies for newborn baby to treat cold and flu, and for 60 years old man from bath recipes to foot massage. They wanted the world to make connections with nature and explore the hidden treasures in it for the benefit of mankind. The herbal remedies handed over from generation to generation are still very useful against many infections, working even better than the modern world cures because modern medicines come at the cost of side effects, while herbal remedies are with benefits, no side effects.

Native American Healers

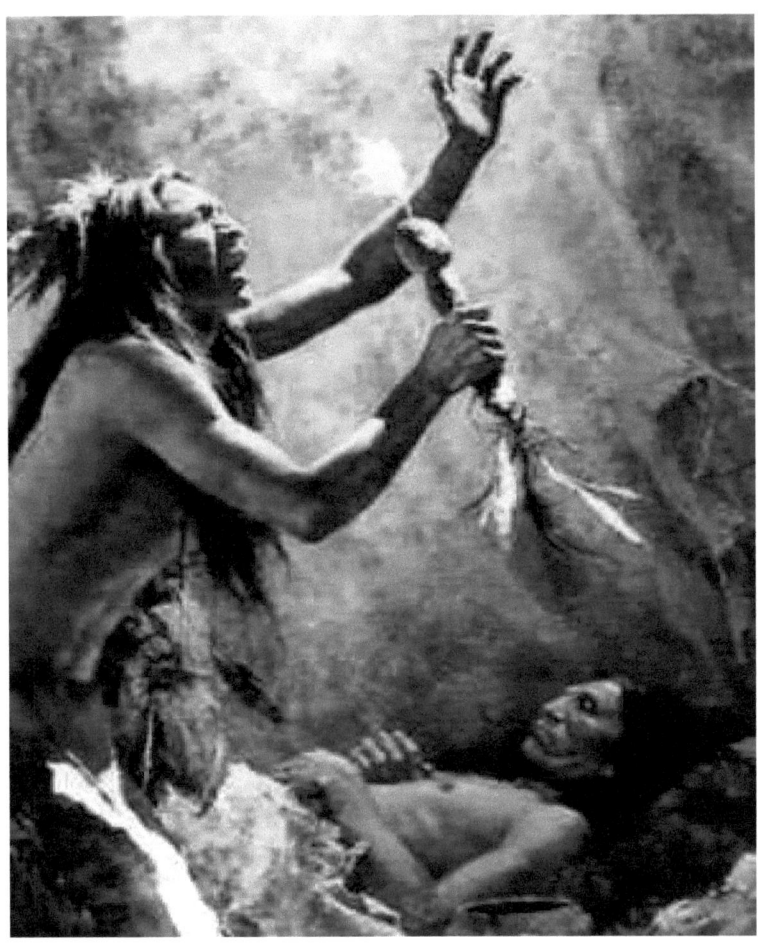

Native healers were older people with great knowledge of animals and plants and using every element provided by nature to treat the most common symptoms. They had to understand the subject. They were well aware that the mind was one with the sick body and that very often, the predominant cause of a body disorder had to be sought in it. Finally, they were in direct contact with the spirit world, from which they drew inspiration to heal any disease. This aspect may make us smile but, it is important to remember that Indian society was deeply imbued with a pantheistic conception of the life in which the relationship with the gods was the basis of every event. Beyond all beliefs and perplexities, the fact remains that for Native Americans, prevention and therapy were held in significant consideration, with positive repercussions that still today are primarily staggering.

What was crucial so as to become a Native American healer was to have a good relationship with nature.

In order for one to have a good relationship with Mother Earth, it was said that "a person must respect the power of Mother Earth and understand how to create balance within themselves. This balance between an individual and nature must be maintained in order to be able to contact the spirit world."

When a person was chosen as a healer, he took his name from one of Mother Earth's four directions. It is said that the name chosen by the healer would also match their personality and character.

"There is a belief that each healer has an attendant spirit who is always present with the healer and who may be visible or invisible to others. As a result of going on a healing journey, it is said a person may become a shaman by having an experience of seeing spirits during a healing ceremony. It has been said that some healers will actually go on a spiritual journey without using any form of medicine or plant to help give them the power to heal."

In order for one to become a Native American healer, they must have visions from their spirit guide. The vision must be accepted before it can be used as power for healing.

In addition, in order for a person to be a Native American healer, they must have been born with the knowledge or be able to obtain it from their spirit guide.

Without this knowledge, the person would not be able to serve as a Native American healer. Native American healers had to be able to make prayer sticks and sacred corn in order to become a "dweller of Mother Earth."

Native Americans believe that Native Americans are a part of Mother Earth's body.

They believe that through ceremony and dance, they can communicate with Mother Earth and learn about her four hearts.

In order for the medicine wheel to work properly, each element must be involved. This includes the earth, water, fire, and wind. Each element has different powers.

The Treatment Approach

Native American medicine is a complete framework that balances every sphere of one's life, including lifestyle and social interactions with one inner world. Native medicine assumes that in the divine realm, the roots of every imbalance lie. In the course of every recovery procedure, spiritual approaches are vital. Including fees and rates, clinical approaches are often clearly and uniquely tailored for the patient. They require, as part of the healing method, the process of fee negotiation.

The Healing Elder is someone who is trained to use plants medicinally. A Healing Elder, or HE, specializes in the use of plants as healing agents for cleansing, strengthening, or bringing balance to the soul. Ancient healing traditions gave rise to the tradition of Alternatives Medicine with its roots deeply rooted in nature's way of dealing with problems.

The Healing Elder seems to have the most healing strength, and the elder practitioner loses his prestige as a powerful healer when treatment fails. The person in need of healing makes a proposition to the doctor of medicine and waits to see if it is approved. They rarely negotiate face-to-face. The customer leaves the bid outside the healer's door, and if it remains there till the morning, it means that it has not been approved, and one can go somewhere else. Once they come to an agreement, therapy will, for example, start with a behavioral prescription, a pledge, a selfless act, genuine repentance, or scaling a holy mountain. Techniques include self-inquiry and discovery to ascertain whether there is a need for a dietary improvement, prayer, herbs, massage, a sweat lodge ritual, or a vision quest.

Theories

The main objective is to alter the patient's comprehension of the world through a healthier self-concept, increased acceptance of others, and behavior adjustments. The healer's goal is not only to treat sickness but to change the patient's overall approach towards life and the world around him. Native American medicine combines science as well as spirit with the onset of new technology. They mostly use herbal interventions and pharmaceuticals. We can explain this by narrating a Native American story on the use of herbal medicine. Barb, a wife, mother, and lawyer, was still fighting breast cancer. Despite doing all she could, the cancer continued to spread. She met with an Indian elder named Big Nose in a sweat lodge. He wanted to understand what she was doing or what hadn't changed in her life. Deep inside, as a mother-wife and lawyer, she thought she was a loser, and now she was healing herself. It was the pessimistic self-talk that needed to end, Big Nose told her. Barb decided to let go of thoughts that she would be not cured and started to enjoy life with her family due to this relationship. Another story tells of a woman who had had extreme arthritis and was desperately looking for the right healer. To facilitate recovery, medicine men go further and beyond the most visible problem and understand that radical improvement is often required. The shifts are primary, and herbs are secondary, along with massage and prayer. Right relationships, the correction of relationships with oneself and with families and members of the society, and the spiritual environment are all effects of disruption of relationships and disease development.

Teaching

Native American healers teach their students through intensive apprenticeship. For preparation, several weeks of testing the purpose and dedication of a student are vital. An apprentice acquires knowledge and gains patience and respect. Native medicine is still an oral tradition and cannot be taught in an academic setting. Students learn the skills required only through experience, and only when the patient is ready does the older instructor encourage them to begin medical practice.

Ceremonies, the Healing Process Scenario

Ceremony is an important part of traditional native healing. Because of the close relationship between physical and spiritual wellbeing, body and soul should heal together. Popular healing rituals encourage wellbeing by representing traditional concepts of the world, the Creator, and spirit. Prayer, drumming, chants, poems, legends, and the use of several religious artifacts may be part of them. Wherever an ill person requires healing, healers perform ceremonies, and the ceremonies are sometimes performed only in sacred places. Special buildings for healing are mostly referred to as Medicine Lodges. Traditional healing rituals are considered holy wherever they occur and are only performed by the native healers and local spiritual facilitators. Non-Natives can participate only by invitation. Native powwows, on the other hand, have grown today into social and cultural activities that include indigenous music, singing, drumming, regalia, and food. Most powwows welcome all persons.

Dream Catchers among Native Americans

Many Native Tribes use a handcrafted willow hoop fashioned into a net as their version of a dream catcher. As a sort of armor and protection, they are often made of feathers and beads and hung from cradles.

Among the original Americans, it was thought that once the sun sets, the night sky is filled with a variety of dreams, both pleasant and evil. For this reason, they utilize a dream catcher made of a medicine wheel or a hoop-shaped dream catcher to keep the sleeper from experiencing terrible nightmares. The dream catcher may also be used as a kind of protection for warriors or those who are on the go. In addition, it is said to harmonize emotions, the mind, and the body as a whole, as well as protect against sickness. Good dreams may be encouraged with the usage of a dream catcher. Dreams and the spiritual world were very important to Native Americans, and this is something that even today's experts are mystified by and still trying to understand.

Native American Traditional Healing Rituals and Ceremonials

Native American healing activities exemplify key cultural perspectives and have an impact on the development of Native American identities.

These healing practices are based on values and experiences that are beyond the norm of western psychological tenets, but they can have a significant impact on Native Americans' sense of well-being.

Through symbolic healing rituals and ceremonies, participants were brought into harmony with themselves, their tribe, and their environment.

Ceremonies were often used to help in the reunification of groups of people, but not for individual healing. Some tribes, such as the Sioux and Navajo, used a medicine wheel and a sacred hoop in ceremonies that lasted days, as well as singing and dancing.

Many plants and herbs were used as medicines or in sacred ceremonies in ancient Indian rituals, creating a link with spirits and the afterlife. In spiritual rites, Sage, Bear Berry, Red Cedar, Sweet Grass, Tobacco, and a variety of other plants and herbs were used.

The healing mechanism in Native American Medicine is very different from what we see today. Religious, philosophical, therapeutic, and ceremonial beliefs and rituals are used for both medical and emotional problems of Native American healing.

Native Americans believe that medicine is more about healing the person than curing diseases.

Traditional healers claimed that most diseases are caused by metaphysical problems, and their goal was to make people "whole."

Sweat lodges were used by many tribes for purification and cleansing of the body, in addition to herbal remedies. In these darkened and heated enclosures, a sick person would be given herbal medicine, smoke, or a rub with sacred plants, and a shaman would use healing ceremonies to ward off angry spirits and invoke the healing powers of a God.

Healing ceremonies could include whole groups of people singing, dancing, and painting their bodies, as well as the use of mind-altering drugs to cause spirits to heal the sick person.

Native Americans' celebration ritual aims to give symbolic meaning to one's life experiences. Counselors must learn from a variety of perspectives in order to gain a deeper understanding of Native American experiences, provide a framework in which to effectively communicate with Native Americans, and cultivate multicultural flexibility in their counseling practices in general.

Furthermore, those raised in the western tradition must form relationships with indigenous practitioners in order to contribute to a wider understanding of the world by listening and exchanging meaningfully.

Many tribes that adopt a pan-Indian ideology use a variety of traditional Native American healing practices.

These customs include powwows, music, smudging, storytelling, sweat lodges pipe ceremonies, and herb. Sweat lodge traditions also include music, smudging, pipe ceremonies, herbs, and occasionally storytelling.

Pow Wow

A powwow is a social and religious assembly of Native American tribes. Native Americans do their singing, drumming, and dancing in a circular arena at powwows. Many of the attendees wear traditional Native American attire, which they usually design and sew themselves.

Wearing regalia and dancing in the arena circle is a traditional Native American symbol of unity, giving sense and expression to Lakota terms like 'mitayuke oyasin', which means "we are all related." At a powwow, attendees can have experiences that are entirely unique to them.

In addition to the dancing and drumming, trade booths are typically set up to sell traditional and modern Native American objects, crafts, artwork, musical instruments, and foods.

Music: Dance, Drum, Flute

For many Native Americans, the drum has a special and sacred meaning because of its circular shape, which represents the entire world, and its rhythmic beat, which represents the world's heartbeat.

Drumming and dancing are traditional features of powwows and other Native American gatherings. Most healing rituals include drumming and singing as part of the ritual. Drumming, according to research, can cause a range of physiological responses that have mystical implications in some spiritual practices.

Traditional sacred songs are written for specific ritual occasions, but new songs may also be written for new and different situations. Music and dance provide a connection between the past, present, and future. Dance at powwows, according to one subject interviewed for this project, is a time when he is accompanied by his ancestors, allowing him to directly experience a timeless bond with those that have gone before him.

One of the most important rites for the Oglala Sioux is the Sundance. It entails a significant effort on the part of those willing to sacrifice themselves and their suffering on behalf of the people in order to increase their appreciation and determination to persevere. This rite symbolizes sacrificing one's comfort for the greater benefit of the group.

Leather thongs are tied to the flesh of a Sundancer's chests, backs, and shoulders, with the other end attached to buffalo skulls. They dance until the flesh is ripped loose, symbolizing freedom from ignorance's earthly chains. Gourd Dances and Spirit Dances are two other religious dances.

Participation in these dances has been linked to a decrease in the use and misuse of drugs and alcohol. Other people who hear the player play the Native American flute tell him they experience feelings of calm while listening.

Smudging

Smudging is the burning of plants and herbs in a ceremonial manner to cleanse and purify bad energy, provide good fortune, and safeguard a person or location. Using a huge feather or your hand, you'll disperse the smoke across all directions as part of your smudging routine. Feather symbolism and significance are added to the ceremony by the feather. In the same way that smoke connects the sky and the earth, so do birds, particularly eagles. A smudge stick may be made first and then used without a container or bowl in certain instances. Dried plants are all that are included in these packages.

Story-Telling

Native American tribes have traditionally relied on oral tradition of storytelling to pass down information from one generation to the next. Storytelling kept tribal and human origins, histories, rituals, and healing practices alive.

As a result, storytelling aids one's sense of self, comprehension of meaning, and healing direction, as well as shapes one's view of reality. Indigenous healing stories are just as real as any modern western medical science, and they provide a way to comprehend the individuality of the healing process.

Such stories will give those who are suffering trust and confidence in the healing process, and the stories themselves can be used as medicine and lead to healing. "A narrative approach helps one to consider the authenticity of people's stories," writes Mehl-Madronna.

The underlying concept is that everything is related, but this takes various forms in different families and cultures.

Inipi/Sweat Lodge

The Inipi rite, also known as the sweat lodge, is a purification ritual.

The Inipi may be performed as a stand-alone ceremony or as part of a larger ritual such as a visual search, wedding, or Sundance.

The lodge is made up of a frame made of willow branches bound together in a dome shape that is only big enough for a few adults to sit around a small pit reserved for heated stones.

Tarps and blankets are then draped over the frame. For entry and exit, a small opening is left, which can be closed during the inipi ceremony.

Prior to entering the sweat lodge, most participants fast (abstain from certain foods). The sweat lodge chief, who oversees the whole ritual, and the fire keeper, who creates a fire to warm the stones, are two important ceremonial participants.

The stones are then brought into the sweat lodge during the ritual. In most cases, a total of 28 stones are heated. The ceremony has four "doors." Seven stones are brought in through each door, the door is closed, and songs and prayers are sung as water, and herbs like sage, cedar, and sweetgrass are sprinkled onto red hot rocks, releasing incredibly hot and aromatic steam that fills the lodge.

The impact of a sweat lodge ceremony on participants was investigated in a pilot study. The findings indicated that participants' mental and spiritual well-being improved as a result of their sweat lodge experience.

The Dances

For Native Americans, dancing has long been an important part of their culture, serving as both a fun pastime and a sacred ritual. As a part of religious rites and celebrations of harvesting and gratitude, several dances were conducted.

The following is just a partial list of some of the dances and variants that were practiced in North America.

Dancing Associations

Several semi-religious festivals or events, in which a vast number of people took part, were passed down from one tribe to the next through dancing. The Grass or Omaha Dance, which was also performed by the Arapaho, Omaha, Pawnee, Crow, Dakota, Assiniboin, Gros Ventre, and Blackfoot, is one of the best-known instances of Plains Indian culture.

In vast circular wooden halls created for this purpose, these groups conducted their meetings at night. In other cases, the dancers donned what was known in the region as crow belts, which were composed of feathers, as well as an unusual headgear of hair. Every now and again, a meal of dog meat was offered. Some of these organizations' members were well-known for their charitable deeds and self-denial.

Fancy Dance

Ponca Indians invented the Fancy Dance in the late 1920s as a way to maintain their religion and culture in the face of racial prejudice. The governments of the United States and Canada had made it a criminal offense to perform Native American sacred dances during this period.

Visitors to reservations and "Wild West" performances were able to see this dance, which was loosely modeled on the conventional War Dance. The dance is quicker, vibrant, and very energetic, frequently including tricks and athletic motions. Feather bustles and headdresses, as well as leggings, beaded bodices, moccasins, and shawls, are all part of the traditional costume. Fringe, feathers, needlework, and ribbon work are all common additions to clothing. Also worn are bracelets, earrings, chokers, and eagle plumes. In addition to being a ubiquitous sight at public events, fancy dancers are also a popular form of competition.

Ghost Dance: A Fulfillment Promise

After years of hardship on Indian reservations, Native Americans turned to the Ghost Dance as a kind of spiritual solace in the late 1880s.

This dance was devised by the Native Americans as a means of resisting European colonization. It may be seen as a kind of opposition to further growth. As a result of Wovoka's spirit search or vision, the general consensus was that the dancing would bring back the spirits of ancestors, bring back the vast buffalo herds, and prevent the whites from wiping out the inhabitants or taking over the remainder of the area.

Gourd Dance

It's very uncommon to see gourd dances done in conjunction with Pow-Wows, but they have their own distinct dance and history. According to Kiowa folklore, a man out alone one day heard strange music coming from the opposite side of a mountain. Upon investigation, he discovered that the music was being performed by a red wolf, who was standing on its rear legs while singing. When the wolf woke him up in the morning, he instructed him to bring back some of the music and dances he had heard all night. Gourd dance songs culminate with a "howl" in honor of the red wolf. "Ti-ah pi-ah" means "ready to go, prepared to die" in the Kiowa language.

Ladies are welcome to join in the fun as well, either dancing behind the males or dancing around the outside of the circular arena. The drummer may be situated to one side or in the middle of the circle, and the dancers normally dance in place as they go around the perimeter. Participants just raise their heels and shake their rattles to the rhythm of the drum. Also, the dancers don't wear a lot of jewelry, but they do wear sashes around their waists or around their necks that reach the ground.

Grass Dance

Grass dancers were responsible for removing the grass from the arena before other major events in Native American culture. However, the term "grass" is not derived from the pounding on the ground but rather from the practice of attaching strands of sweetgrass with the dancer's belts, which caused the dancers to sway. The Dakota Sioux and Omaha-Ponca are said to have been the originators of the dance, which is traditionally performed exclusively by males. According to an ancient tradition, it was invented by a disabled Northern Plains youngster who had a deep yearning to dance. He was told by a Medicine Man to look for inspiration in the wide-open spaces of the prairie. While wandering over an open field on the plains, he had an epiphany on how to dance like grass. A legend has it that after returning home to convey his vision, he finally stood on his feet for the first time and performed the very first grass dance.

With their flowing movements and bending poses, dancers' postures mimic those of grass waving in the breeze. The inter-tribal nature of the dance is due in part to the modernization of rites caused by the persecution of the early 20th century and it is believed that it isn't only the dancers that benefit from these special privileges.

Hoop Dance

The Hoop Dance (Storytelling dance) utilizes up to 40 hoops, creating both dynamic and static forms. The motions of many animals and other components of the tale are represented by these structures. According to legend, the dance was originally part of a curing ritual aimed to return the planet to its natural state. The hoop symbolizes life's never-ending cycle since it has no beginning or end. Reed or wood-based hoops, shaped into various symbols, are often seen in the art of Mongolian carpet-weaving.

In most cases, a single hoop is used to represent the beginning of the dancer's journey through life. Humans, wind, animals, seasons, and water are all represented by additional hoops. To create wings and tails, the hoops interlock and are stretched from the body in a series of quick movements.

Snake Dance

For the Hopi, the Snake Dance, which takes place every year in August and features artists dancing with real snakes in their mouths, was the most well-known ceremony. Because snakes were considered to be the ancient protectors of springs, many believe the dance had its origins in a water ritual. Hopi ancestors are mostly honored in the rain ritual today. To the gods and ancestors of their ancestors, the snakes are regarded as "brothers" who convey their rain-requesting prayers.

A sedative herb is apparently used to induce vomiting before the dance, which is subsequently followed by a snake-in-the-mouth performance by the performers. With an Antelope Priest in the audience, snakes are often stroked with feathers, or their weight is supported. In addition to swaying and rattles, the dance included guttural chanting and snakes encircling the plaza in a circle. The dancers' prayers are carried out by the snakes, which are released into the four directions after the performance. Snake Dance rituals are complex and take place over a long period of time, with the majority of them taking place in kivas away from the public eye.

Rain Dance

The Rain Dance is a ritual used by many agricultural peoples, particularly in the southwest, since summers would be severely dry. For the tribe's crops, the ritual was a way of asking the gods or spirits for rain. The dance is generally held in April before crops are harvested. It was, of course, also done when there was a dire need for rain.

In contrast to several other ceremonial dances, men and women both engage in rain dances. There are many different dances and ceremonies among different tribes. The rain dance required the use of ceremonial attire and decorations that were not normally worn throughout the year. Instead, they were kept in reserve for this one-time event. In contrast to other ritual dances in which participants stand in a circle, most dance moves involve zigzagging back and forth.

Stomp Dance

It is a religious and social rite to perform the Stomp Dance. The "shuffle and stomp" moves of the dance are referred to as "Stomp Dance" in English. "Drunken," "wild," or even "inspired" are among the terms used to describe the dance in the Muskogee language of Opvnkv Haco, which refers to how the medication and dance affect participants. The Cherokee, Muscogee Creek, and other Southeastern Indian tribes perform this dance at night as part of the Green Corn Ceremony.

During the summer, these dances are usually done a number of times to keep the community healthy. Men and women perform together, and there may be 30 or more acts on the bill. Those who desire to participate follow the leader around the holy fire in a single line. Participants sing, shake rattles, and beat their feet while they dance counterclockwise around the fire. The line of dancers is arranged by age and competence, with the youngest and most inexperienced dancers at the end.

Sun Dance

This Dance is mostly done by people in the Rocky Mountains and Upper Plain regions. This annual ritual takes place in the summer with preparations starting up to a year in advance. The Eagle is a major metaphor in the dance, assisting in bringing body and soul together in peace, as is the buffalo, because of its crucial role in clothing, plains Indian food, and shelter, which is why the dance is conducted differently by various tribes.

War Dance

On the eve of an assault, several tribes would perform a War Dance to in turn perform particular religious procedures to assure victory. Warrior after warrior performed a war dance in preparation for combat while pondering revenge. The dance-inspired strong feelings in the braves, who then went into battle with a clear sense of purpose.

Typically, drums, rattles, and whistles are the only instruments used in these events. Rituals were commonly performed with people clothed and disguised as representations of different deities or supernatural animals, such as the Woodlands Iroquois, in the Pacific Northwest, Southwest, and elsewhere.

Other Ceremonies

Painting the Body of a Native American

Throughout the North America's continent, Native Americans used a wide array of body art to express themselves. In the social and religious lives of Native American tribes people, body ornamentation ranged from simple motifs painted on the skin to intricate jewelry made of symbolic materials.

There are several cultures that revered tattooing and painting on the skin as an art form. Despite the fact that soldiers painted their bodies in preparation for combat, this practice was not limited to war paint. Tattoos and painted body art have long been used to denote a person's age, standing in society, marital status, or, in the case of males, and their prowess as warriors.

Pipes of Peace for Native Americans

Various types of steam and smoke are often used in Native American rituals. Symbolic of a link between the world and the celestial home, it appears in the sky. During these rituals, several tribes make use of a variety of pipes, which they pass around or deliberately smoke in the four cardinal directions.

In addition to holy pipe and calumet, peace pipes go by many other names. To make it, elders of the tribes used bone or wood-like cigars, but longer. A disagreement may be put to rest by smoking a peace pipe, and the herbs are used as a therapeutic ritual to do so.

The Sacred Pipe Ceremony

The pipe is an undeniably important sacred object for all the Native American tribes. It was used in many healing and sacred ceremonies; its presence enhanced the effect of the medicine and called to gather all the spirits of the earth.

The pipe, in all its parts, has a deep meaning: the bowl represents the female nature of life, the nurturing, the Mother Earth; the stem represents the male part, the Father Sky; the tube that connects stem and bowl represents the connection between the visible and material world with the invisible and spiritual one.

As a complete object, it represents the thin line man must walk to live in balance with nature. Once assembled, the pipe is the joining of all the aspects of life in one single object; it reconnects the multi-faced aspects of reality into a single entity.

The healer had the right to choose the herbs to be smoked during the ceremony (usually they were tobacco, uva ursi, sage, thyme, raspberry, and willow).

Before smoking, the healer offered small pinches of tobacco to the four directions, the plants and the animal kingdom, the sky, the earth, the mother, the sun, and the moon. With this, all the elements were witnessed and invited to the ceremony.

The one who carried the pipe was not its owner, but rather the keeper. He was entrusted by the whole tribe to be the intermediary with the Great Spirit, and due to this power, he was taken into great consideration. Smoking was praying: each inspiration of smoke was a prayer to the Great Spirit and all its manifestation in the world.

The keeper and the pipe were deeply connected. The pipe spoke to him and created the connection between the material and the spiritual world. The more experienced the keeper, the stronger was this connection.

The Sacred Pipe Ceremony is a moment of profound reconnection with the deepest nature that lies within ourselves. During the ceremony, we surpass our senses and achieve a deeper sense of meaning.

Although each tribe has its own specific rituals and peculiarities regarding the sacred pipe ceremony, the essence is very similar between all of them. Each part of the ceremony has a proper etiquette, motivated by an important, sacred meaning.

The first step of the ceremony is smudging: the bundle is lit and the participants (pipe keeper first) are smudged using a bird feather.

When all the people have been smudged, it is the turn of the parts that will be assembled to form the pipe: first the stem north to south and then west to east, then the bowl in the same way.

Smoke must penetrate all the cavities of the stem and the bowl to purify the pipe in each of its parts.

This part of the ceremony is very evocative and it gives you the possibility to concentrate on the healer and to calm your inner dialogue so that you are prepared for what comes next.

Once the smudging is completed, the bowl and stem are held high, respectively in the left and in the right hand, and permission to smoke is requested to the Great Spirit.

Here the pipe keeper acts as an intermediary between the spiritual and the material world for the first time: he evokes the Spirit and attunes with it, looking for signs of the granted permission. It might be a light breeze rising up, or a rustling of leaves, or just the feeling that permission is granted by an experienced pipe carrier.

Granted permission, the healer joins the two parts of the pipe. As already stated, this is a very important and sacred moment because it represents the joining of all the parts of life and the reconciliation of all dualisms. The entire universe becomes one single entity.

After the junction of the two parts, comes the filling part. The stem is laid down on the lap of the healer and the bowl on the ground.

The healer takes four pinches of the smoking mixture one at a time, he holds them up and puts them inside the bowl with the right hand.

Each time he fills the bowl, he asks an entity to join the Sacred Pipe. In order, he calls for the Great Spirit, the spirits of trees and greens, the spirits of the animals that walk, swim, or fly, and finally the four elements of fire, water, air, and stone.

With each pinch, he invites a part of the material and spiritual world to join the ceremony.

A lot of experience and practice is required from the carrier to actually feel these elements joining the ceremony and to be able to talk with them.

In the next phase, each one of the attendants places his prayers into the pipe holding the bowl of the pipe with the left hand. The first is the pipe keeper, and then the person on his left, and so on until the circle is completed. Prayers might not be necessarily requests or desires but also thanks or worries that the participants wants to share with others and the spirits.

Once the circle is completed, the pipe comes back to the healer who lights it with big puffs of smoke without inhaling. Then, the carrier holds it up, stem higher, and offers the pipe to the Creator, the first to smoke.

Also in this phase, the sensitivity of the carrier is vital because he must sense the Creator to come and smoke the pipe. Once the Creator accepts the first smoke, the pipe is lowered down and passed to Mother Earth, and then to the four directions.

Once all the spirits have their smoke, it is the healer's turn to smoke, and subsequently, the others, starting from the left.

The inhalation of the smoke is a moment of deep connection between the one who smokes and the Spirit: each prayer that has been placed inside the pipe becomes smoke and it blends with the smoker. With the exhalation of smoke, the prayer diffuses in the universe, towards the Creator, but a part of it remains with the one who expressed it.

The pipe passes to the left until all the smoking mixture is gone. Once the pipe is empty, the carrier expresses his final thanks to the Great Spirit for generously giving them permission to smoke and then he cleans and puts the pipe away.

Totems and Animal Medicine in Native American Culture

A person or group's totem is a spirit, holy item, or emblem of that group. Some Native American tribes believe that each individual is linked to nine distinct animals that serve as his or her personal guardians during the course of his or her lifetime.

Depending on where we're going and what we need to accomplish along the way, different animals serve as power animals and/ or spirit guides in our life.

They believe that a totem creature is one that will accompany you throughout your whole life, both in this world and the hereafter. This one totem creature serves as the primary guardian spirit for humans throughout their lives, even if they identify with other animals.

Conclusion

This book is a complete elaboration of the spiritual history of the Native Americans and how they used to carry out their spiritual practices and help themselves survive in the difficult world of that time. To review what you just covered, here is a systematic flow of the entire book, which ranges from the spiritual understanding of the history of Native Americans to their herbal medicine outreach.

The Native Americans were known for all their religious beliefs. They were not just smart in discovering healing aids by exploring the plants around them, but they also followed some impactful sacramental practices, irrespective of their tribes. All of the indigenous peoples of Native America were following the religions and beliefs taught to them during their time. All of these traditions did lack the sacred texts and fixed all of the moral codes and doctrines.

These codes were then embedded into the tribes or societies without the necessity of writing them and even without wealth. There were no recognizable systems of justice, politics, or any usual civilization. But as of today, the situations are turned around, and there are students of the ecological sciences, scholars of religion, individuals keen to expand the religious lives of themselves and others. The histories of Native Americans didn't get complete justice or success.

All of the traditions, culture, and beliefs were hampered by economic and political rules intervening in the system. With the small and complex ceremonies becoming extinct, the community members mourned the loss of their tradition. But the people who tend to believe in their ancestors and their traditional ceremonies can still continue with their beliefs and hold onto them.

The Native Americans used to believe in many different deities as having control over different elements on Earth. Some such things include the weather, the underworld, and others. Some of the Native Americans had a belief that there was a deity who used to control the mountains as well. This is the idea of a singular and Great Spirit with a sense of Spirituality within the Native Americans of different tribes. The Dakota, Sioux, and Lakota tribes call this Wakan Tanka.

It is a concept that is quite different from that of the concept of gods and goddesses of today! Wakan Tanka means a great or sacred mystery! It encompasses the belief in spirits that interacts with the world in several ways. It is often accountable as the great force which exists within all humanism, animals, plants, and all of the other objects around the world. This concept is similar to that of animism, which is practiced mostly in the pagan religions across the world.

There are different groups of Native Americans who counted on this supreme force to be the creator of all things around the world. All of the older cultures across the globe have their own stories about the creation of this world and how the people came to existence. The Native Americans also had their own story on how they believed that spiritual power exists. Hence, they had complete faith in their spiritual beliefs that is even passed onto the generations of today.

The Native American concept upon death was similar to that of all of the other paths of religions across the world. The belief they had was of a spirit that continues to live even after physical death has stopped the body. It is said that the soul of a person will travel onto another realm or the spirit world, where the person will be born again in a different body. The concept of journeying onto the other world makes ideal sense because the Native American tribes did spend a lot of time traveling to different places in the early days.

The Native Americans see the journey as a usual progression of life, for which they count death with the same belief. But they also believed in a concept that, in some cases, the spirit gets stuck on Earth itself and fails to enter the spiritual realm. The ceremonies and funeral rites were carried out in order to facilitate the profession of spirit to the next life. It is again similar to that of most of the religions across the world. The Last Rites or prayers at funerals offer eternal peace to the spirit of the dead. This is what the Native American tribes believed about death.

They had a strong sense of survival, for which they started their own agricultural efforts. The thoughtful discovery of ideas and implementations pushed them to grow their own food! There were celebration for the growth of new food for a fresh season, which was a sign of early agricultural civilization. These celebrations are often carried out in communities and groups for embedding Spirituality.

Some Native American tribes were engaging in agriculture around the Eastern and Southern parts of the US. Some of the celebrations, such as the Green Corn Festivals, had a special significance. This ceremony was all about picking the corn at the end of the growing season and waiting until it gets ready to be used as food. These agricultural ceremonies were carried out by the Creek, Cherokee, and Iroquois nations of Native Americans.

These rituals include ritual cleansings, feasts, dancing, and many other such ceremonies that were not just fun but were meaningful as well. Every special occasion within these Native American tribes was carried out in between these ceremonies. Some such occasions include sports, games, baby naming, and council meetings! Following agriculture, the Native Americans soon realized that herbs or plants around them have medicinal properties in them.

They realized this when they saw animals eating the plant leaves and getting healed. The Native Americans took the initiative to explore and experiment with the plants in their possession or the ones that they used to grow! Soon, they collected every alternate plant that they could find and ran their experimentations on healing different medical adversities. This is what pushed them towards the idea of utilizing herbs for healing the human body.

These approaches inspired later generations to adapt natural healing methodologies and all of the spiritual beliefs of the Native Americans. There were ceremonies for cleansing the soul, mind, and body in the past, which are still being carried out in some form of tradition such as Sun Dance, The Ghost Dance, Smudging, Pipe Ceremony, sweat Lodges, and others. Along with the traditions, this generation adapted the healing beliefs from the sacred plants of that time.

Amidst all these spiritual traditions, the Native Americans showed their spiritual belief in some sacred plants which they believe had healing properties. Research on these plants and their medicinal properties is still going on. There are very few plants that have been discovered with medicinal properties so far in the world. There are still more herbs and plants out there in the world that still need to be discovered. The era is already begun by the Native Americans in the past. But, the latter discovery and experimentations are still in process.

The world has many gifts for humans on this planet. There are sufficient plants and herbs with medicinal properties to heal almost any health problem. Native Americans were not just popular for their belief in God, but they also worked upon finding out the gifts of that supreme almighty. There might come a time in the near future when there will be plant or herb-based medicine for all critical medical conditions such as cancer, tumors, and others. It is a possibility that Herbalism intends to explore!

Soon, there were some changes imposed upon the Native American religion. These changes did not begin due to the arrival of European settlers on the eastern shores. Rather, it was the nations and tribes within the country that affected each other through battles and assimilation. If there was more than one group of tribes, they tried to influence one another in some way or another. This is how t change in tradition and beliefs started amongst the Native Americans. However, it was the European settlers who encouraged the change of name for the country to the US later after their arrival.

The most cherished discovery of the Native Americans and their spiritual beliefs are the plants and herbs they used to heal. Apart from these brilliant revolutions and teachings to the world, some traditions are not understandable at all by the modern world. From the outside perspective, the American Indians were forced out from their ancestral homes and pushed towards the reservations, a deplorable act.

This is something that didn't justify their sense of Spirituality in the past. There were ghost stories of sacred lands, holy ground, and other such places involved within the various religious practices and beliefs of the Native Americans. Just like these assumptions, there were many other beliefs that were accountable as the spatial truth. People also believed in a sacred mystery that existed in the mountains; fish, stones, people, and the land itself were part of the spiritual existence of the Native Americans.

Everything in this world is alive and is subject to a degree of consideration. And with this understanding, the idea of moving people out of their ancestral home and following myths becomes a destructive measure to that of their Spirituality. Native Americans have contributed quite a number of lessons for the modern world to adapt and utilize! And the modern day scientists are leveraging the potential of technologies and tools to derive more information on the historical traditions, beliefs, and plant-based medications.

This book is now complete with all of the instances referred to as the spiritual history of Native Americans. Every possible piece of information that you can gather about the existence of Native Americans and their traditions is available within this book. So, thank you again for downloading it. I hope this helped you get impactful insight into the spiritual and medicinal practices for attaining inner peace and healthcare

BOOK 3: HERBALISM ENCYCLOPEDIA VOL. 1

Introduction

Before modern medicine, we relied heavily on "unrefined" herbal medicine to treat different illnesses we came down with. The herbs weren't even put through any pharmaceutical modification before we, at that time, took them for one ailment or another. We either cooked or ground the herbs to break the plant components down making them edible before consuming them, and they always worked.

Fast forward to today, herbal medicine remains one of the only few highly effective medicinal remedies to the medical conditions we develop. Pharmaceutical companies even still use them in modern medicines for their scent, flavor and healing properties. If you walk into any pharmacy today and buy a drug, there is a high chance you'll find these herbs in the tablets, capsules, powders, teas, extracts, etc. that you will but over the counter. These herbs are used in drug production because they contain strong substances that stimulate vigorous physiological and, certainly, medicinal activities in our body when we consume them.

The herbs found in Native America, particularly, have been confirmed to possess highly therapeutic substances and these have been further categorized, by experts, into the following: Alkaloids, Anthocyanins, Anthraquinones, Cardiac Glycosides, Coumarins, Cyanogenic Glycosides, Flavonoids, Glucosilinates, Phenols, Saponins, Tannins, etc.

All these substances have the power to repair our tissues and organs and also provide the body with a long-lasting protection against recurring diseases and ailments.

Native American medicine had been a major influence on modern medicine, even long before the Europeans came into Native American territory. It served as remedies to many of the illnesses and conditions the natives experienced. These herbs still serve us today, and will continue to do so. It is for this reason that I have decided to dedicate a body of extensive research—and a period of thorough inquiry into the therapeutic properties of these herbs—to provide you with the necessary information about Native American herbs and their immense benefits to you when you use them as medicine.

I'd like you to see this book as a definitive guide to all the Native American herbs you can ever find, anywhere. The fact you're holding this book at the moment suggests you already understand how powerful Native American medicine is and that you would like to explore the healing powers they provide. Well, you've done the right thing by acquiring this book and I'd like to congratulate you.

Native American Herbalism is the master key you need to unlock the deep secrets about the tremendous power Northern American herbs possess. I implore you to make continued use of it. Trust me; at the end of this book, you'll be so glad you devoured its contents. Not only is it informational, but it is quite an interesting read as well.

So, I wish you a happy reading.

The Twelve Categories of Herbs

There are over three hundred different types of herbs in the world. Each kind has its own unique properties and healing benefits, and though these herbs all carry some positive power, they're not all equal.

Here we'll explore the twelve different categories of herbs that can be found in today's world.

Let's look at these twelve groups of herbs mentioned in this book using this fundamental understanding of energetic concepts. Keep in mind that any given herb could fall under multiple categories.

1. Pungent Herbs

Pungent herbs have a spicy or fiery flavor and a characteristically strong scent. Capsicum (cayenne pepper), ginger, mustard, and onions are examples of plants that spice up recipes. The presence of resins, alkamides, allyl sulfides, or monoterpene essential oils give these herbs their strong flavor. They are warming and drying herbs with a strong flavor. They transport blood and energy from the body's interior to the skin and mucous membranes and from its exterior to the skin and mucous membranes. This implies they aid in removing stagnation, the induction of sweat, and the stimulation of blood circulation. They boost intestinal peristalsis and increase hunger by stimulating the production of digestive fluids. Excessive consumption of spicy herbs depletes the body's energy reserves and causes it to chill. Some people's digestive tracts are irritated by these herbs. Aromatic herbs should not be used by hot, flushed, irritable, or those who have a reddish complexion.

2. Herbs with Volatile Oils

Aromatic herbs have volatile oils in them (also called essential oils). When volatile oils are exposed to heat and light, they evaporate. Many aromatics, like pungent herbs, are utilized as culinary spices. Dill, peppermint, and lemon balm are among the aromatic herbs found in the mint and carrot families. Warming and drying properties are common in aromatic herbs; however, they have a softer effect than pungent herbs. They usually have a powerfully relaxing or energizing effect on the nervous system. Because many essential oils are antibacterial, aromatic herbs can help fight illnesses. When ingested as hot teas, aromatics can cause perspiration, stimulate blood circulation, and expel intestinal gas. Aromatic herbs are extremely safe to use. On the other hand, pure essential oils should be used nearly exclusively for topical applications, and even then, they should be considerably diluted. Essential oils are concentrated extracts that are considerably more prone to cause adverse reactions than whole herbs.

3. Nonalkaloidal (Simple) Bitters

Simple bitters are plants that are bitter due to what is known as bitter principles in traditional herbal textbooks. These chemicals are now known as diterpenes and different glycosides. Stimulant laxatives, which are a subtype of simple bitters, are controlled by anthraquinone glycosides. Artichoke leaf, gentian, wild lettuce, kale, and hops are examples of nonalkaloidal bitters. Cascara sagrada, Turkey rhubarb, buckthorn, butternut bark, and aloe leaf are stimulant laxatives (not the gel). The majority of nonalkaloidal bitters have a cooling and drying effect. Dong Quai and turmeric, for example, have aromatic components that make them warming and drying. Bitters encourage energy to flow inward and downward (toward the eliminative organs) (toward the digestive organs). Nonalkaloidal bitters have a detoxifying effect. Some have sedative or soothing properties, while others are anodynes or pain relievers. They stimulate the synthesis of hydrochloric acid, bile, and pancreatic enzymes, among other things. Bitter herbs that are sweetened or ingested in capsules do not promote digestive secretions; thus, this only happens when they are tasted. Cooling bitters can deplete digestion over time. Warming bitters, aromatic or pungent herbs are used in traditional digestive tonics to counteract the depleting effects of cooling bitters. Thin, weak, malnourished, and dry people should avoid bitters.

4. Alkaloidal Bitters

Due to the presence of alkaloids, alkaloidal bitters have a bitter flavour. Caffeine, nicotine, and berberine are examples of chemicals with names ending in -ine. Alkaloidal bitters include coffee and chocolate. Goldenseal, Oregon grape, and California poppy are examples of alkaloids-containing herbs. Alkaloidal bitters, like nonalkaloidal bitters, are cooling and drying. Many of them are detoxifying and help to stimulate the digestive and liver systems. Goldenseal and Oregon grape are alkaloidal bitters that contain berberine and are used to treat infections. Alkaloids can imitate hormones and neurotransmitters, activating or sedating specific biological processes. Nonalkaloidal bitters and alkaloidal bitters both have broad contraindications. People should be aware that they can be drying and depleting when these are used excessively. Keep in mind the indications and contraindications for each herb in this category.

5. Fragrant Bitters

Fragrant bitters are a hybrid of aromatics and simple bitters. Sesquiterpene lactones and triterpenes are the main components. Elecampane, black walnut hulls, wormwood, tansy, and wormseed are examples of fragrant bitters. Bitters with a floral aroma are both warming and drying. They are used in tiny doses to help with digestion and appetite. Many of them are used to get rid of parasites. The use of most fragrant bitters is not recommended during pregnancy, and many are not suitable for long-term use. They have the same general contraindications as the other bitters groups.

6. Acrid Herbs

Acrid herbs have a bitter, unpleasant, and burning flavor similar to the taste of bile. Resins (like aromatic herbs) and alkaloids are found in these plants (like alkaloidal bitters). Lobelia and kava-kava are the strongest examples of this flavor, but black cohosh, skunk cabbage, and blue vervain have it to a lesser extent. Acrid herbs are calming, which means they are diffusive, allowing blood, lymph, and energy to flow freely. They have the potential to be both cooling and drying. Their main effect is antispasmodic, which means they help to relieve cramps. In some traditional medical systems, they are used to treat what are known as wind illnesses. Fever and chills, as well as diarrhea and constipation, are examples of alternating symptoms. Wind diseases are characterized by pains that travel from one place of the body to another. Excessive doses or long-term usage of acrid herbs can cause vomiting, and large doses or long-term use can harm the nerves.

7. Astringent Herbs

Herbs that contain tannins are referred to as astringent herbs. Tannic acid has a slightly bitter flavor and causes a drying, puckering sensation in the mouth when consumed. Green tea has astringent properties. White oak bark, uva ursi, and sage are all astringent plants. Herbs that are astringent constrict and dry tissues. Excessive secretions are stopped, loose tissue is tightened, oedema is reduced, and blood coagulation is aided. When used topically to bites and stings, they are anti-venomous. Internally, they tone up intestinal membranes and slow intestinal peristalsis (which helps to prevent loose, watery stool). Astringents are best used between meals since they slow digestive secretions and may interfere with mineral absorption. Constipation can occur in large doses, and long-term use might irritate the skin and mucous membranes.

8. Sour Herbs

The presence of several fruit acids (citric, malic, and ascorbic acid), as well as flavonoids, gives many berries and fruits a sour flavor. Flavonoids are anti-inflammatory and anti-fever agents. Herbs with a sour taste are both cooling and nutritious. They might be balanced, moistening, or drying in nature. They're utilized to minimize tissue inflammation, irritation, and damage from free radicals (which cause ageing and degenerative disease). They can improve capillary integrity and tone weak tissues. The liver and eyes, which use more antioxidants than any other organ, benefit from sour herbs. They are safe foods with no known side effects.

9. Salty Herbs

Plants don't have the same salty flavor as table salt. It has a more delicate flavor, with a grassy or green undertone. Consider the taste of celery or spinach. Mineral salts like magnesium, potassium, sodium, and calcium give these foods a slightly salty flavor. Green herbs like alfalfa, mullein, and seaweeds are salty herbs. Salty herbs are both balanced and nourishing. They can both moisten and dry damp tissues. They are nutritious because they include minerals that aid in tissue toning and healing. They stimulate lymph flow, remove mucus and often swollen lymph nodes by clearing the lymphatic system. Many salty herbs are diuretics that do not irritate the kidneys and nourish and promote renal function. They are generally non-addictive and have no known side effects.

10. Sweet Herbs

Sweet herbs don't have the same sweetness as sugar or honey. It reminds me of the sweetness of a dark chocolate bar. Polysaccharides or saponins are responsible for sweetness. Licorice and stevia are obvious examples of sweet herbs, but many tonics and adaptogenic treatments, such as American or Korean ginseng, codonopsis, and astragalus, are also sweet. Sweet herbs are moisturizing and neutral, but they might be somewhat warming or cooling. Sweet herbs help to strengthen weakened conditions, prevent wasting, strengthen glands, and refill energy reserves. They combat tissue dryness and ageing, and they frequently work as immune tonics, stimulating or balancing immunological activities. The majority of sweet herbs are highly safe and can be used in tiny dosages for a long time. Larger doses can overstimulate the body and be abused in the same way that stimulants like coffee are abused, especially by teenagers. They are often more effective when used as part of a formula than when used alone.

11. Mucilant Herbs

Although most literature refers to these herbs as mucilaginous or demulcent, we prefer the term "mucilant." Mucilants have a bland or mildly sweet flavour, but their texture is their most defining feature. They have a slimy, slippery texture when wet. Gums, mucilage, and pectin are examples of water-loving polysaccharides or mucopolysaccharides. Glycosaminoglycans may also be present. Okra is a mucilant vegetable. Aloe vera, slippery elm, and kelp are some examples of herbal remedies. Mucilants are hydrating, cooling, and nourishing to the skin. They are used to relieve hot, red, dry, and irritated tissues. When taken internally, they add water-soluble fibre to the stool, and when taken with enough water, they act as bulk laxatives. They can also assist in stopping diarrhea. Mucilants nourish and nurture beneficial gut flora while also promoting overall intestinal health. They help lower cholesterol and remove toxins from the body by absorbing bile from the gallbladder and liver. Mucilants protect mucous membranes and are used topically as poultices to soothe and cure irritated or injured skin. Mucilants should be administered separately from nutrients and drugs because they are absorbent. Excessive use can cause the gastrointestinal function to slow and cool, but this is easily remedied by adding a tiny amount of an aromatic or spicy plant. To operate efficiently, mucilants must be taken with plenty of water.

12. Oily Herbs

Due to fatty acids, oily herbs, especially seeds, have an oily flavor and texture. Flaxseed, evening primrose seed, and coconut are all oily plants. Herbs that are rich in oil are both nutritious and cooling. They give fatty acids to the body, which are needed for energy synthesis and immunological, neurological, and glandular function. (Both borage and evening primrose oils are sold as treatments for affecting prostaglandin function.) Dry tissues are moistened, and tissue flexibility is increased by using oily herbs. Some are moderate laxatives that lubricate the stool to make it easier to pass. There are no real contraindications to using oily plants.

Native American Herbs

Agave

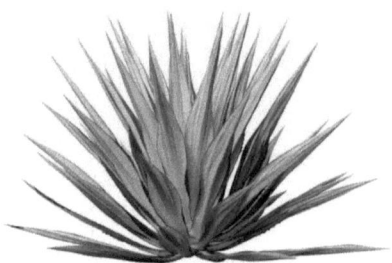

Common Names: Century Plant, Maguey, American Aloe

Scientific Name: Agave Americana

Family: Asparagaceae

Origin: Native to semi-arid and arid regions of America, particularly the Caribbean and Mexico.

About Agave

This plant takes a lot of time to grow – about 5 to 7 years. It also possesses a low glycemic index which helps to keep blood sugar levels in check. It is good for boosting the immune system.

Medicinal Parts:

- The sap
- The leaves
- The seed

Habitat and Foraging:

- The agave plant is a monocarpic plant that dies after fruiting.
- It only blossoms once after 10 years in a warm climate or 35 years in a cool climate.
- In its native range, this plant blooms from June to August

Influence on the Body:

- Antiseptic
- Wound healing
- Anti-inflammatory

Traditional uses:

- The sap poultice was used as a wound healing agent and as a hand skin treatment.
- The root and leaves poultice was used to treat toothache.

Possible Side Effects:

- Digestive system irritation if taken in large quantities.
- Allergic reactions for those who are allergic.

Alder

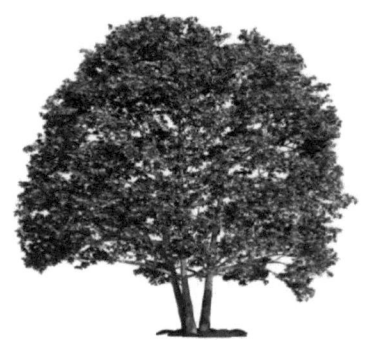

Common Names: Mountain Alder

Scientific Name: Alnus Incana

Family: Betulaceae

Origin: Native to Northwest America (California)

About Alder

The leaves and barks of the alder tree are used to make medicine for sore throats, rheumatism, swellings, and fever. Anyone can take alder medications but dosage depends on age and severity of health condition. Those on other medications need to be careful when using alder.

Medicinal Parts:

- The bark
- The leaves

Habitat and Foraging:

- Alder grows on open woodland.
- It grows in most soil types with a flowering period between March to April.

Influence on the Body:

- Fever
- Constipation
- Bleeding

Traditional uses:

- tea made from the bark was used as a gargle to treat toothaches and bleeding gums.
- Poultice from the leaves was used to treat wounds, burns and hemorrhoids.

Possible Side Effects:

- None

Alfalfa

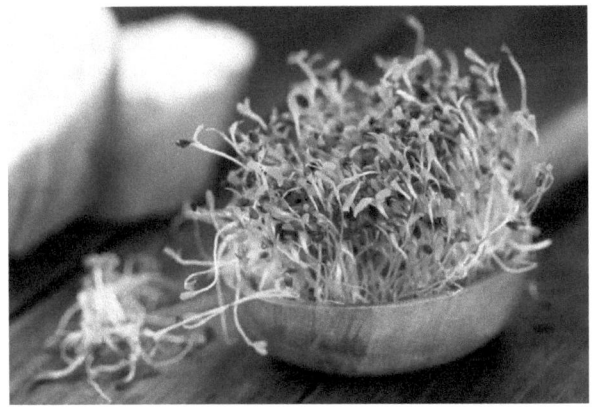

Common Names: Buffalo Herb, Lucerne

Scientific Name: Medicago Sativa

Family: Fabaceae

Origin: Native to Asia and introduced to North America

About Alfalfa

Alfalfa is a native of Asia but only got to North America in 1860. This deep growing plant can beseen around Virginia down to Maine and westward to the Pacific coast of the United States. Its seeds, sprouts, and leaves are used to make medicines mostly for kidney, bladder, and prostate conditions. It contains many essential nutrients, which makes it popular for constant use.

Medicinal Parts:

- The seeds
- The leaves

Habitat and Foraging:

- The alfalfa plant is usually found in vacant lots, abandoned fields, and railroads.

Influence on the Body:

- It helps improve metabolism.
- It lowers cholesterol levels.
- It contains healthy antioxidants.

Traditional Uses:

- Relieving menopause symptoms

Possible Side Effects:

- It should not be used by pregnant women.
- It should not be used by those who take blood thinners or have autoimmune disorders.

Aloe Vera

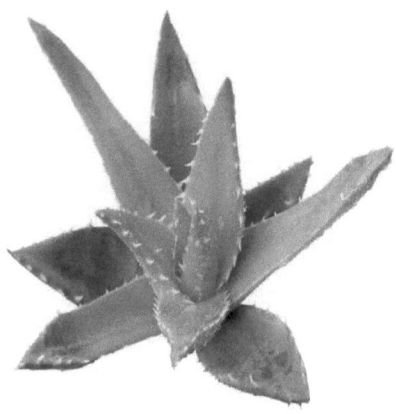

Common Names: Cape aloe, Barbados Aloe

Scientific Name: Aloe Vera

Family: Asphodelaceae

Origin: South-east Arabian Peninsula

About Aloe Vera

At the base of this plant is a basal rosette of long, pointed succulent leaves with toothed edges. It is olive green in color and sometimes mottled in yellow. It creates a group of red or yellow tubular flowers from a central spike.

Medicinal Parts:

- The leaves are used for juice
- The leaves are also used for gel

Habitat and Foraging:

- Ornamental plant
- Low natural rainfall areas

Influence on the Body:

- It is good for most skin conditions.
- It is used as a tonic.
- Vermifuge
- It is cathartic

Traditional Uses:

- Skin treatment for wounds, burns, frostbite and rashes.
- The fresh leaves poultice was used to treat wounds and insect bites.

Possible Side Effects:

- Oral ingestion is potentially toxic.
- Dangerous for people with aloe allergies.
- Do not use in case of pregnancy, liver or gallbladder conditions, or hemorrhoids.

Angelica

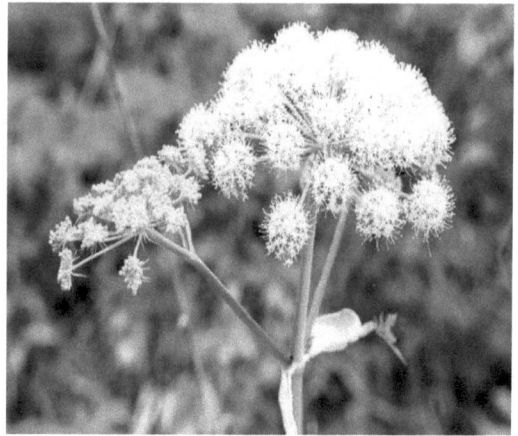

Common Names: Angelica

Scientific Name: Angelica Californica

Family: Apiaceae

Origin: Northern California and occasionally in southern Oregon. Dry, low-elevation foothills.

About Angelica

Angelica is a plant that grows from three to nine feet tall and has thick, purple stems. Its leaves are large and divided into three to five minor, smaller, oval-shaped leaves. Its flowers are grouped in umbels and are small and white. It is like hemlock but is poisonous so, to be sure it is the one, one must smell its roots and or the seeds. If these have the typical angelica smell, almost like celery, it is angelica. Another method for double-checking it is to break a branch or a leaf and smell it. If it smells like urine, then it is hemlock.

Medicinal Parts:

- The roots
- The leaves
- The flowers
- The seeds

Habitat and Foraging:

- Biennial and perennial plant

Influence on the Body:

- Carminative
- Expectorant
- Diuretic
- Emmenagogue

Traditional uses:

- Poultice from the fresh roots of this plant was used to treat swollen joints for an anti-inflammatory and pain relief effect.
- The leaves and flowers decoction was used to cure rheumatism, sore throats, fever, ulcers, urinary tract infections, and headaches.
- Raw leaves were used to treat diarrhea.

Possible Side Effects:

- None

Arsemart

Common Names: Smartweed, Water Pepper, Marshpepper knotweed

Scientific Name: Persicaria hydropiper

Family: Polygonaceae

Origin: All over the United States, in wet environments.

About Arsemart

This annual plant can grow up to 30 inches and likes wet environments such as marshes and alluvial meadows. Its taproot sinks into the ground up to 3 feet in general, so it is difficult to eradicate. The green-reddish, smooth stems emerge straight from the ground with alternate, lance-shaped leaves covered with thin hair. The inflorescence is located at the top of the stem as a vertical cluster of small pink flowers, and it blooms in summer. After pollination, the plant produces a small, triangular black seed at the base of each dried flower.

Medicinal Parts:

- The whole plant

Habitat and Foraging:

- Annual plant
- Several active ingredients

Influence on the Body:

- Diuretic
- Diaphoretic
- Tonic
- Vermifuge
- Analgesic

Traditional uses:

- The poultice and juice were used to treat ulcers and swollen joints.
- Chewing the root treats toothache.
- The leaves and flower tea were used as a cure for sepsis and intestinal worms.

Possible Side Effects:

- Wild arsemart produces oils that cause skin irritation.

Amaranth

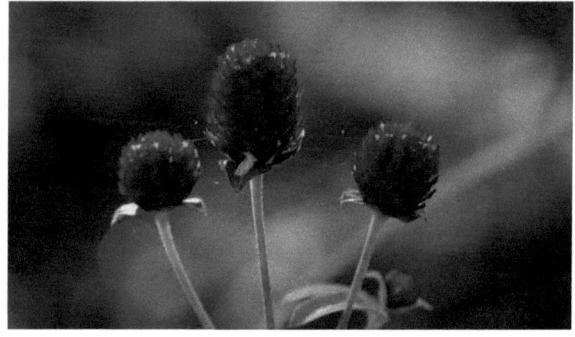

Common Names: Wild Amaranth Pigweed, Purple Amaranth

Scientific Name: Amaranthus

Family: Amaranthaceae

Origin: Native to Central America (Mexico)

About Amaranth

Amaranth is a group of grains of more than 60 species. This ancient grain gives a healthy dose of protein, fibers, and other important macronutrients. The leaves are also rich in soluble and insoluble fiber, which helps to reduce weight. The seed is easily prepared by soaking it in water for about three days when it begins to germinate. This makes it easy for it to break down and for all the ant nutrients to be digested. It can be used for different tasty dishes.

Medicinal Parts:

- The leaves
- The seeds

Habitat and Foraging:

- Amaranth is easy to plant.
- It is found in North America and South Asia.
- It needs to be planted for close to 120 days for a long season.

Influence on the Body:

- Lowers cholesterol levels
- It contains antioxidants
- Reduces inflammation

Traditional uses:

- The oil obtained from leaves and seeds was used for weight loss.

Possible Side Effects:

- None

American Licorice

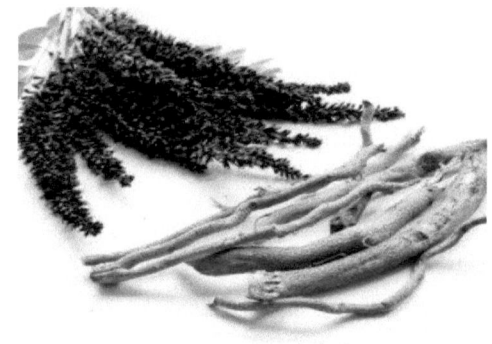

Common Names: Wild Licorice

Scientific Name: Glycyrrhiza Lepidota

Family: Fabaceae

Origin: Native to Canada and Northwest America (Texas-California)

About American Licorice

The root of the American licorice is one of the oldest herbal remedies in the world. It has been popularly used to treat coughs, viral infections, hot flashes, heart burns, and acid refluxes. It also helps to manage sore throats and clears difficult skin conditions. Even though it has no standard dosage, it is advised for people to take no more than 100 grams a day.

Medicinal Parts:

- The leaves
- The roots

Habitat and Foraging:

- American licorice is mostly found in prairie and other grassland communities.
- It grows to 16-39 inches high.
- It is grazed in summer and early fall.

Influence on the Body:

- It protects against cavities.
- It helps treat peptic ulcers.

Traditional uses:

- The root infusion was used to treat cough, diarrhea, and chest pains.
- Also, the infusion was used as a wash on swellings.
- Chewing the root was known to relieve toothaches and sore throats.

Possible Side Effects:

- Not good for pregnant and breastfeeding women.
- Bad interaction with certain drugs.

American Mistletoe

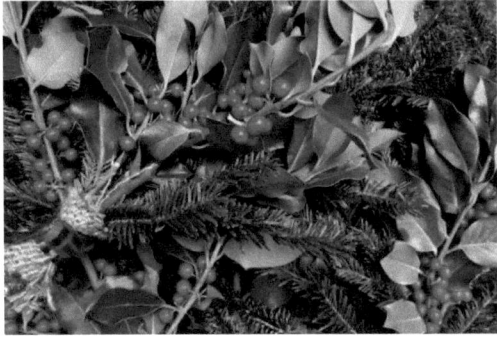

Common Names: Eastern Mistletoe, Oak Mistletoe

Scientific Name: Phoradendron Leucarpum

Family: Santalaceae

Origin: Native to North America (New Mexico, Florida, Illinois)

About American Mistletoe

The American mistletoe has been used since the early 1920s and is an important plant with numerous uses. Every part of this plant is medicinal from the stem, leaf, fruit, and flower. The chemicals in the American mistletoe plant affect the muscles and treat low blood pressure and constipation. While it is considered a great and healthy herb, it is however advisable to take the berries and leaves in small quantities to avoid complications.

Medicinal Parts:

- The flower
- The root
- The stem
- The leaves

Habitat and Foraging:

- American mistletoe grows on a host of trees like lime, blackthorns, willows, and apple.
- It grows best in open spaces with a lot of light.

Influence on the Body:

- Constipation
- Low-blood pressure

Traditional uses:

- Easy emptying of the system.

Possible Side Effects:

Taking a lot of berries or leaves can lead to complications such as:

- Diarrhea
- Heart problems
- Vomiting
- Nausea

American Raspberry

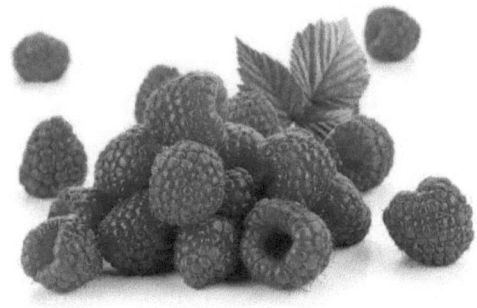

Common Names: American Red Raspberry, Blackberry, Dewberry

Scientific Name: Rubus Strigosus

Family: Rosaceae

Origin: Native to Europe and introduced to North America

About American Raspberry

The American raspberry is found in different colors, and it packs a lot of nutrients that help lower blood pressure. This herb contains Omega-3 fatty acid, which helps prevent heart complications and even stroke. With constant but healthy consumption, American raspberry helps keep the body healthy, protecting the skin and the bones. Each of the American raspberries has distinctive tastes – according to the color – and to get all the nutrients from them, you can use them as toppings for cereals, muffins, and fruit salads. Countless recipes are designed to help you get the best out of your raspberries.

Medicinal Parts:

- The fruit
- The leaves

Habitat and Foraging:

- American raspberries are found in most temperate regions of the world.
- It is found in many North American regions, and it grows for most of the year.

Influence on the Body:

- It contains numerous healthy nutrients like folate Vitamin C and fiber.
- It has antioxidant properties which protect against cancer and other complicated diseases.

Traditional uses:

- It is used as a face mask for protecting the face.

Possible Side Effects:

- None

Arnica

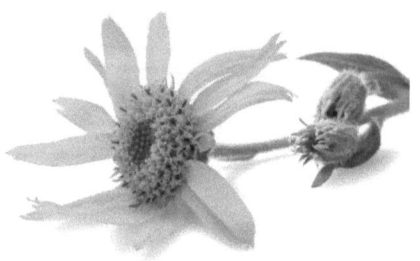

Common Names: Wolf's Bane, Mountain Arnica, Mountain Tobacco

Scientific Name: Arnica Montana

Family: Asteraceae

Origin: Native to North America (Alaska, Montana, Nevada, Oregon, Utah)

About Arnica

Arnica is commonly used for treating bruises. The leaves are also used to treat certain muscle-related conditions. It is usually administered orally but is also applied as a gel. Arnica has often been taken topically to help prevent overdosing on the drug. The best way to take arnica is through homeopathic solutions; let it dissolve slowly until it is completely diluted before ingesting it as it is actually bad to take it directly. Arnica is useful for pain management and, compared to other drugs; is not addictive.

Medicinal Parts:

- The flower
- The leaves

Habitat and Foraging:

- Arnica grows best in partial shade and in open woods of higher elevations.
- This hairy flower blooms in the flowering season in central Europe, which is between May to August.

Influence on the Body:

- It helps to reduce inflammation.
- It helps bring down joint pains and swellings.

Traditional uses:

- Aches and pain relief.
- As a cure for bruises.

Possible Side Effects:

- It can cause skin irritation if left on for too long.
- It can cause allergic reactions for hypersensitive people.
- It is not advisable for pregnant women.

Arrowwood

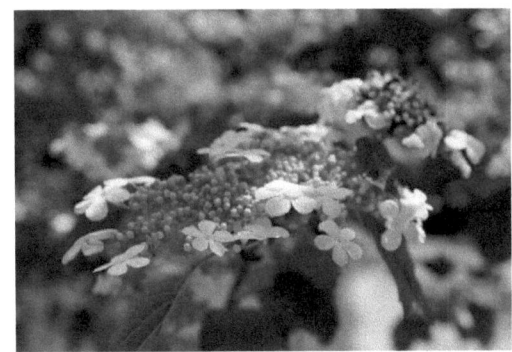

Common Names: Southern Arrowwood, Roughish Arrowwood

Scientific Name: Viburnum Dentatum

Family: Adoxaceae

Origin: Native to Canada and North America (Texas, Florida)

About Arrowwood

The Arrowwood, also known as Arrowwood Viburnum, is a native of Southern Minnesota and Georgia. Native Americans named it after the arrow shafts they used to make with its roots.

The fruit of this plant is taken either boiled or raw for its sweet flavor and for calming the stomach. The fruit is small but works effectively in small doses, so you do not have to take too much. On the other hand, the stem of the arrowwood is applied on swollen legs of women who have just given birth for fast relief.

Medicinal Parts:

- The fruit
- The stem

Habitat and Foraging:

- This herb grows on most soils.
- It can be propagated using the seed. It takes some time to germinate even up to 18 months.
- Propagation takes place between July and August.

Influence on the Body:

- It is useful for calming body pains.

Traditional uses:

- The strong shoots were traditionally used for making arrow shafts.

Possible Side Effects:

- None

Ashwagandha

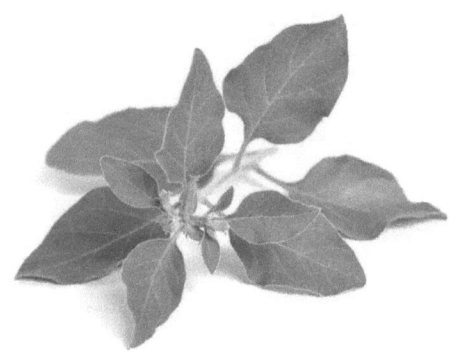

Common Names: Indian Ginseng, Poison gooseberry, Winter Cherry

Scientific Name: Withania Somnifera

Family: Solanaceae

Origin: This plant is not Native American, but it is widely diffused and cultivated in India, Nepal, Pakistan, and some Mediterranean regions.

About Ashwagandha

This woody shrub can grow up to 2 feet and 7 inches in shadowy but dry environments like deep forests. From the root, a thin, single hairy stem bears many other sub branches that spreads radially. Leaves are elliptic, dark green and 5 inches long. From the green, bell-shaped flowers, the red, round fruit evolves.

Medicinal Parts:

- The root (dried)

Habitat and Foraging:

- Prefers dry soil.
- It can be grown from seed in the early spring.

Influence on the Body:

- Used to treat stomach aches.
- Indigestion.
- Used as an antibiotic.
- Treats wounds.

Traditional uses:

- The tea obtained from the powdered root was used as an effective stomachache and indigestion treatment.
- Poultice from the fresh leaves was used as an anti-inflammatory remedy for topical applications on wounds.

Possible Side Effects:

- Due to its sedative characteristics, it may interact with the following drugs: Anticonvulsants, Antipsycotcs, Benzodiazepine, Sedatives, Fenitonine, Antidepressive drugs

Aspen

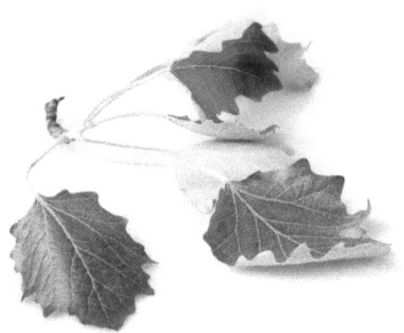

Common Names: Trembling Aspen, American Aspen, Álamo Temblón

Scientific Name: Populus Tremuloides

Family: Salicaceae

Origin: Native to Canada and Central America (Mexico)

About Aspen

Aspen thrives in cool summers and cold regions – mostly high mountains, plains, and high altitudes. Many people in North America refer to the aspen tree as the trembling or quaking aspen because of how it quakes in the wind.

This tree is dominant in regions with other coniferous tree species. It does not thrive in well-shaded regions as the seeds find it difficult to grow and develop. One popular use of aspen bark is making paper and match sticks. The bark as well as the leaves have medicinal properties for treating joints, nerves, and the bladder. It contains a chemical similar to what is found in aspirin, known as salicin, and this is known to help reduce inflammation.

Medicinal Parts:

- The bark
- The leaves

Habitat and Foraging:

- Aspen reproduces both by seeds and root, and it germinates within a few days of planting.

Influence on the Body:

- It helps treat rheumatoid arthritis.
- It helps to manage nerve pain.

Traditional uses:

- It helps treat swellings that come from infections.

Possible Side Effects:

- Skin reactions to the leaves or bark.

Balsam Fir

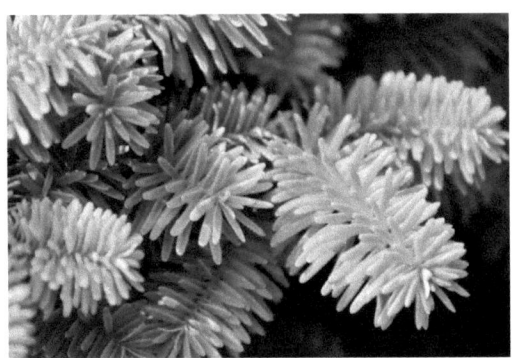

Common Names: Evergreen Tree

Scientific Name: Abies Balsamea

Family: Pinaceae

Origin: North of the United States or South of Canada in forests.

About Balsam Fir

Evergreen tree grows to 65 ft. tall. The gray bark frequently leaks sap and changes its appearance depending on the age of the plant: smooth for younger trees and coarse for older ones. The leaves are like needles, green on the upper part, white on the bottom, and the cones are 4 inches long and red/purple.

Medicinal Parts:

- The sap
- The roots
- The barks
- The leaves

Habitat and Foraging:

- Grows in cool climates.

Influence on the Body:

- Analgesic
- Antiseptic
- Vitamin C

Traditional uses:

- The barks decoction was used to reduce fever and stimulate sweating to detoxify the body.
- Needle tea to cure respiratory systems and colds.
- Use the sap to treat burns and close wounds.

Possible Side Effects:

- None

Balsam Poplar

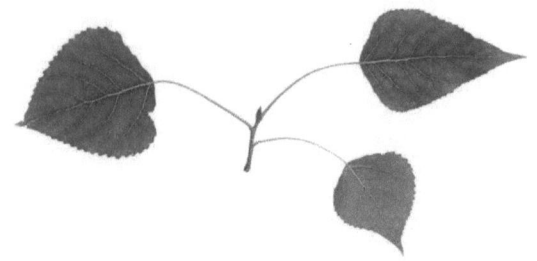

Common Names: Bam, Tacamahac Poplar, Hackmatack Tacamahaca

Scientific Name: Populus Balsamifera

Family: Salicaceae

Origin: Native to Canada and North America (Alaska)

About Balsam Poplar

This tree species and North American Hardwood grows on floodplains s where it attaches itself. It is a fast-growing tree that is generally short-lived except in special situations. It has a sweet and strong fragrance that comes from sticky buds. The smell is so profound that it has been compared to the balsam fir tree. The softwood of this tree is used for construction. Animals use the twigs for food. Balsam poplar is good for the body for numerous reasons like coughs, injuries, sunburns, and frostbites.

Medicinal Parts:

- The leaf
- The buds

Habitat & Foraging:

- The balsam poplar tree is usually found in waterways and floodplains.

Influence on the Body:

- Hemorrhoids – direct application
- Frostbite cure – direct application
- Chest congestion
- Cough

Traditional uses:

- Relieving skin injuries – direct application.

Possible Side Effects:

- It can be bad for pregnant women.

Balsam Root

Common Names: Arrowleaf balsamroot

Scientific Name: Balsamorhiza Sagittata

Family: Astraceae

Origin: Foothills of Rocky Mountains in North America

About Balsamroot

This is a small plant (one to two feet tall). The leaves are arrow-shaped and hairy to the touch and are concentrated on the bottom part of the plant (basal). Its flowers are yellow both on the petals and on the florets, with protruding stamens.

Medicinal Parts:

- The whole plant.

Habitat and Foraging:

- Can be found in many types of habitats from mountain forests to grassland to desert scrub.

Influence on the Body:

- Antibacterial
- Antiseptic

Traditional uses:

- It was consumed raw to stimulate the immune system.
- Poultice from the leaves was used to cure wounds and burns.

- The sticky sap was used to glue together two edges of a wound.

Possible Side Effects:

- Roots are very bitter but boiling them removes the bitter taste.

Black Alder

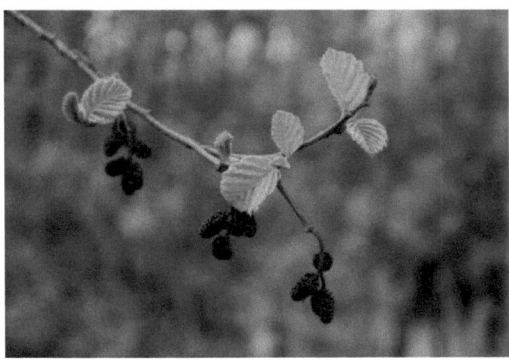

Common Names: Canada Holly, Fever bush, Coralberry, Winterberry holly

Scientific Name: Ilex Verticillata

Family: Aquifoliaceae

Origin: Mostly thrives in wet environments (but also in sandy soils) of North-Eastern to the Central States and South-East of Canada.

About Black Adler

This deciduous shrub can grow up to fifteen feet tall. It has glossy, alternate leaves, which fall during autumn. Leaves are lance-shaped and with serrated margins. Flowers are very small and are made of five small white-greenish petals that encircle a green calyx. Fruits are glossy red berries that persist during winter, becoming a food resource for birds and animals in general.

Medicinal Parts:

- The berries
- The leaves

Habitat & Foraging:

- Can be found in wetland habitats but also on dry sand dunes and grassland

Influence on the Body:

- Emetic
- Febrifuge

Traditional uses:

- The leaves decoction was used to reduce fever

Possible Side Effects:

- The raw consumption of the berries or leaves induces nausea and vomit and was used in food poisoning.

Blueberry

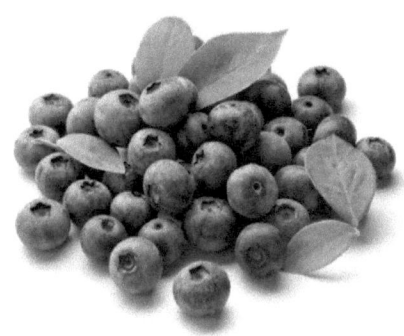

Common Names: Blue Huckleberry, High Blueberry, Swamp Blueberry, Tall Huckleberry, Swamp Huckleberry

Scientific Name: Cyanococcus

Family: Ericaceae

Origin: Native to North America

About Blueberry

The blueberry is a perennial flowering shrub that produces blueberries. When used fresh, blueberries are taken as fruits, and they can be used as a great additive for cereals and other exciting meals in the home. They can be used to produce homemade entities like juices and wine for personal enjoyment.

It contains many healthy nutrients like protein, fat, and water, all in the right quantities. They also contain the right amount of micronutrients like manganese Vitamin C and K, which is great for healthy living.

Medicinal Parts:

- The entire fruit

Habitat and Foraging:

- Blueberries can be found in rocky or sandy soil with a pH level of 4.5 to 5.5.

Influence on the Body:

- It reduce the cholesterol in the body.
- It helps to prevent heart complications.

Traditional uses:

- Preventing cataract and glaucoma.
- Treating ulcers and urinary infections.
- Chronic fatigue syndrome, colic, and fevers.
- Improving varicose veins and circulation.

Possible Side Effects:

- It causes mild side effects like weight gain and headaches.

Black Locust

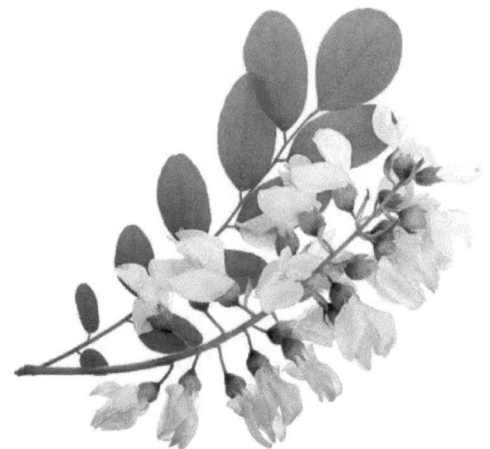

Common Names: Common Locust, False Acacia

Scientific Name: Robinia Pseudoacacia

Family: Fabaceae

Origin: Native to North America (California)

About Black Locust

The black locust is a native of Northern America but was brought to Western America by gold miners who needed trees for mining timber. This was a great way to get good timber and was then taken over to France for making ships. They also used the flower for cooking and the fruit as a substitute for coffee.

The black locust is a medium-sized melliferous tree found in North America. Native Americans have used the dried leaves of the black locust for treating burns and wounds. It can likewise be used to treat internal conditions like stomach burns and for individuals who have stomach conditions.

It simply helps with digestion and covers some of the digestion-related complications. It also has sedating and calming effects on the body, and this is great for adults and children who have insomnia and overall difficulty falling asleep.

Medicinal Parts:

- The leaves
- The flowers
- The fruit

Habitat and Foraging:

- Black locus is native to the Appalachian Mountain, and it grows fast.

Influence on the Body:

- It helps to improve the digestion.

Traditional uses:

- Pain reliever
- Easing digestion

Possible Side Effects:

• Reaction with certain medications.

• Toxic if not heated.

Black Walnut

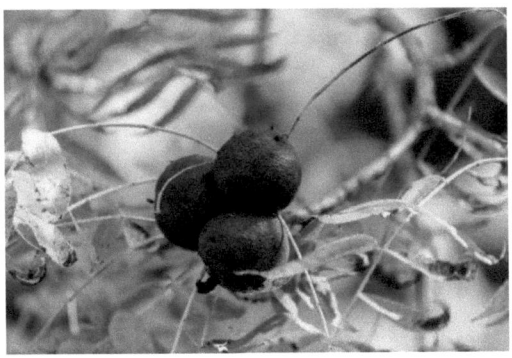

Common Names: Persian Walnut, English Walnut, Carpathian Walnut, Madeira Walnut, American Black Walnut

Scientific Name: Juglans Nigra

Family: Juglandaceae

Origin: Native to North America (Florida, South Dakota, Ontario)

About Black Walnut

Compared to the usual nuts we know; the black walnut is not grown in orchards, but grows in most Native American locations. It is rich in protein and contains many other vitamins, minerals, and fiber. It contains many antioxidants that make the body healthy, preventing some of the worst complications to the immune system, like diabetes and cancer.

The great thing about this is that it can easily be incorporated into the diet by adding it to other dishes for tasty and healthy diets.

Medicinal Parts:

• The nut

Habitat and Foraging:

• The black walnut grows in rivers and valleys as well as the base of the lower slopes of bluffs.

Influence on the Body:

• Reduces risks of diabetes, cancer, and even heart complications.

Traditional uses:

• Beauty and radiance support.

• Digestive support.

Possible Side Effects:

• None

Blazing Star

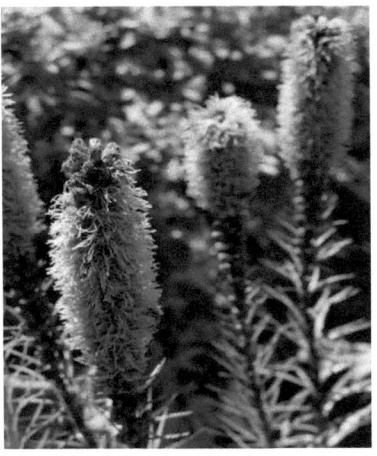

Common Names: Cattail Blazing Star, Gay-Feather

Scientific Name: Liatris pycnostachya

Family: Asteraceae

Origin: Native to Central United States

About Blazing Star

The blazing star is a perennial flowering herb that is a member of the sunflower family. This herb blooms fast and usually in mid-summer. The blooming process of this plant starts with a new flower with other offshoots coming up after the first one, and this process lasts until early fall. The blazing star is a big target for numerous pollinating insects in North America.

This herb is also useful for humans to relieve health challenges like earaches and headaches. The root of the blazing star also helps with more complicated diseases like smallpox and measles. The leaves are also useful for treating upset stomachs while it is used by others as antiseptic washes.

Medicinal Parts:

- The root

Habitat and Foraging:

- It thrives in sunset's climate zones.
- The herb grows best in well-irrigated soils.

Influence on the Body:

- It helps treat kidney disorders.
- It helps to treat gonorrhea.

Traditional uses:

- It is used to improve blood flow.

Possible Side Effects:

- Nausea

Boneset

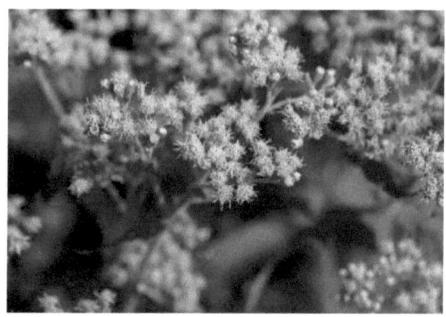

Common Names: Common Boneset, Agueweed, Sweating-plant, Feverwort

Binomial Name: Eupatorium Perfoliatum

Family: Asteraceae

Origin: All over the Eastern United States and Canada, in wet environments.

About Boneset

This perennial shrub can grow up to 39 inches tall. The stems that emerge from the ground bear opposite, long, pointed leaves with teethed margins. It almost seems as if the stem is piercing one wide big leaf. The white-pinkish flowers are grouped in clusters at the top of the stems.

Medicinal Parts:

- The leaves
- The flowers

Habitat and Foraging:

- Do not consume in large amounts.

Influence on the Body:

- Febrifuge
- Diaphoretic
- Carminative

Traditional uses:

- Tea from dried boneset leaves was considered a powerful febrifuge.
- It was used to treat malaria, pneumonia, arthritis, and gout.
- The double infusion of the roots was used as emetic in case of food poisoning.

Possible Side Effects:

- May cause vomiting and liver damage if taken in large quantities.

Borage

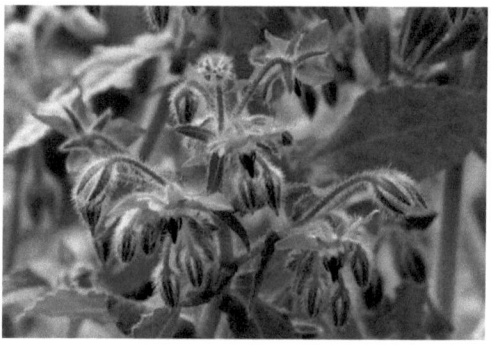

Common Names: Starflower

Scientific Name: Borago Officinalis

Family: Boraginaceae

Origin: Native to the Mediterranean region and introduced to America

About Borage

The borage is a plant with seed oils, flowers, and leaves used for numerous medical purposes. It is known as the starflower of North America and the annual herb in the flowering plant family Boraginaceae. This plant can easily be grown in home gardens, and it can likewise be commercially cultivated to extract the borage seed oil. It also contains alkaloids that are carcinogenic and healthy.

The oil derived from the borage seeds treats skin disorders like rashes, eczema, and other topical skin conditions. It can also be used for other inflammation-related internal conditions like pains and swellings. Likewise, it is added to infant formulas for added fatty acids, which are required for the development of pre-term infants. The leaves and the flowers help with coughs and even hormonal problems, which help to purify the blood. It can be eaten in salads and other tasty meals to get the best of the herb.

Medicinal Parts:

- The flower
- The leaves
- The seeds

Habitat and Foraging:

- Borage grows in pastures and woodlands but can likewise be cultivated in gardens.

Influence on the Body:

- Preventing inflammation.
- Treats coughs and fevers.

Traditional uses:

- It helps to dress and soften the skin.

Possible Side Effects:

- It can be dangerous when taken in high quantities.

Buckthorn

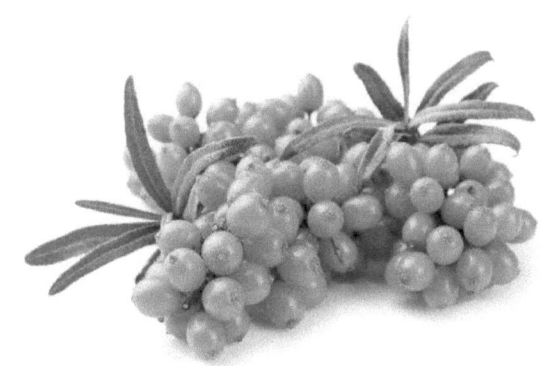

Common Names: European Buckthorn, Common Buckthorn, Purging Buckthorn

Scientific Name: Rhamnus Cathartica

Family: Rhamnaceae

Origin: Native to Europe and introduced to America

About Buckthorn

Buckthorn contains vitamins, minerals, and amino acids that are useful for healthy living. The buckthorn's leaves, flowers, seeds, and berries make oils and teas healthy for many medical complications. It has antioxidant properties, which help cleanse the body and remove any free radicals in the blood.

This helps treat intestinal problems, regulate overall blood pressure, and prevent any heart challenges meaning improved immune functions. It is also applied topically as sunscreen or as a cosmetic for keeping the skin healthy.

Medicinal Parts:

- The leaves
- The flowers
- The berries
- The seed

Habitat and Foraging:

- The buckthorn grows in forested upland habitats but can thrive in grasslands.
- Buckthorn grows from May to June and matures from July through September.

Influence on the Body:

- Combats stomach upsets.
- Prevents heart diseases.
- Improves blood cholesterol.

Traditional uses:

- Treats obesity.
- Improves dry eyesight.

Possible Side Effects:

- None

Buffaloberry

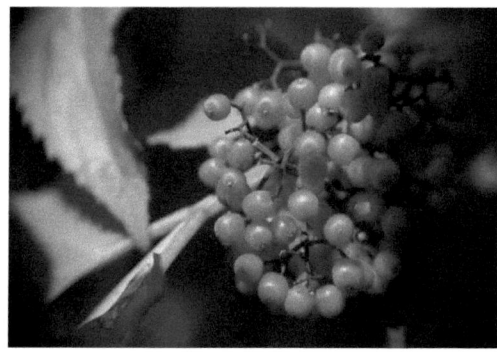

Common Names: Bull Berry, Graise De Boeuf, Rabbit Berry, Silver Buffaloberry, Thorny Buffaloberry

Scientific Name: Shepherdia Argentea

Family: Elaeagnaceae

Origin: Native to Canada and North America (Arizona, California)

About Buffalo berry

The buffalo berry is a rugged shrub that thrives in many growing conditions. The fruit of the buffalo berry is edible, and some people tag it "the super fruit." The buffalo berry has a red and tart color for easy identification.

This super fruit is useful for treating a couple of health conditions like cuts, arthritis, fever, body aches, and stomach cancer. The red-colored fruits from this plant are rich in antioxidants which help to keep people healthy.

Medicinal Parts:

- The roots
- The berries

Habitat and Foraging:

- The buffalo berry grows on moist or rocky soils with low elevations.

Influence on the Body:

- It helps with the treatment of constipation.
- It helps to manage tuberculosis.

Traditional uses:

- Treating swellings
- Covering deep cuts

Possible Side Effects:

- None

Burdocks

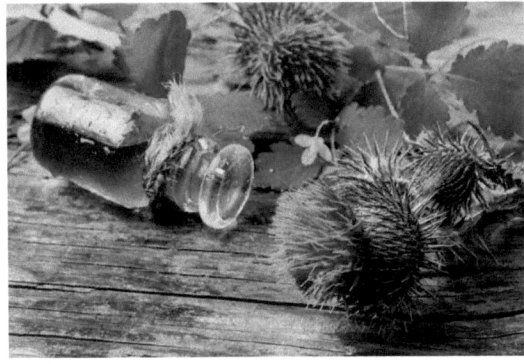

Common Names: Great Bur, Edible Burdock, Fructus Arctii, Great Burdocks

Scientific Name: Arctium

Family: Asteraceae

Origin: Native to Europe and introduced to North America

About Burdocks

Burdock is a weed covered in spores that can grow up to 4 feet tall. It is a genus plant that is part of the daisy flower, and it has many health benefits.

The Burdock is native to North America but is found in various other places in the world. Its root, leaves, and seeds are used as medicine, but the root is sometimes consumed..

Medicinal Parts:

- The leaves
- The flowers
- The stalks
- The roots

Habitat and Foraging:

- It grows in plains pastures and fields.

Influence on the Body:

- It is used in the treatment of colds
- It helps to soothe joint pains

Traditional uses:

- It was used to treat skin conditions like psoriasis.
- It helps to reduce syphilis.

Possible Side Effects:

- None

California Poppy

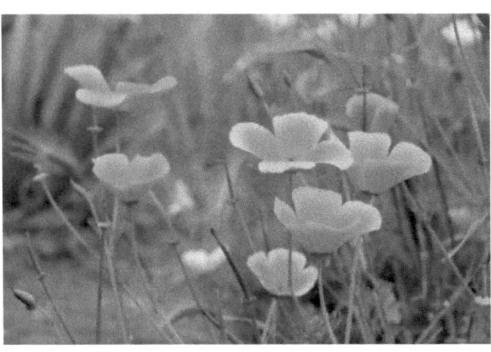

Common Names: Cup of gold, California sunlight, Golden Poppy

Scientific Name: Eschscholzia Californica

Family: Papaveraceae

Origin: Western Coast of the United States and Canada, in dry environments.

About California Poppy

This is a small flowering plant, 30 inches tall on average. It does not have many leaves and is divided into many thin blue-green and pointed leaflets. The single flower that emerges from the ground and has four bright yellow-orange petals, and small black seeds are contained.

Medicinal Parts:

- The whole plant

Habitat and Foraging:

- It is drought-tolerant
- It is se lf-seeding

- and is an annual plant, that grows in full sun and sandy, well-drained soil.

Influence on the Body:

- Sedative
- Diuretic
- Analgesic

Traditional uses:

- Tea from the dried leaves was used to reduce anxiety and soothe panic attacks.
- The tea was also used as a hair wash in case of head lice.
- The sap was used to reduce toothache pain

Possible Side Effects:

- Avoid during pregnancy

Catnip

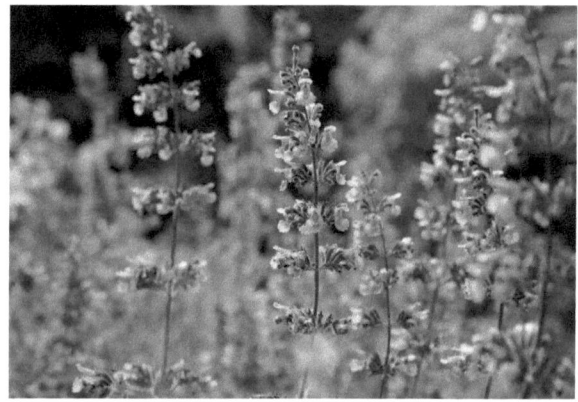

Common Names: Catswort, Catmint, Catwort

Scientific Name: Nepeta Cataria

Family: Lamiaceae

Origin: Diffused all over North America

About Catnip

This perennial, many-branched shrub grows up to 4 feet tall. The leaves are small, ovate, and gray white, with serrated margins. Flowers are small and lilac, and they appear from the top of the stem in large clusters.

Medicinal Parts:

- The leaves
- The stems
- The flowers

Habitat and Foraging:

- The catnip is a short-lived, drought tolerant perennial plant.
- Easy to cultivate as ornamental plant

Influence on the Body:

- Carminative
- Tonic
- Diaphoretic
- Emmenagogue

Traditional uses:

- The whole plant infusion was used for intestinal problems.
- The tonic effect reduces intestinal spasm and inflammation related to diarrhea and dysentery.
- Another use of the tea was related to its diaphoretic character: increased sweating would help in reducing fever states and in promoting overall detoxification of the body.

Possible Side Effects:

- Do not use during pregnancy

Cattail

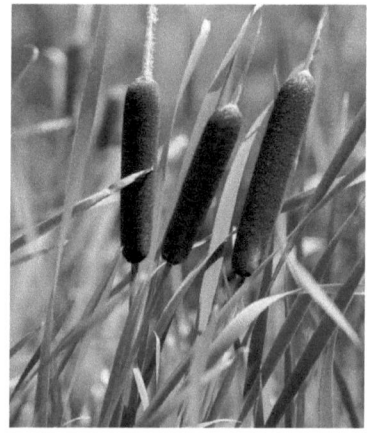

Common Names: Broadleaf cattail, Great reedmace, Cumbungi, Reed

Scientific Name: Typha Latifolia

Family: Typhaceae

Origin: Cattail is diffused all over North America, in wet environments (lakeshores, bogs, streams…)

About Cattail

Cattail is a long, spear-shaped plant growing up to 8 feet tall. It produces two flowers during spring that resemble hot-dogs on a stick. The thicker one, located in the lower part of the plant is the female one while the upper one is the male which disappears after the dispersion of all the pollen.

Medicinal Parts:

- The roots
- The leaves

Habitat and Foraging:

- It is always found near water.
- It grows in flooded areas

Influence on the Body:

- Anodyne
- Emollient

Traditional uses:

- The roots decoction was used as topical treatment for sunburns
- The flowers were used to treat wounds and to absorb moisture

Possible Side Effects:

- None

Chamomile

Common Names: Camomile, Rayless mayweed

Scientific Name: Matricaria discoidea

Family: Asteraceae

Origin: Diffused all over North America

About Chamomile

Chamomile is a small flower, 20 inches in height at the maximum while grown in the wild. It grows mainly along the pathway. The flower has yellow pollen and a corolla of white petals, and leaves are bright green and oblong, with narrow laciniae.

Medicinal Parts:

- The flower
- The whole plant

Habitat and Foraging:

- Annual herbaceous plant

Influence on the Body:

- Nervine
- Sedative
- Antispasmodic
- Carminative

Traditional uses:

- The fresh or dried plant infusion was used to soothe stomachache and cure excessive intestinal gas, menstrual cramps, dysmenorrhea, and relieve skin inflammations, acne, and eczema.
- The tea was used to calm anxiety and panic attacks.

Possible Side Effects:

- Do not use during pregnancy
- May cause allergic reactions

Corn

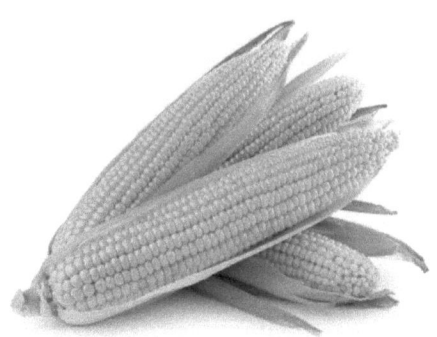

Common Names: Maize

Scientific Name: Zea mays

Family: Poaceae

Origin: Diffused all over the North-Eastern and the Central United States and the whole of the Central and South American continent.

About Corn

Corn belongs to the Poaceae family. It is one of the most ancient cereals cultivated by men. Corn is a six to nine feet long, spear-shaped, plant that produces two types of flowers. The lower ones are female and are widely known as the corncobs; the ones on top of the plant are male.

Medicinal Parts:

- The green pistils
- The cornsilk

Habitat and Foraging:

- It was the first domesticated cereal grain.
- Corn is the most cultivated plant around the world.

Influence on the Body:

- Diuretic
- Emollient

Traditional uses:

- There are a number of well-known uses as food such as boiling and roasting.
- The green pistils' decoction, known as "young silk", was used in treating urethra and kidney problems.
- The tincture obtained from the maceration of minced fresh silk with 50% alcohol solution is a panacea against any urinal tract infections.

Possible Side Effects:

- None

Candle Bush

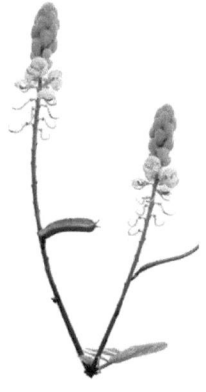

Common Names: Ringworm Shrub, Craw-Craw Plant, King of the Forest, Candle Stick Cassia , Christmas Candles

Scientific Name: Senna Alata

Family: Fabaceae

Origin: Native to Central America (Mexico)

About Candle Bush

Candle bush, also known as Senna Alata, is an important flowering tree inherent in the tropical region of America. Native to America, it is found in other locations like Jamaica, where the barks, leaves, and roots are used as herbal medicine for different ailments.

It has antimicrobial and anti-inflammatory properties, which allows it to help with many medical conditions. The fungicidal properties of this plant help against fungal infections on the skin and even ringworm. The leaves and pods are cooked and eaten as vegetables.

Medicinal Parts:

- The leaves
- The roots
- The barks

Habitat and Foraging:

- It is found in diverse locations of North America and on different types of soils.

Influence on the Body:

- It has anti-inflammatory properties for improved health.
- It was used for the treatment of ringworm.

Traditional uses:

- It was used for treating fungal infections

Possible Side Effects:

- Dehydration
- Cramps

Cat's Claw

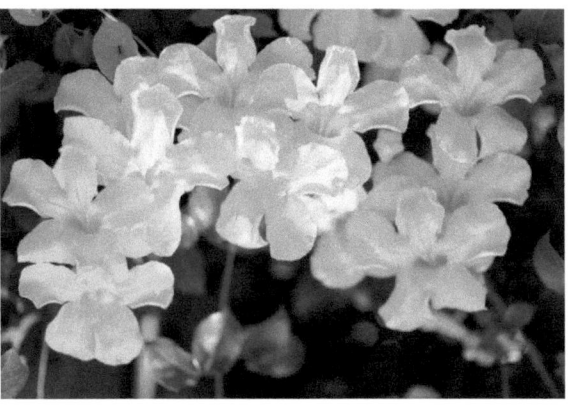

Common Names: Uña de Gato

Scientific Name: Uncaria Tomentosa

Family: Rubiaceae

Origin: Native to Central America (Mexico)

About Cat's Claw

Cat's claw is a tropical vine found in the tropical areas of North America. It gets its name from how it looks, that is like the claws of a cat. For a long time now, the bark and the roots of cat's claw have been used to make traditional medicines for infections and inflammations.

It can be taken as tea, powder, capsule, or as liquid extracts and – not by direct ingestion. Some of the major health benefits are that it has immune-boosting properties, it gives relief from symptoms of osteoarthritis and rheumatoid arthritis.

Medicinal Parts:

- The root
- The bark

Habitat andForaging:

- This is a tropical and sub-tropical herb found in warmer temperate regions.

Influence on the Body:

- Alzheimer's disease
- Arthritis
- Cancer

Traditional uses:

- It was taken traditionally for the treatment and management of anxiety.

Possible Side Effects:

- Nausea
- Stomach issues in case of consumption in large quantities.

Chaga

Common Names: Siberian Chaga, Clinker Polypore, Birch Canker Polypore

Scientific Name: Inonotus Obliquus

Origin: Native to Canada and North America (Alaska)

About Chaga

Chaga mushrooms have been extensively used for many centuries now, mostly for their immune-boosting properties. The mushroom has a rough and sturdy outlook, but people still love to use it because it is packed with antioxidants.

It helps with the treatment of heart diseases, cancer, and diabetes. Taking chaga with hot or cold water helps to release these medicinal properties helping the body fight external factors that might cause harm in the first place.

Medicinal Parts:

- The entire mushroom

Habitat and Foraging:

- Chaga grows predominantly in cold habitats and predominantly on birches.

Influence on the Body:

- It helps to improve the immunity of the body.
- It reduces cholesterol and blood sugar levels.

Traditional uses:

- As a mosquito repellant when burnt.
- It was also used as a medicinal tea.

Possible Side Effects:

- Not to be used by people on anti-diabetes drugs like insulin.

Chaparral

Common Names: Creosote Bush, Greasewood

Scientific Name: Larrea Tridentata

Family: Zygophyllaceae

Origin: Native to North America (Oregon, California, Alaska)

About Chaparral

Chaparral, also known as greasewood, is native to North America. It is a desert shrub with bright yellow flowers and thick green leaves. It is a very controversial herb and while it is found and planted in America, it is banned in certain countries like in Canada.

It has antioxidants and is used for curing several diseases like the common cold, tuberculosis, and skin conditions. However, there needs to be proper regulation when it comes to dosage because if it is not taken the right way, it can lead to disorders in the liver, which people need to avoid at all costs.

Medicinal Parts:

- The leaves

Habitat and Foraging:

- This a coastal biome that functions in hot, dry summers and in rainy winters.

Influence on the Body:

- Tuberculosis
- Common cold
- Complicated skin conditions

Traditional uses:

- Stomach pains
- Snakebite pains

Possible Side Effects:

- Not to be taken by mouth to prevent damage to the kidney and liver.
- Weight loss.

Chicory

Common Names: Wild Endive, Blue Daisy, Blue Weed, Bunk, Coffee Weed

Scientific Name: Cichorium Intybus

Family: Asteraceae

Origin: Native to Europe and introduced to North America

About Chicory

Chicory is a root fiber from a bright blue flower from the dandelion family. Native to North America and enjoyed for many years now, this root fiber is known for its medicinal properties and common use as a coffee alternative. The fiber is extracted for use as a supplement or a food additive.

Chicory contains insulin that inspires healthy gut bacteria growth, relieves constipation, increases stool frequency, and likewise helps to improve blood sugar control. One of its major uses long ago was for weight loss, as it helped reduce appetite and curb the intake of calories.

Medicinal Parts:

- The root
- The leaves

Habitat and Foraging:

- Chicory grows in fields and waste areas

Influence on the Body:

- Stomach upsets
- Constipation
- Gall bladder disorders

Traditional uses:

- It was traditionally used for treating cuts, bruises, and sinus problems.

Possible Side Effects:

- When taken by mouth, it causes gas bloating, belching, and abdominal pains.

Cow Parsnip

Common Names: American cow parsnip, Pushki, Indian Rhubarb

Scientific Name: Heracleum Maximum

Family: Apiaceae

Origin: Diffused all over the North American continent, both in the United States and Canada, in the inland regions.

About Cow Parsnip

This perennial plant can reach six to eight feet tall. It has various vertical, hollow, and hairy stems that pop up from the ground, with opposite and large leaves, divided in pointy lobes. The small white flowers are grouped in umbels, like other apiaceae.

Medicinal Parts:

- The whole plant

Habitat and Foraging:

- It is herbaceous perennial plant.
- It can be found at sea elevations over 9000 ft., especially in Alaska.

Influence on the Body:

- Anti-inflammatory

Traditional uses:

- Stems and leaves can be consumed raw for food.
- Before any use of the plant, remove the outer skin to reduce the level of toxicity.
- The plant poultice was used for direct topical application on eczemas and rashes.
- The roots poultice was used to reduce swellings, especially on the feet.

Possible Side Effects:

- The use of this plant is not advised in any case, especially during pregnancy and lactation.

Cranberry

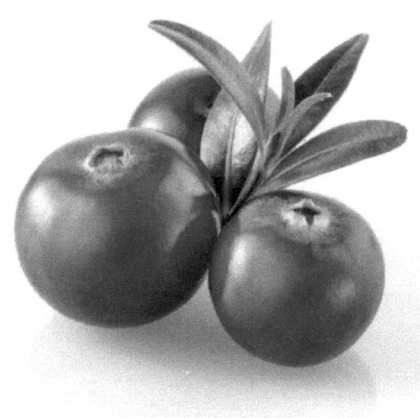

Common Names: Large Cranberry

Scientific Name: Vaccinium Macrocarpon

Family: Ericaceae

Origin: North of the Unite States, in wet environments.

About Cranberry

This small evergreen plant is located at the base of the forests' ground. It can grow up to 15 inches tall at maximum. The woody branches have smooth, dark brown bark. The flowers are often solitary and located at the end of the branches. They are white-pinkish, and bell-shaped with petals curled inward. Its fruits are round and deep red.

Medicinal Parts:

- The bark
- The fruits

Habitat and Foraging:

- It can be found in Central to Eastern Canada, and Northeastern to North-Central United States.
- Cranberries grow in open bogs, swamps, and lakeside.

Influence on the Body:

- Diuretic
- Astringent
- Tonic

Traditional uses:

- It was used to treat urinary tract infections.
- Tea from the bark was used as an extremely effective treatment for menstrual pain and dysmenorrhea, and as a topical wash for infected wounds and skin ulcers, due to its astringent properties.

Possible Side Effects:

- None

Dandelion

Common Names: Common dandelion

Scientific Name: Taraxacum Officinale

Family: Asteraceae

Origin: Diffused all over the South-Eastern United States.

About Dandelion

In Europe, it is also known as "lion tooth". This perennial plant can grow up to 20 inches in height. It has a taproot and a crown of basal big, green, and deeply-toothed leaves. The stems from the basal leaves are straight and green, bearing flowers on top. These are round, yellow, and with a multitude of petals. Each flower is a hermaphrodite, which has both male and female characteristics. The flower head, when pollinated, evolves into spherical clusters called blow balls, where seeds are grouped. Seeds are dry and umbrella-shaped to be easily moved by wind.

Medicinal Parts:

• The roots

Habitat and Foraging:

• This plant grows as a wildflower.

Influence on the Body:

• Diuretic
• Deobstruent
• Tonic

Traditional uses:

• The root decoction was used for cleansing and detoxification in liver and gallbladder conditions.
• With its antispasmodic properties, the decoction was also used to treat menstrual cramps.

Possible Side Effects:

• None

Devil's Club

Common Names: Devil's Walking Stick

Scientific Name: Oplopanax Horridus

Family: Araliaceae

Origin: The North-Western States, in wet, shaded environments

About Devil's Club

This bushy shrub is a close cousin of ginseng. The central stem and the minor ones are full of pointed thorns. Leaves spread in spirals from the stems. They are many-lobed and have thorny peduncles. The small, white flowers are arranged in spherical umbels at the top of the plant. The fruits are bright red drupes.

Medicinal Parts:

• The root
• The barks

Habitat and Foraging:

• It can be found in moist, dense forest habitats.
• It is more common in conifer forests.

Influence on the Body:

• Tonic

Traditional uses:

• The root bark decoction was used as a tonic for nerves due to its qualities which are similar to those of ginseng.
• The plant was used as a dye for tissues and as a traditional body painting for warriors.

Possible Side Effects:

• None

Echinacea

Common Names: Coneflower

Scientific Name: Echinacea Purpurea

Family: Asteraceae

Origin: Widely spread on flatlands of the Eastern and Central United States.

About Echinacea

Echinacea isa single stem, 3 feet tall. The single flower is purple and umbrella shaped. The stem is covered with a thick pelt of tiny thorns. The leaves are large and rough to the touch. The roots are yellow on the inside with black spots.

Medicinal Parts:

- The flower
- The leaves
- The roots

Habitat and Foraging:

- It is mostly found in dry and moist prairies and open wooded areas.

Influence on the Body:

- Febrifuge
- Sialagogue
- Analgesic
- Diaphoretic

Traditional uses:

- The root decoction was used as an analgesic for sore throat, toothache, and stomach pain.
- The decoction was also used to induce sweat, thus cleansing the body and reducing fevers.
- The poultice obtained by pounding its flowers and leaves was used to treat wounds, acne, and other skin conditions.
- Its raw leaves help fight microbial and fungal infections (such as candida) and have been proven to be good antivirals.

Possible Side Effects:

- Do not use during pregnancy.

Elderberry

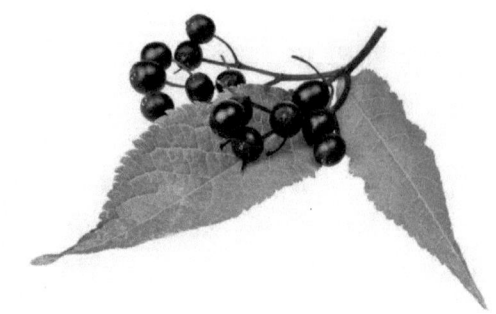

Common Names: Elder, Sambucus

Scientific Name: Sambucus

Family: Adoxaceae

Origin: Diffused all over the United States and Canada

About Elderberry

This bushy shrub can grow up to 33 feet. The stems that emerge from the ground have dark brown bark, often with vertical fissures. The leaves are oval shaped with a pointy end, bright green, with serrated margins and hairy at the bottom part. The white (or cream depending on the species) flowers are arranged in large clusters at the top of the plant. Fruits are round berries whose color may vary from one species to another: red for the racemose, blue for the cerulean, and almost black for nigra.

Medicinal Parts:

- The whole plant from root to flowers and fruit.

Habitat and Foraging:

- It can be found near homesteads and farms.
- Also, generally found near places of disposal of organic waste.

Influence on the Body:

- Vomit inducing

- Cathartic
- Diaphoretic
- Diuretic
- Demulcent
- Febrifuge

Traditional uses:

- Tea from the flowers was used to reduce fever and stimulate diuresis. This tea was used for respiratory problems, asthma, and sinusitis It was also used in topical application to treat skin conditions such as urticaria or rash.
- The bark decoction had different effects, promoting bowel movement for a laxative action.

Possible Side Effects:

- Excessive consumption of berries can be poisoning.

Evening Primrose

Common Names: Sundrops, Suncups

Scientific Name: Oenothera Biennis

Family: Onagraceae

Origin: Native to North America (Alberta, South Florida, Texas)

About Evening Primrose

The Evening Primrose is becoming popular today, especially since all the parts are edible. Many Native Americans in Nevada and Utah consumed the seed and used the leaves for raw salads. It was cooked in different ways to remove the extra bitterness.

The Evening Primrose is a great herb used to reduce and relieve symptoms related to premenstrual syndrome, mood swings, tenderness, and breast pains. It contains healthy essential fatty acids, amino acids, vitamins, and minerals. Taking it gives the body all the healthy minerals that it cannot produce itself except through healthy diets.

Medicinal Parts:

- The entire plant

Habitat and Foraging:

- The Evening Primrose grows mainly in open woods and dry open fields alongside the road.

Influence on the Body:

- Reduces blood pressure.
- Eases breast pain.
- Is good for heart health.

Traditional uses:

- It was traditionally used for treating atopic dermatitis – a certain type of eczema.

Possible Side Effects:

- Mild nausea
- Diarrhea
- Headaches

False Unicorn

Common Names: Devil's Bit, Helonias, Blazing Star Root

Scientific Name: Chamaelirium

Family: Melanthiaceae

Origin: Native to North America (Florida, New York)

About False Unicorn

The false unicorn is a healthy natural herb whose roots and underground stem are used to make medicine. It was used to treat women with menstrual problems, symptoms of menopause, and ovarian cysts. It helps to normalize hormones when women stop using birth control pills.

The False Unicorn is also good for treating problems related to digestion. It also helps increase urine flow for individuals with kidney issues. It can be taken as a worm expellant. Since it has properties that stimulate the uterus, killing the worms in the intestine and helping with urine production in the process.

Medicinal Parts:

• The underground stem
• The roots

Habitat and Foraging:

• This root prefers shady meadows, acidic and moist soils.

Influence on the Body:

• Menopause
• Pregnancy
• Hormones

Traditional uses:

• It was traditionally used for normalizing hormones in women.
• It can help stop vomiting during pregnancy.

Possible Side Effects:

• It can irritate the intestine and stomach.
• It is not good for breastfeeding mothers.

Fendlerbush

Common Names: Yerba desierto, Utah fendlerella, Cliff fendlerbush

Scientific Name: Fendlera Rupicola

Family: Hydrangeaceae

Origin: Diffused all over the Southern United States.

About Fendlerbush

This plant is a small shrub two to three feet tall. Branches are deeply tangled together and are covered with a gray-brownish bark. The small leaves are opposite and oblong. Flowers are made of four white, arrow-shaped petals and a central part with stamens and styles. Fruits are egg-shaped.

Medicinal Parts:

• The inner bark

Habitat and Foraging:

• It is found in the south, in dry locations.

Influence on the Body:

• Cathartic

Traditional uses:

• The inner bark decoction was used as a laxative or as a hair wash in case of head lice

Possible Side Effects:

• None

Feverfew

Common Names: Chrysanthemum

Scientific Name: Tanacetum Parthenium

Family: Asteraceae

Origin: Diffused all over the United States and southern Canada in gardens and meadows.

About Feverfew

This small flower can grow up to 20 inches in height at maximum in the wild. It is a very simple plant with a flower with yellow pollen and a corolla of white petals. The leaves are yellow-greenish and pinnate.

Medicinal Parts:

• The flower

- The herb

Habitat and Foraging:

- Perennial herbaceous plant

Influence on the Body:

- Nervine
- Sedative
- Antispasmodic
- Carminative

Traditional uses:

- The tea from the flowers was used to reduce fever, since the plant is a powerful febrifuge, and to treat headaches due to its mild sedative action.

Possible Side Effects:

- May cause allergic reactions

Geranium

Common Names: Cranesbill

Scientific Name: Geranium

Family: Geraniaceae

Origin: Diffused all over the Eastern United States.

About Geranium

This plant produces many branches with single flowers emerging from a central root and two feet maximum height. The leaves are usually palate and have seven lobes, each with serrated edges (depending on the specific species). Flowers have five wide petals of different colors from species to species: purple, pink, red, white.

Medicinal Parts:

- The leaves
- The flowers
- The roots

Habitat and Foraging:

- Great plant for greenhouse, city growing because of the colorful flowers.

Influence on the Body:

- Astringent
- Anti-hemorrhagic

Traditional uses:

- The poultice from the pounded whole plant was used on deep wounds to stop bleeding.
- Chewed to create the poultice.
- The root poultice was used to treat hemorrhoids.
- The root decoction was used to treat toothache.

Possible Side Effects:

- None

Ginseng

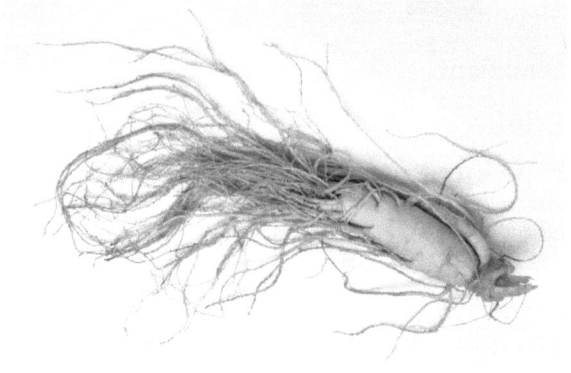

Common Names: Quinquefolius

Scientific Name: Panax

Family: Araliaceae

Origin: Diffused wild on the South-Eastern part of Canada and in the Eastern part of the United States up to Mississippi. It needs a dry and shaded environment, such as big forests of trees with big canopies.

About Ginseng

This small perennial plant grows in shaded and well-drained zones. The single stem can reach up to 20 inches in height from the basal rhizome. It divides into three basal leaves, arranged in whorls. Each leaf is made by five, smaller leaflets lance-shaped and finely serrated margins. At the top of the single stem, a cluster of small, yellow/green flowers develops into a group of bright red round seeds.

Medicinal Parts:

• The roots, especially when dried.

Habitat &Foraging:

• Perennial plant
• The ginseng is considered a vulnerable plant species.

Influence on the Body:

• Emollient
• Nervine
• Stimulant
• Febrifuge

Traditional uses:

• The dried roots decoction was used as a febrifuge.
• The drink was also used as a cleansing agent due to its diaphoretic properties.
• Lastly, the decoction had an anti-stress and nervine effect on the nervous system and was used to treat trauma.

Possible Side Effects:

• Excessive consumption (more than .01 oz. per day) will cause dysentery and insomnia.
• To be avoided during pregnancy and if breastfeeding.

Hawthorn

Common Names: Quickthorn, Hawberry, May-Tree, Thornapple

Scientific Name: Crataegus Laevigata

Family: Rosacea

Origin: Diffused in wet environments and forests, all over the North American continent, both in the United States and Canada.

About Hawthorn

This shrub can grow up to ten feet tall in an intricate entanglement of branches. These are thorny and widely populated by green-yellowish leaves, five-lobed with serrated margins. The flowers are located at the end of the branches in white clusters of ten to twenty. After pollination, they evolve into round glossy black or red Fruits.

Medicinal Parts:

• The leaves
• The fruits

Habitat and Foraging:

• It can be found in old hedgerows and old woodlands.

Influence on the Body:

• It treats diarrhea
• It helps with heart diseases.

Traditional uses:

• The leaves were simply chewed, and the poultice applied on wounds and burns for easy emergency medication.
• The seeds decoction was used to treat diarrhea.
• It was also used to treat tachycardia and hypertension.

Possible Side Effects:

• Do not use during pregnancy or if breastfeeding.

Herbal Alphabetic Index

Agave; 73
Alder; 73
Alfalfa; 74
Aloe Vera; 75
Amaranth; 77
American Licorice; 78
American Mistletoe; 78
American Raspberry; 79
Angelica; 75
Arnica; 80
Arrowwood; 81
Arsemart; 76
Ashwagandha; 81
Aspen; 82
Balsam Fir; 83
Balsam Poplar; 84
Balsam Root; 84
Black Alder; 85
Black Locust; 86
Black Walnut; 87
Blazing Star; 88
Blueberry; 85
Boneset; 88
Borage; 89
Buckthorn; 90
Buffaloberry; 91

Burdocks; 91
California Poppy; 92
Candle Bush; 95
Catnip; 93
Cat's Claw; 96
Cattail; 93
Chaga; 97
Chamomile; 94
Chaparral; 97
Chicory; 98
Corn; 95
Cow Parsnip; 98
Cranberry; 99
Dandelion; 100
Devil's Club; 100
Echinacea; 101
Elderberry; 102
Evening Primrose; 102
False Unicorn; 103
Fendlerbush; 104
Feverfew; 104
Geranium; 105
Ginseng; 105
Hawthorn; 106

Conclusion

Herbs are plants that have been used for centuries and are still used for their nutritional values which have been identified through scientific research.

Previously, these herbs were preferred because ancient people had discovered that they could be used to treat illnesses which began the whole concept of herbs as medicines. Today, people all over the world are aware of the nutritional value of vegetables which, although being very good for one's health, are very different from herbs.

Some people prefer to get all their facts before they say anything wrong. They refer their preferred diet with herbs as "Eating Green." The habit of eating green has proven to have great impact as it is continuously making people realize the benefits of a healthy have lifestyle.

So far, we have discovered that herbs have great health benefits and that herbalism is a very vast study which has been carried down to our generation from very old times, times almost as old as humanity itself. But herbalism has never been used to its fullest potential, even now.

Fortunately, a lot of research has been carried out using new technologies.

This has helped us in some ways, for example in making us understand how people in ancient times survived without medicines. This chapter has also made us realize that it is better to use nature-based medicines (that are herbs) and not synthetic medicines because herbs have proven to be more beneficial. The biggest advantage of herbs is that one can easily produce them in large quantities, quantities that are large enough for daily use for the whole family.

Hope you become a green head too!

BOOK 4: HERBALISM ENCYCLOPEDIA VOL. 2

Introduction

Unlocking the secrets behind the great health practices of the ancient tribes could be the key to curing many of the diseases and illnesses that plague us today.

Native Americans are maybe most famous for their comprehension of the healing forces of plants, an area where they were relatively revolutionary. Therapeutic herbs are presently a billion-dollar business. Today, a considerable number of Americans use herbs, and more doctors are suggesting them for their patients.

Today, herbal remedies are one of the most popular ways for people to maintain good health. The use of herbal remedies is useful when you want to maintain or improve your overall health.

There is no need to create dependency on prescription drugs. Going herbal is much safer and healthier most of the time.

These herbal methods have been carefully developed, researched and preserved over thousands of years so they can be useful for generations to come. However, modern civilization and its many complexes and views about the right standards for human existence changes most of that.

Herbal remedies do not contain any chemicals or pharmaceuticals and in fact, use natural ingredients rather than chemicals or prescription medications to treat any illnesses.

Much like people today are using herbal remedies for many different health conditions, ancient people used herbal remedies to cure illnesses and treat ailments. In fact, in ancient societies, it was common to find remedies for illnesses made with natural plants and plant extracts.

Our intention is to make you understand why it is important to seek alternative medicine for your ailments.

You don't need to put the delicate natural balance of your body at risk by taking chemical drugs and medications if easily available natural solutions are just outside your door. Harvest carefully or grow your own herbs, learn to know your body and what works best for you. Communicate with the nature surrounding you, and you will in a small way bring back a culture that for too long has been treated as inferior.

This book will teach you how to find and treat the herbs the way the Native American tribes did: from the forest to your herbalist table, but you will have to find your own way to listen to your body and the plants around you.

As with all herbal remedies, consult with a qualified health care practitioner before using any herbal products and take particular care for any patients who are pregnant or nursing and on any other medications for children.

In the Native American view, health was more than just a physical state. It therefore emphasized an individual's internal agreement with the forces of nature. Native Americans accepted that neglecting to show sufficient regard for Mother Earth and the effects that made her could negatively affect physical health. A significant number of our remedies are as such manufactured adaptations of herbal concentrates that Native Americans utilized with extraordinary achievement.

The book will explain in depth the different Native American Herbs and how they can be used for medicinal purposes.

Tips for Using Native American Herbs Safely

In collecting, harvesting, and preparing herbs, there must be safety protocols followed. Even if herbs are beneficial to people, they come with various disadvantage, and ignorance would not save anyone. The following are the safety tips given on how herbals are consumed safely:

- Before purchasing any herbal medicines, make sure to validate its legitimacy. Look for stores, practitioners, or suppliers that are well known for herbal medicines. Search for good reviews.
- Make sure to buy products that are named in English, or any language you understood well. This assures that you know exactly what they are buying. For a given reset, make sure that the name, batch number, date, quantity, dosage, directions, information, and the practitioner's name is labeled.
- Before acquiring any herbal medicine, make sure you know all about it; how it was prepared and how it is used. Herbal plants are also medicines and taking too much of it could be harmful. Know the right count to make a dosage.
- Try using herbs as food supplements at first to test the waters and to set the mood. The journey to herbs could start with consuming garlic, ginger, nettle, dandelion greens, shiitake mushrooms, burdock root also known as gobo, and rosehips. These are usually used in preparing food, but they are unlikely to be acknowledged as herbally aiding. Or you could try commonly used plants first such as thyme, oregano, turmeric or cayenne. Thirdly, you could try externally applied herbs; compresses, poultices, and salves. You could then proceed to infusions and making teas. Extracting herbs could also be started together with various preparations.
- Beware that apply herbal medicine to the skin could result into an allergy reaction. It must therefore be done with caution; one must know whether a plant can cause skin irritations which in turn can cause asthma, skin rash, fever, stomach upset, and life-threatening anaphylaxis.
- Extra care should be taken if one is taking drugs for medication. If an herbal medication interferes with drug medication, it could result in harm or conflict. A benefit could be disregarded when too many benefits are at hand. This is the possible body reaction of humans.
- When Herbal Medicine is suggested to kids, it must be studied thoroughly. Six month old are babies not allowed to intake any medicinal herb. However, a small amount of herb is permitted, as long as it is applied externally such as salves, oils, baths and compresses. For kids who are older than six months, dosage intake is calculated by their weight. Nonetheless, proper caution and study is advised.
- Like previously mentioned, pregnant women must also be conscious. It is advised that they must not apply or intake any kind of medicinal plant. However, herbs that are tied with food are allowed, this is the best choice a pregnant woman can take.
- Before purchasing online, make sure that the product is made locally. Avoid trusting imported products because they are not required to follow the country's protocols about safety. Scamming could also happen.
- A person must also know when to seek guidance from a practitioner. When a one feels indifferent with its intake or application, they are advised to seek for professional help quickly, to prevent further damage.

- Essential oils are one of the most used herbs. However, they come with too much power, resulting to too much impact. They are not advised to be applied on one's mucous membrane like mouth, ears, nose, eyes, vagina, or rectum. If essential oils are undiluted, they must not be applied on skin. The usual drops listed under dilution for essential oils is ten to twelve drops. For younger people, half of this is their limits. If you have existing diseases like asthma or skin conditions, applying or inhaling essential oils is not recommended.
- Lastly and actually the most important thing, a person must educate herself or himself about herbs. It is important to be aware of how these medicinal plants work. They must be taken seriously because they could affect various aspects of one's health.

These are just a few reminders to help anyone intending to use herbal medicine. They are actually safety tips, advice and guidelines. There is nothing to lose if followed and a lot to gain.

Native American Herbs

Honeysuckle

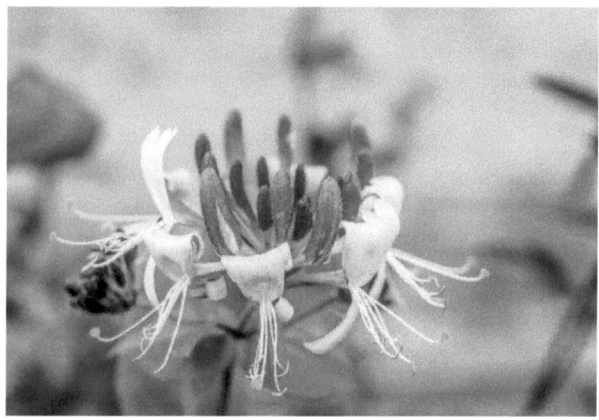

Common Names: Canada Fly Honeysuckle, American Fly Honeysuckle

Scientific Name: Lonicera canadensis

Family: Caprifoliaceae

Origin: Diffused all over the United States and Canada. Being invasive, it is widely diffused at the edges of forests and streams.

About Honeysuckle

This small plant is a climbing vine. The leaves that populate the green-reddish branches are oblong and lance-shaped. Flowers have the shape of white or red trumpets, depending on the species with many protruding white/yellow stamens. Fruit obtained after the pollination is round and black.

Medicinal Parts:

- The whole plant

Habitat and Foraging:

- Can be found in upland woods, growing along streams, and sometimes found in coniferous swamps

Influence on the Body:

- Febrifuge
- Astringent
- Antimicrobial

Traditional uses:

- The tea from the flowers was used to treat diarrhea and fever.
- The tea was also used as a gargle to treat sore throat and laryngitis.
- The bark tea was used to treat urinary tract infections.

Possible Side Effects:

- None

Hops

Common Names: Seed Cones, Strobiles

Scientific Name: Humulus lupulus

Family: Cannabaceae

Origin: Diffused in the inland zone of Northwest of the United States and Southwest of Canada.

About Hops

This climbing perennial plant is the main aromatic ingredient in preparing beer. The climbing green stems are populated by opposite leaves, with three to five lobes with serrated edges. The female flowers are small and made of numerous florets, while the male ones are small and yellow. Female flowers evolve into fruits (strobili) with conical shape and are gray yellowish in color.

Medicinal Parts:

- The female flowers

Habitat and Foraging:

• Hops are a perennial and herbaceous climbing plant, that can be found in a hop yard

Influence on the Body:

• Diuretic

• Nervine

• Sedative

• Febrifuge

Traditional uses:

• The tea from dried cones was used to reduce fever and calm nerves.

Possible Side Effects:

• May cause allergy

Horsetail

Common Names: Puzzlegrass, Snakegrass, Candock

Scientific Name: Equisetum Arvense

Family: Equisetaceae

Origin: Diffused all over the United States and southern Canada, alongside water shores.

About Horsetail

This perennial plant can grow up to five feet tall. It is a leafless, segmented stem with an apothecium on top, from which spores can diffuse. It seems to change into a different plant in summer: many thin, long, needle-like branches grow for the stem in whorls.

Medicinal Parts:

• The leaves

• The root

Habitat and Foraging:

• The plant dies in winter

• The plant has non-photosynthetic cone bearings, produced early in spring.

Influence on the Body:

• Emollient

• Astringent

• Diuretic

Traditional uses:

• The tea obtained with the needle-like branches was used to treat painful urination.

• The bath obtained by infusing the branches in hot water was used to treat gonorrhea and syphilis.

Possible Side Effects:

• Excessive consumption may be poisonous

Hyssop

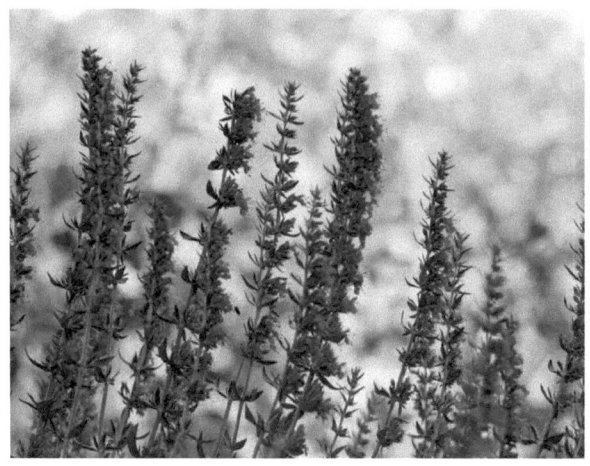

Scientific Name: Hyssopus Officinalis

Family: Lamiaceae

Origin: Diffused in South-Western States of North America and North-East Mexico, in deep forests and moist environments.

About Hyssop

This perennial plant belongs to the mint family. The stems emerge straight from the underground rhizome, to reach up to 3 feet tall.

The lance-shaped leaves are bright green, aromatic, and with serrated edges.

Medicinal Parts:

• The whole plant.

Habitat and Foraging:

• It is resistant to drought, chalky and sandy soils, but grows well in full sun and warm climates.

Influence on the Body:

• Anti-inflammatory
• Expectorant
• Febrifuge

Traditional uses:

• The salves and oils obtained from the whole plant were used to treat coughs.
• The tea obtained from the whole plant is used to reduce fever.

Possible Side Effects:

• None

Ironwood

Common Names: Creambush, Oceanspray

Scientific Name: Holodiscus discolor

Family: Rosaceae

Origin: Widely diffused throughout the Pacific Coast of the United States (especially in California) and Canada. The plant can grow in various habitats, from the coastal moist environments to dry mountain ones.

About Ironwood

This shrub can be three to five feet tall. It has small, alternate leaves, lance-shaped, and with serrated margins. From May to July, white clusters of white, sweet-scented flowers droop down from the edge of the branches. Fruits are small and covered by hair.

Medicinal Parts:

• The flowers
• The leaves
• The berries

Habitat and Foraging:

• Can be found from coastal moist to dry mountain environments.

Influence on the Body:

• Astringent

Traditional uses:

• The decoction of flowers was used to stop diarrhea.
• The decoction of berries was used to stop diarrhea, along with using it as a wash in case of smallpox and chickenpox among children.
• The poultice of leaves was used to treat wounds and burns.

Possible Side Effects:

• None

Juniper

Common Names: Common Juniper

Scientific Name: Juniperus Comunis

Family: Cupressaceae

Origin: Widely diffused all over the North American continent, both in the United States and Canada.

About Juniper

This evergreen shrub can grow up to 50 feet tall at its best. Thorn-like green leaves assembled in whorls densely populate the branches of this plant. Female flowers are small, spherical, and green; male ones are small, yellow and grow in three groups. They have a catkin shape with whorls of stamens. The highly aromatic berries are deep blue and hard.

Medicinal Parts:

• The berries

Habitat and Foraging:

• The cones need more than a year to become ripe.
• They are found in the northern hemisphere.

Influence on the Body:

• Contraceptive
• Antiseptic
• Diuretic

Traditional uses:

• The berries' decoction was used to ease premenstrual pain and dysmenorrhea.

Possible Side Effects:

• Do not use during pregnancy and lactation.
• Do not use in case of kidney disease.

Lady's Slipper

Common Names: Moccasin Flower, Steeple Cap, Venus' Shoes, Slipper Orchid

Scientific Name: Cypripedioideae

Family: Orchidaceae

Origin: Native to Central America

About Lady's Slipper

The Lady's slipper is found in many locations in North America and Canada. The flower of this herb is large and has pale yellow labellum with reddish spots on the inner side. Lady's slipper originated from the blue ridge mountains of Virginia in thinly wooded bluffs along the river forested bogs.

It is useful for treating anxiety-related conditions, emotional tension, and even insomnia. For children, Lady's Slippers can be used to reduce hyperactivity. Adults can also apply it topically to relieve cramps, twitches, and muscle spasms. This root is beneficial when used, but it can have allergic reactions. It is not good for pregnant women.

Medicinal Parts:

• The root

Habitat and Foraging:

• This root comes from rocky and mossy slopes.

Influence on the Body:

• Insomnia
• Anxiety
• Nervous tension

Traditional uses:

• It was traditionally used for tooth pains and muscle spasms.

Possible Side Effects:

• Giddiness
• Restlessness
• Headache

Larch

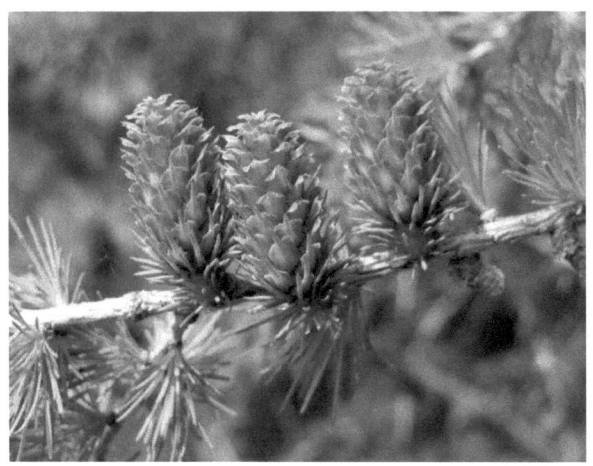

Common Names: Hackmatack, Eastern Larch, Red Larch, Tamarack Larch, American Larch

Scientific Name: Larix Iaricina

Family: Pinaceae

Origin: Native to Canada and Alaska

About Larch

Larch is a conifer in the genus Larix and the family Pinaceae, which grows up to about 40 meters long. It grows better in cooler temperatures of the northern hemisphere on the high mountains. It is used for treating the common cold, flu, ear infections, and other health conditions.

It contains fibers that ferment in the intestine, which causes the intestinal bacteria to increase, and this helps to improve your digestive health. It also helps boost immune functions, preventing cancer in the body and liver, allowing them to function well at full capacity.

Medicinal Parts:

- The bark
- The resin
- The shoots
- The needles

Habitat and Foraging:

- This is a forest tree that requires a reasonably humid climate and a cool temperature

Influence on the Body:

Asides from treating problems with digestion, it helps with the following health conditions:

- Ear conditions
- Common cold
- Asthma
- High cholesterol

Traditional uses:

- Menominee tribe used larch to treat burns

Possible Side Effects:

- Simple bloating
- Intestinal gas

Lemon Balm

Common Names: Honey leaf

Scientific Name: Melissa Officinalis

Family: Lamiaceae

Origin: Diffused in gardens and meadows all over the United States and Canada.

About Lemon Balm

This perennial, low-lying plant reaches roughly three inches tall. While growing, it has many stems widely populated with oval-shaped, bright green leaves with serrated margins. Flowers are small, tubular, and white. The main characteristic of this plant is the intense fragrance of lemon that it emanates from leaves and flowers, hence the name.

Medicinal Parts:

- The leaves
- The flowers
- The stems

Habitat and Foraging:

- The plant grows easily from seed
- It grows best in moist, rich soil

Influence on the Body:

- Carminative
- Febrifuge
- Analgesic

Traditional Uses:

- The tea prepared from aerial parts was used to treat intestinal gas, calm nerves, and menstrual cramps.
- The diaphoretic properties induce sweat and promote cleansing of the body.

Possible Side Effects:

- Do not use during pregnancy and lactation.
- Do not use if there is a hypothyroidism condition.

Licorice (Wild American)

Common Names: Sweet wood

Scientific Name: Glycyrhizza glabra

Family: Fabaceae

Origin: Widely diffused in wet, moist environments of the Western United States or Canada.

About Licorice

This plant grows in intricate root stalks and spreads in width rather than growing in height. It can reach up to 5 feet in height at its best, but it can occupy a wide surface on the ground. Odd-pinnate, flat leaves with smooth edges populate the root stalks and, at the top of the stalk, the green-yellowish flowers are grouped in vertical clusters, like red clover. Seeds are contained inside pods, like peas, and are shiny black.

Medicinal Parts:

- The roots (dried)
- The leaves

Habitat and Foraging:

- Can be found in heavy, moist, or sandy soil

Influence on the Body:

- Purgative
- Expectorant
- Febrifuge

Traditional uses:

- The peeled, dried root decoction was used as a laxative.
- Another use of the decoction was to reduce fever.
- The raw consumption was used for toothache and sore throat.
- The leaves' tea was used as a treat for earache.

Possible Side Effects:

- Not advised in hypertension, since it increases blood pressure

Mayapple

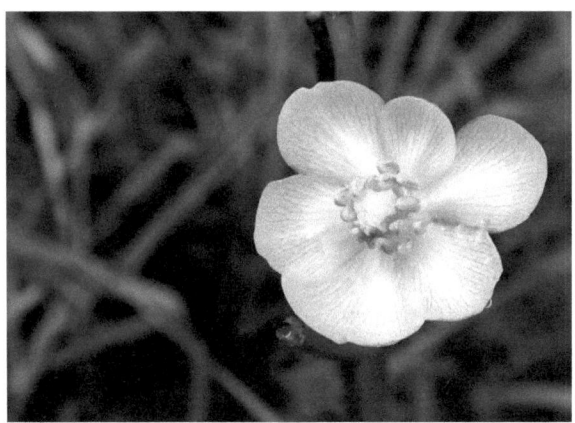

Common Names: American mandrake, Ground lemon, wild mandrake

Scientific Name: Podophyllum Peltatum

Family: Berberidaceae

Origin: Diffused in the deep forests in the Eastern United States and Canada.

About Mayapple

This perennial flower grows in the deep, shaded woods. Each stout has two wide and five-lobed leaves. The single flower that grows underneath the leaves is white and with six petals surrounding a central group of yellow stamens.

The edible fruit ripens in the latest part of summer.

Medicinal Parts:

- The sap
- The roots

Habitat and Foraging:

- Can be found in woodlands. The flower appears in May
- The apple ripens in the late summer.

Influence on the Body:

- Purgative
- Cholagogue

Traditional uses:

- The roots poultice was used to treat warts.
- The leaves decoction was used as a strong emetic and laxative.

Possible Side Effects:

- Use only strictly under medical supervision

Milkweed

Common Names: Butterfly flower, Virginia silkweed, Silky swallow-word

Scientific Name: Asclepias Speciosa

Family: Apocynaceae

Origin: Diffused mainly near the cultivated fields, all over the North American continent, both in the United States and Canada.

About Milkweed

This perennial plant is made by a single stem emerging from the ground to reach three to five feet tall. Leaves are opposite, large, and oval-shaped. The pink flowers are concentrated in spherical clusters that grow from the leaf axils. Seeds are contained in seedpods and have a pappus to move by the wind easily.

Medicinal Parts:

- The flowers
- The leaves
- The roots

Habitat and Foraging:

- Can be found in sandy soils in sunny areas

Influence on the Body:

- Pregnancy
- Skin Conditions

Traditional uses:

- The flowers were used as food, after boiling them.
- The dried roots decoction was used to increase lactation.
- The sap from leaves was used to treat warts, urticaria and insect bites.
- The leaves poultice was used to treat wounds.
- The dried leaves infusion was used to treat stomach problems.

Possible Side Effects:

- The use is strictly forbidden without medical advice and supervision because it contains toxic substances for the heart.
- It may cause infertility

Mullein

Common Names: Greater mullein, Great mullein

Scientific Name: Verbascum Thapsus

Family: Scrophulariaceae

Origin: Common plant widely diffused all over the mountain areas of the United States and Canada, from coast to coast.

About Mullein

The Mullein is a biennial straight plant, two to eight feet tall. The single stem is populated by leaves that grow in whorls around it. The lower ones are wide, long, and hairy. Leaves size decrease from the bottom to the top of the plant. At the top of the spike, there is a vertical cluster of yellow flowers with red pistils.

Medicinal Parts:

- The flowers
- The leaves

Habitat and Foraging:

- It can be found in uncultivated lands, near roads
- It needs a lot of light and excessive drought
- Indicated for beginner gardeners because it can easily grow in yards

Influence on the Body:

- Diuretic
- Astringent

Traditional uses:

- The leaves and flowers' decoction was used to treat mild respiratory conditions, from cough to nasal congestion.
- The fresh leaves poultice was used to treat wounds, swellings, and skin ailments.

Possible Side Effects:

- None

Mexican Yew

Common Names: Ciprecillo Colorado, Pinabete Colorado

Scientific Name: Taxus Globosa

Family: Taxaceae

Origin: Native to Mexico

About Mexican Yew

Mexican yew is an evergreen shrub and one significant yew species. This herb grows to the height of about 15 feet. Mexicans and North Americans make use of the branch tip, bark, and needles for making medicine. Many scientists have reservations, but the Mexican Yew has been used for a long time to treat tapeworm, seizures, and liver illnesses.

Mexican and Native American women used this herb to start their periods.

Medicinal Parts:

- The barks
- The leaves
- The fruits
- The flowers
- The roots
- The stems

Habitat and Foraging:

- It is usually found in tropical to subtropical cloud forests.

Influence on the Body:

- Liver conditions
- Urinary tract conditions
- Seizures

Traditional uses:

- It was traditionally used to make longbows

Possible Side Effects:

- Heart rate reduction or increase.
- Pregnant women and nursing mothers are advised to avoid Mexican Yew to prevent unnecessary complications.

Mint

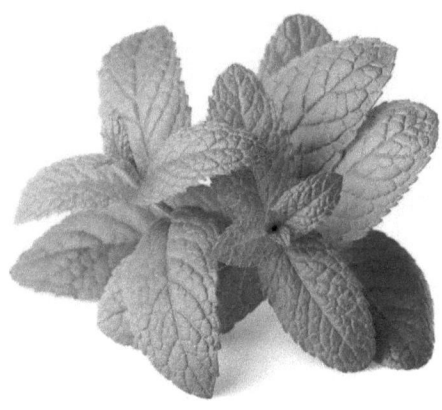

Common Names: Native Spearmint, Scotch Spearmint, Cornmint, Apple Mint

Scientific Name: Mentha

Family: Lamiaceae

Origin: Native to North America

About Mint

Mint is the name of a plant species like the spearmint and peppermint, all belonging to the Mentha genus. Everyone loves mint because of the cooling sensation it brings to the table, and it can be used in various recipes in its dried or fresh form.

Mint grows in wet environments and moist soils, and it can reach a height of 4-45 inches tall and spread across a big expanse of land. Consuming mint has many health benefits, such as improving irritable bowel syndrome, relief from digestive problems, and improved brain functions.

Medicinal Parts:

- The leaves
- The flower
- The stem
- The bark
- The seeds

Habitat and Foraging:

- Mint grows in moist places along streams and shorelines

Influence on the Body:

- It helps to relieve indigestion.
- It helps to improve brain functions.
- It reduces breastfeeding pains.

Traditional uses:

- Traditionally used for treating irritable bowel syndrome

Possible Side Effects:

- None

Nettle

Common Names: Stinging nettle, Common nettle, Nettle leaf, Stinger

Scientific Name: Urtica Dioica

Family: Urticaceae

Origin: Widely spread all over the United States and Canada, near cultivated fields, marshes, and wetlands in general.

About Nettle

Leaves are dark green, ovate, opposite, and deeply serrated margins. Dioica means that the male and female flowers are located on different plants: female ones are drooping raceme, while the male flowers are erect ones. Male and female flowers have four tepals that enclose the reproductive organs (stamens or ovary). The female flower evolves, after pollination in an egg-shaped achene. Pay attention when handling the nettle, since it has many stinging hairs that produce a stinging sensation upon contact

Medicinal Parts:

- The roots
- The leaves

Habitat and Foraging:

- Can be found in places with high density of rain

Influence on the Body:

- Diuretic
- Astringent
- Expectorant

Traditional uses:

- The fresh leaves and stems' infusion was used to treat allergies, cough, or even asthmatic conditions.
- The dried and powdered plant was used on wounds and burns in topical application to stop bleeding and as a disinfectant.
- The dried leaves' tea was used to treat the urinary tract infections.
- Fresh, stinging stems were beaten on the swollen joints to create a counter-inflammation that would recall blood and relieve some of the pain due to the swelling.

Possible Side Effects:

- None

Oak

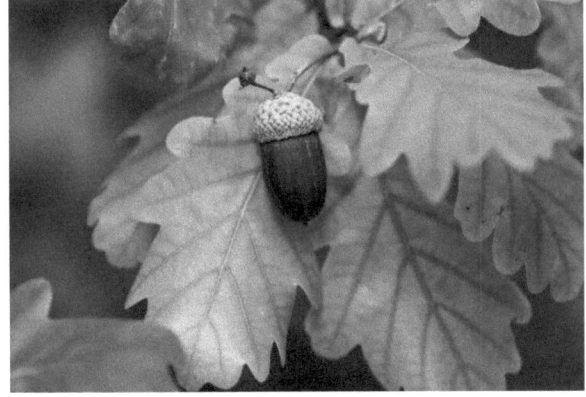

Common Names: Silky oak, She-oak

Scientific Name: Quercus

Family: Fagaceae

Origin: Widely diffused throughout the United States and Canada, from coast to coast, in forests and yards.

About Oak

This family includes many trees that can grow up to one hundred feet high. The leaves that populate the branches of these towering trees are alternate. Lobes, cuts, margins, and overall shape of the leaves change from species to species. Male flowers are yellow amentia throughout the species while female flowers are small and green, located at the base of the leaves. After pollination, they evolve into acorns.

Medicinal Parts:

- The barks
- The acorns

Habitat and Foraging:

- The Oak blossoms in May.
- It can be found in plains, rarely on hills, in forests of oaks or in a mix with other trees.

Influence on the Body:

- Antiseptic
- Astringent

Traditional uses:

- The barks' tea was used as a wash for mouth, wounds, and burns'
- The red oak barks decoction was used to treat diarrhea and abdominal pain'

Possible Side Effects:

- None

Oregon Grape

Common Names: Holly leaved barberry

Scientific Name: Mahonia Aquifolium

Family: Berberidaceae

Origin: Evergreen shrub widely diffused at the edge of the forests in the north-western United States.

About Oregon Grape

This evergreen shrub can reach up to seven feet tall. Leaves are pinnate, pointed, and bright green. Flowers are small and yellow greenish with purple sepals and evolve into blue berries after pollination. Roots are bright yellow on the inside.

Medicinal Parts:

- The fruits
- The inner bark
- The roots

Habitat and Foraging:

- It can be easily grown as a decorative plant.
- It can be found in forests.

Influence on the Body:

- Purgative
- Cathartic

Traditional uses:

- The fruits were used to induce vomiting to treat food poisoning.
- The stems' decoction was used to detox the liver and gallbladder.
- The bark decoction was used as an eyewash for conjunctivitis.
- The roots decoction was used to treat upset stomach.

Possible Side Effects:

- Do not use during pregnancy or lactation.

Oshà

Common Names: Wild Parsnip, Indian Root, Empress of the Dark Forest, Porter's Lovage, Porter's Licorice-Root, Wild Lovage

Scientific Name: Ligusticum Porteri

Family: Apiaceae

Origin: Native to Canada and North America (British Columbia, New Mexico)

About Oshà

Oshà is a special plant that has been used historically as medicine in Mexico for many years now. It is special for improving coughs, common cold, swine flu, influenza, and other viral infections. It is even great for people with irregular digestive systems, improving how the body digests food.

It is usually applied on the skin for topical application to help keep wounds safe and free from infections. People always confused Osha with Hemlock, which is poisonous in ancient times, so you must be careful.

Oshà grows in high elevations in Northern America, making it difficult to cultivate. Without easy cultivation and the level of popularity, oshà has become an endangered species.

Medicinal Parts:

- The root

Habitat and Foraging:

- This herb grows on moist soils with partial shade

Influence on the Body:

- Cough
- Sore throat

- Bronchitis
- Pneumonia

Traditional uses:

• It is traditionally used as a decongestant.

Possible Side Effects:

• Liver pain

Partridge Berry

Common Names: Running Fox, Squaw Berry, Two-Eyed Berry

Scientific Name: Mitchella repens

Family: Rubiaceae

Origin: Native to North America (Texas, Minnesota, Florida)

About Patridge Berry

Partridgeberries are small red berries that taste just like cranberries. This berry has numerous names like cowberry and foxberry, and it has great nutritional value, which helps keep the heart healthy and control weight.

It is high in antioxidants and contains essential minerals like Vitamin C and Vitamin E. It also helps to improve gut bacteria which is a key factor for good health. It likewise helps to improve blood sugar levels, which is a significant cause of many health complications like diabetes. It also helps eliminate free radicals that damage the eye cells, improving eye health overall.

Medicinal Parts:

• The entire berry

Habitat and Foraging:

• It is found in rocky upland woodlands and the edges of red maple swamps.

Influence on the Body:

• It promotes a healthy gut.
• It supports heart health.
• It protects eye health.

Traditional uses:

• It was traditionally used for soothing menstrual cramps.

Possible Side Effects:

• A buildup of fluid in the body

Pasque Flower

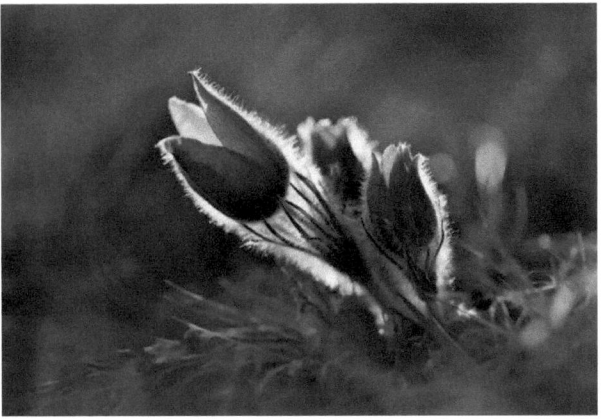

Common Names: Easter Flower, Meadow Anemone, Windflower

Scientific Name: Pulsatilla Patens

Family: Ranunculaceae

Origin: Native to North America (South Dakota)

About Pasque Flower

The Pasque flower is a slow-growing herbaceous perennial plant that blooms in spring and is a member of the buttercup family. This plant has a short stature and requires many drainages, so it grows mainly at rock gardens around hillsides.

It was traditionally useful for medical conditions like calming pains in the testicles and the female reproductive organs, ovaries, and menstrual cramps. It is also useful for insomnia, asthma, boil, nerve pains, asthma, and urinary tract disorders. It is also applied topically on the skin for inflammatory diseases and boils.

Medicinal Parts:

• The entire plant

Habitat and Foraging:

• The Pasque flower typically grows in open areas like rocky outcrops.

Influence on the Body:

• Nerve pains
• Insomnia
• Boils
• Asthma

Traditional uses:

• It was traditionally used to treat anxiety and nervousness.

Possible Side Effects:

• Skin irritations

Passionflower

Common Names: Yellow Passionflower, Giant granadilla, Passion vines

Scientific Name: Passiflora

Family: Passifloraceae

Origin: Native to North America (Alabama, Georgia, Florida, North Carolina, Kentucky)

About Passionflower

The passionflower is a flower from the Passiflora family and is native to Central America. Native Americans traditionally used this flower for treating various health conditions like liver problems, wounds, and boils. Spanish explorers named this plant because it resembles the crucifix, where the word passion comes in.

On colonization in Europe, this herb was mostly used for treating anxiety-related conditions, while the fruits were used as flavors in many delicious beverages. One of the significant reasons this flower is great for anxiety is its calming effect on the mind. It helps boost the level of gamma-aminobutyric acid (GABA) in your brain, which helps to calm the mind, helping you sleep better.

Medicinal Parts:

• The above-ground parts

Habitat and Foraging:

• The passionflower is common in open and cultivated fields.

Influence on the Body:

• It helps to relieve insomnia.
• It helps to relieve anxiety.

Traditional uses:

• It was traditionally used to treat seizures and anxiety.

Possible Side Effects:

• Dizziness
• Drowsiness
• Confusion

Plantain

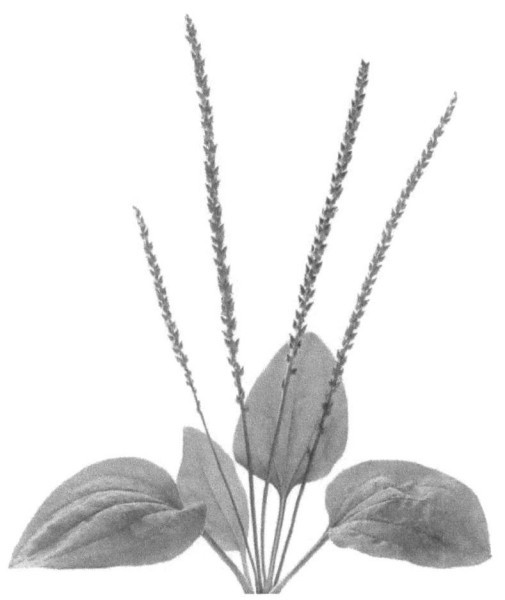

Common Names: Fleawort, Broadleaf plantain, Greater plantain

Scientific Name: Plantago Major

Family: Plantaginaceae

Origin: Native to North America

About Plantain

Plantain is a low-growing plant with medium and broad leaves that sprout out of the soil in flat rosettes. When you let it flower, thin spikes grow alongside tiny flowers. These flowers later transform into seeds which quickly spread to other parts of the soil. This perennial plant has a thick taproot, allowing it to grow rapidly in well-groomed lawns.

Medicinal Parts:

- -The leaves
- -The seeds

Habitat and Foraging:

- -It can be found anywhere in America

Influence on the Body:

- Diarrhea
- Yeast infection
- Cough
- Baby Rash

Traditional uses:

- Bee bites
- Eczema
- Dye for fabrics

Possible Side Effects:

- None

Prickly Pear

Common Names: Pear Cactus

Scientific Name: Opuntia

Family: Cactaceae

Origin: Diffused in dry environments, all over the Southern United States, alongside cultivated fields.

About Prickly Pear

This plant belongs to the cactus family and has large, drop-shaped, light green pads covered with black dots from which thorns emerge. Flowers are large and yellow, fruits are egg-shaped and in various colors within the same plant (yellow, green, purple, orange).

Medicinal Parts:

- The pads
- The fruits
- The flowers

Habitat and Foraging:

- It can be usually found in sandy soils.
- Resistant to drought

Influence on the Body:

- Astringent
- Antiseptic

Traditional uses:

• The flowers' tea was used for irritable bowel syndrome and dysentery to calm the and soothe the inflammation .

• The peeled pads were used as topical applications on burns and wounds.

Possible Side Effects:

• Nausea

• Diarrhea

Queen of Meadow

Common Names: Mead Wort, Meadowsweet

Scientific Name: Filipendula Ulmaria

Family: Rosaceae

Origin: Native to Europe and naturalized to North America

About Queen of Meadow

The meadow plant has a long history of medicinal use. It is rich in salicylic acid, which is great for relieving pains and has been used traditionally for moderating pain, especially in certain parts of the body like the head, where it prevents headaches.

It has anti-inflammatory properties, which makes it great for tackling conditions related to inflammation. The salicylic acid and other compounds in this plant help reduce inflammation and likewise helps to calm the digestive system lining. It also helps to build overall immune functions, promoting healthy living.

Medicinal Parts:

• The leaves

• The flowers

• The stems

Habitat and Foraging:

• The queen of meadow grows in rich, moist, and well-drained soils.

Influence on the Body:

• Colds

• Stomach upsets

• Peptic ulcers

• Joint disorders

Traditional uses:

• It was traditionally used for treating rheumatism.

Possible Side Effects:

• When taken in large amounts, it can lead to nausea and stomach upsets.

Red Clover

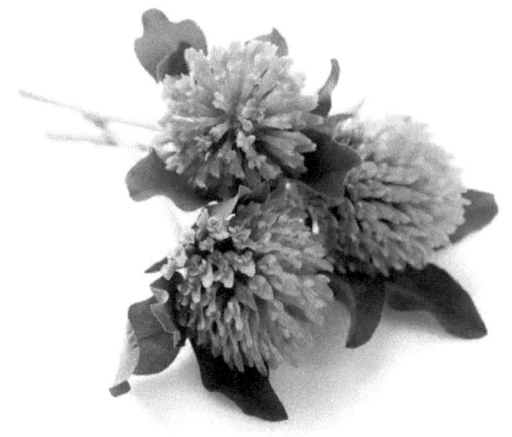

Common Names: -

Scientific Name: Trifolium Pratense

Family: Fabaceae

Origin: Diffused all over the United States, in sunny plains and meadows.

About Red Clover

This perennial plant is made by a single, hairy stem emerging from the ground. It can reach ten to twenty inches in height. The alternate compound leaves are trifoliate. The lower compound has long petioles which are absent in the upper compound. Leaves are oval-shaped, hairy, and with smooth margins. The leaves have the characteristic arrow-tip-shaped "stain" of light green toward the middle. The plant terminates with a spherical cluster of red or purple tubular flowers that bloom from July to September.

Medicinal Parts:

- The leaves
- The flowers

Habitat and Foraging:

- It blooms from July until September.

Influence on the Body:

- Sedative
- Expectorant
- Antiseptic
- Anti-Inflammatory

Traditional uses:

- The dried flowers' tea was used as a tonic for all the respiratory conditions from asthma to coughs.
- The decoction was used as a wash for wounds and burns.

Possible Side Effects:

- Do not consume during menstruation. It may cause excessive bleeding

Sagebrush

Common Names: Great basin sagebrush, Big Sagebrush

Scientific Name: Artemisia Tridentata

Family: Asteraceae

Origin: Diffused in dry and almost desert environments, all over the Western Unites States, from California to Washington State, from Texas to Montana.

About Sagebrush

This strongly aromatic plant can grow up to seven feet tall. Its leaves are spatula-obovate with a smooth margin, connected to the branch at the narrow end. The bigger ones usually have three lobes towards the end. Each leaf is covered by thin hair that allows the plant to increase the heat transfer surface and be cool even in the hottest desert environments. Leaves send out a strong sage-like scent but the two plants are not even remotely related. This silvery hair gives the plant its typical silver-green color. The plant blooms in late summer with bright yellow flowers that grow in vertical clusters at the end of each stem.

Medicinal Parts:

- The leaves

Habitat and Foraging:

- It can be found in semi-arid conditions, in a range of environments from desert to mountain.

Influence on the Body:

- Febrifuge
- Astringent
- Sedative
- Antiseptic

Traditional uses:

- The leaves decoction was used as a powerful febrifuge, and to help the uterus during childbirth and to treat stomachache.
- Also, the decoction was used as a gargle to treat sore throat and bronchitis.

• The leaves' tea was used as a wash for the eyes in case of conjunctivitis.

Possible Side Effects:

• None

Sassafras

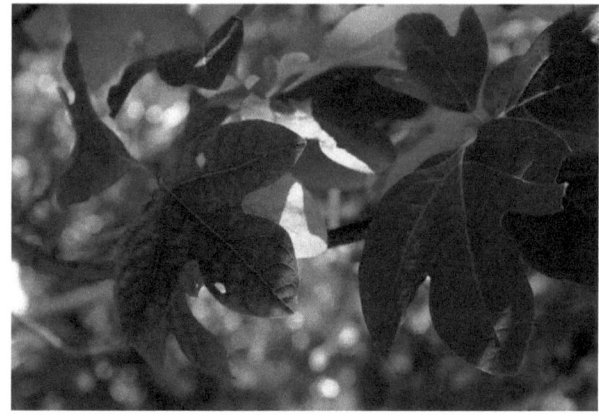

Common Names: White sassafras, Silky Sassafras

Scientific Name: Sassafras Albidum

Family: Lauraceae

Origin: Meadows and edges of forests in the Eastern and Midwestern United States. It needs dry areas to grow and thrive.

About Sassafras

This tree can grow to almost fifty feet tall. Its leaves are three-lobed and with irregular edges. The roots have been used as natural aromas in many drinks and beverages as the root beer. When broken, the roots smell exactly like that. Flowers are green-yellowish with six petals that encircle a crown of yellow pistils.

Medicinal Parts:

• The root
• The barks
• The leaves

Habitat and Foraging:

• It grows the best in moist soil

Influence on the Body:

• Detox
• Anticonvulsant
• Diaphoretic

Traditional uses:

• The roots' decoction was used as a tonic and for its detoxifying effects.

• Also, the decoction was used to treat stomachache, menstrual pain, and cramps.

• The bark tea was used as a febrifuge.

Possible Side Effects:

• Sassafras roots produce a substance called safrole, which is carcinogenic.

• For this reason, it must be taken after consulting with a practitioner and in moderation.

Saint John's Wort

Scientific Name: Hypericum Perforatum

Family: Hypericaceae

Origin: Widely diffused all over the United States and Canada, in gardens and meadows.

About Saint John's Wort

This officinal, perennial plant can grow almost four feet tall from the creeping rhizome. The red-brown stems are woody at the base of the plant and become more "tender" towards the top.. Opposite and stalkless leaves populate the branches. They are bright green and oblong with many small glands attached to the bottom. These can be easily seen in the backlight. The flowers that originate at the end of each stem are made by five ovate, yellow petals that encircle a cluster of long yellow pistils. Seeds are shiny-black and cylindrical, two millimeters long.

Medicinal Parts:

- The whole plant

Habitat and Foraging:

- The flowers can be harvested in the summer.

Influence on the Body:

- Considered a heal-all plant
- Astringent
- Anti-inflammatory
- Antiseptic

Traditional uses:

- The whole plant decoction was used to treat menstrual problems.
- The stimulating effect on uterus contraction was also used to induce abortions and facilitate difficult childbirth.
- The tea obtained from flowers was used as a mild sedative to calm nerves and induce sleep in case of traumatic events.
- The poultice of the whole plant was applied over wounds to facilitate healing.

Possible Side Effects:

- Do not use during pregnancy.
- Do not use if suffering from bipolar disorder or depression.
- Gastrointestinal irritation
- Allergic reactions

Sarsaparilla

Common Names: Jamaican Sarsaparilla, Honduran Sarsaparilla

Scientific Name: Smilax Ornata

Family: Smilacaceae

Origin: Native to Central America (Mexico, Jamaica, Honduras)

About Sarsaparilla

The sarsaparilla is a tropical plant from the smilax genus, and it grows in woody and deep rainforests. It is native to Mexico, Jamaica, and South America and is a healthy plant. For many years, people used the root of the sarsaparilla plant for skin problems and the treatment of arthritis. It was later brought into European countries, where it was adopted for treating syphilis.

It contains phytochemicals with anti-inflammatory properties that help with joints and all types of body pains. It is wise for those who have underlying medical conditions to consult their physician before taking any steps concerning usage.

Medicinal Parts:

- The roots

Habitat and Foraging:

- This plant prefers sandy and clay soils

Influence on the Body:

- It is used for treating skin diseases.
- It is used to increase urination and fluid retention.

Traditional uses:

- It was traditionally used for treating leprosy and syphilis.

Possible Side Effects:

- Stomach irritation

Saw Palmetto

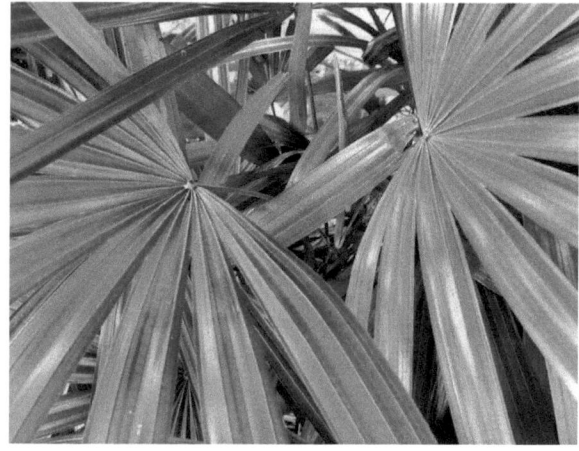

Common Names: Dwarf Palm

Scientific Name: Serenoa repens

Family: Arecaceae

Origin: Diffused all over the South-Eastern United States. It typically grows in dense colonies, in plains and sandhills, especially near the coastline. It can also be found in woods under pines.

About Saw Palmetto

This fan palm is also called Dwarf American Palm and can grow up to 13 feet tall to its best. From the central trunk, deeply scaled, depart many leaves, composed by a long petiole, full of thorns at its side, which terminate with a fan ten to twenty long leaflets. The leaflets are two to three feet long and pointed. Vertical panicles of flowers with three white petals and six yellow stamens appear between the leaves in spring. Fruits are large red or black drupes, a small olive.

Medicinal Parts:

- The leaves

Habitat and Foraging:

- It's a plant that grows extremely slow.
- There are some known exemplars that are 700 years old.

Influence on the Body:

- Digestive

Traditional uses:

- The leaves decoction was used to treat digestive problems.

Possible Side Effects:

- None

Skullcap

Common Names: Marsh Skullcap, Hooded Skullcap

Scientific Name: Scutellaria

Family: Lamiaceae

Origin: Native to North America and Canada

About Skullcap

Skullcap, also known as the American skullcap, is a Native American plant cultivated also across Europe and has been used for more than 200 years now. The skullcap has antioxidants and helps prevent and protect against neurological conditions like Parkinson's disease and depression. It is also scientifically proven to reduce the symptoms of an allergic reaction.

Adults can take the skullcap as tea, fluid extracts, tincture, or dried herbs for healthy consumption. On the other hand, children should not be given this herb no matter the circumstances. Even adults should take precautions when using it, mainly because it can react with specific supplements and drugs. Consult your trusted herbalist.

Medicinal Parts:

- The flower
- The leaves

Habitat and Foraging:

- It grows in marshes and meadows.

Influence on the Body:

- It promotes relaxation.
- It reduces your response to stress.
- It supports healthy sleep patterns.

Traditional uses:

- It was traditionally used as anxiety and tension therapy

Possible Side Effects:

- Anxiety
- Irregular heartbeats

Skunk Cabbage

Common Names: Swamp Cabbage, Meadow Cabbage, Clump Foot Cabbage

Scientific Name: Symplocarpus Foetidus

Family: Araceae

Origin: Native to North America (Minnesota, Tennessee, North Carolina)

About Skunk Cabbage

The skunk cabbage is a herbal medicine known for its unpleasant smell. The rhizome and the root treat breathing challenges like coughs, asthma, and swollen airways. It also has other benefits like preventing excessive bleeding, improved fluid retention, and anxiety prevention.

It is used traditionally and topically for skin sores, wounds, swellings, and splinters. It was also applied to the body for immediate relief whenever a person was bitten by a snake. People used the leaves, stock, and root back then, boiling off the foul smell and immediately eating it.

Medicinal Parts:

- The root
- The underground stem

Habitat and Foraging:

- It grows on wetlands and hilly slopes

Influence on the Body:

- Asthma
- Cough
- Swollen airways

Traditional uses:

- It was traditionally used for treating worms, ringworms, and scabies.

Possible Side Effects:

- Diarrhea
- Vomiting

Slippery Elm

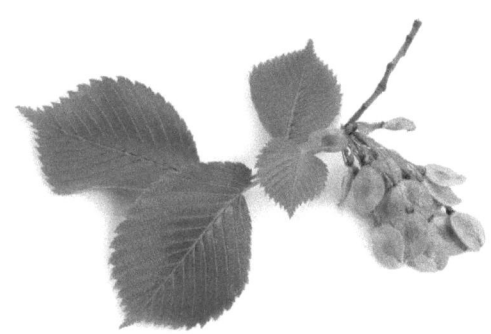

Common Names: Elm

Scientific Name: Ulmus Rubra

Family: Ulmaceae

Origin: Widely diffused in forests and fields all over the North-Eastern United States and Quebec.

About Slippery Elm

The deciduous tree can grow up to 50 feet on average. The leafy branches spread widely around the central trunk made of reddish wood. The dark green leaves are oblong to obovate-shaped (depending on the species) and serrated margins. They are rough to the upper part and velvety on the bottom. Flowers have no petals and are produced in fifteen to twenty dome clusters each. Fruits are ovoid samaras that can be easily diffused by wind, bearing a red, hairy seed.

Medicinal Parts:

• The bark, both inner and outer

Habitat and Foraging:

• It can be planted as ornamental plant.
• It can grow in dry soils and can be found in moist uplands.

Influence on the Body:

• Expectorant
• Emollient
• Diuretic

Traditional uses:

• The dried inner bark decoction was used to treat gastritis and ulcers.
• It was used as a wash, can treat wounds and burns.
• The outer bark decoction was used to induce uterine contraction and causing abortions or helping difficult childbirths.
• The salve obtained by thickening with beeswax the oil of outer bark was useful to treat colds, sore throat, and bronchitis by dissolving it in boiling water and inhaling the steam.

Possible Side Effects:

• None

Sumac

Common Names: Sicilian sumac, Elm-leaved sumac

Scientific Name: Rhus coriaria

Family: Anacardiaceae

Origin: Sumac thrives in forests and fields all over the South-Eastern United States.

About Sumac

This shrub can grow up to 30 feet high from the underground rhizome. The branches grow twisted from the ground and spread in many lesser red-brownish branches. Leaves are pinnately compound, lance-shaped, and bright green with serrated margins. The five-petaled, red flowers are arranged in vertical panicles, densely populated. After pollination, they evolve into red drupes.

Medicinal Parts:

• The bark, both inner and outer

Habitat and Foraging:

• It can be found in any type of soil that is well-drained and deep.

Influence on the Body:

• Astringent
• Anti-inflammatory

Traditional uses:

• The bark decoction was used as a wash to treat conjunctivitis and gargle to treat sore throat.
• The decoction was also drunk to treat dysentery and diarrhea.
• The fresh leaves poultice was used as an anti-inflammatory on skin rash.

Possible Side Effects:

- None

Tobacco

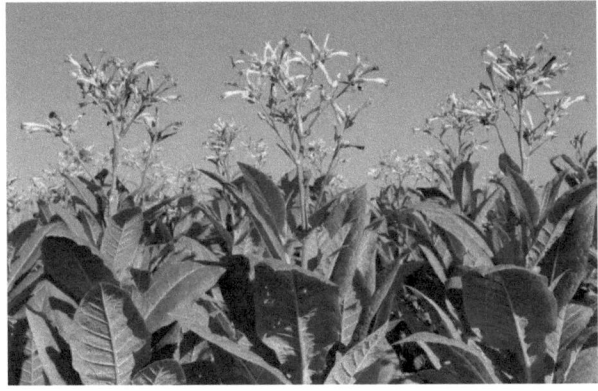

Common Names: Night Queen, Tabaco Flower.

Scientific Name: Nicotiana Tabacum

Family: Solanaceae

Origin: It grows wild in the South-Western United States, in desert environments.

About Tobacco

This shrub can grow up to thirteen feet tall. Leaves are lanceolate (typical dimensions are 12 inches long by 4 inches wide at the base) and yellow greenish. Leaves dimensions reduce from basal to upper leaves. The flowers are located on top of the plant and are trumpet-shaped and pink. They emanate an unpleasant flavor.

Medicinal Parts:

- The leaves

Habitat &andForaging:

- It blossoms from June to October.
- It can be grown as an ornamental plant.
- It needs a well-drained soil.

Influence on the Body:

- Antispasmodic
- Cathartic
- Emetic
- Analgesic

Traditional uses:

- The fresh leaves' poultice was used on joints swelling and scorpion stings.
- Also, the poultice was used as a panacea for skin conditions.

Possible Side Effects:

- Highly addictive stimulant

Toothwort

Common Names: Bittercresses, Crinkle Root, Twoleaf toothwort

Scientific Name: Cardamine Diphylla

Family: Brassicaceae

Origin: Widely diffused in the moist woodlands of the Eastern United States and Quebec.

About Toothwort

This plant belongs to the mustard family; thus, it is edible. The single, thin stem, which can grow up to 12" in height, holds lance-shaped leaves with serrated edges, grouped in triplets. At the top of the plant, there is a cluster of white flowers with four petals.

Medicinal Parts:

- The roots

Habitat and Foraging:

- It blooms from April to June.
- It can be found in moist woodlands.

Influence on the Body:

- Febrifuge
- Analgesic
- Carminative

Traditional uses:

- The root infusion was used to reduce fever and as a gargle to treat sore throats.
- This infusion was also used to treat syphilis and gonorrhea.
- The root consumed raw was used to reduce headaches and reduce stomach gas.
- The root poultice was used topically on swellings and arthritic joints.

Possible Side Effects:

- None

Turtlehead

Common Names: Fish Mouth, Shellflower, Bitter Herb, Cod head

Scientific Name: Chelone Obliqua

Family: Plantaginaceae

Origin: Native to North America (Georgia, Mississippi)

About Turtlehead

Turtlehead is a North American herb with the parts above the ground used for medicine. Its classification has been controversial, but recently, DNA studies have demonstrated that it belongs to Plantaginaceae.

Initially, this plant was used for blood purification and to remedy eczema and chronic rheumatic conditions. Abenaki people used flowers as a method of birth control. Turtlehead is not edible, but it has numerous medicinal benefits once the flower is harvested and dried. And it even has healing powers for indigestion. It is mainly used as tea or tincture to prevent issues with constipation.

Medicinal Parts:

- The parts of the plant that grow above the ground.

Habitat and Foraging:

- It grows perfectly on swamps, rich fens, and marshes.
- Be careful and avoid the red turtlehead, which can be deadly.

Influence on the Body:

- Indigestion
- Stimulation of appetite
- It relieves inflammation

Traditional uses:

- It was traditionally used for treating fever and jaundice.

Possible Side Effects:

- Possible interaction with other drugs.
- Not recommended for pregnant women and nursing mothers.

Usnea

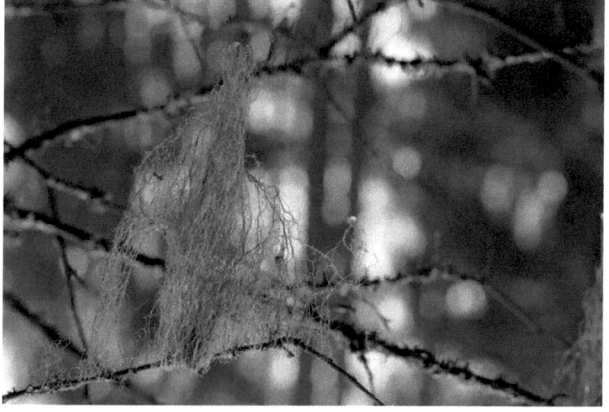

Common Names: Beard Lichen, Old man's beard

Scientific Name: Usnea Florida

Family: Parmeliaceae

Origin: Wild lichen thrives in wet environments, especially in the North-Western United States and British Columbia.

About Usnea

This lichen is a symbiont of pines, junipers, cypresses, and many others. It grows on their branches and feeds on the tree lymph, giving in exchange nitrogenous substances. It is easy to accurately detect the Usnea (also called "old man's beard"): Usnea has a white central core that departs the many filaments. Other lichens that may be poisonous do not have this central white axon, so be sure to check before risking picking venomous look-alikes.

Medicinal Parts:

- The whole lichen

Habitat and Foraging:

- It can be found on old trees.

Influence on the Body:

- Carminative
- Antiseptic
- Emollient
- Antifungal

Traditional uses:

- The whole lichen poultice was used to treat wounds and skin infections.
- Alcohol tinctures were used to treat infections..
- The dried lichen tea was used to treat tuberculosis and other pulmonary conditions.
- The tea was also used as a vaginal wash to treat any fungal or yeast infection like candida.

Possible Side Effects:

- None

Valerian

Scientific Name: Valeriana Officinalis

Family: Caprifoliaceae

Origin: This plant belongs to the mountain climate. It can usually be found in the north face of hills and mountains, all over the United States and Canada.

About Valerian

This small plant grows to almost sixty inches. From the ground emerges a single green stem with nodes at regular intervals. Two opposite small branches depart each node and carry seven to nine long, lance-shaped, and smooth-edged leaves. At the top, it divides into three lesser vertical branches with a cluster of small white flowers on top. Flowers are bell-shaped with four white petals and a protruding central stamen. It blooms from April to July.

Medicinal Parts:

- The root

Habitat and Foraging:

- It can be found in moist, full of minerals soils.

Influence on the Body:

- Sedative
- Nervine
-
- Traditional uses:
- The root tea was used as a mild sedative and stress-relieving drink.
- Its sleep-inducing property was used to treat insomnia.
- The root decoction was used to treat diarrhea and colds.
- The root poultice was used to treat wounds and burns.

Possible Side Effects:

- Headache
- Dizziness

Verbena

Common Names: Verveine

Scientific Name: Verbena Officinalis

Family: Verbenaceae

Origin: Native to Europe and naturalized to North America

About Verbena

Verbena is a well-used herbal medicine used all over the globe for the treatment of numerous diseases. Its benefits include protecting the nerve cells, reducing convulsion, and preventing tumors. It also treats ear infections and can even be used as solar cream. Verbena is used to stimulate and increase milk production while breastfeeding. It is advisable to take verbena in processed forms such as powder, tea, or tincture.

Medicinal Parts:

- Parts above the ground.

Habitat and Foraging:

- It grows as roadside weed.

Influence on the Body:

It is used for treating the following:

- Digestive disorders
- Trouble sleeping
- Agitation

Traditional uses:

- It was used for treating chest pains and related conditions.

Possible Side Effects:

- It is not recommended for people on blood-thinning drugs.

Water Birch

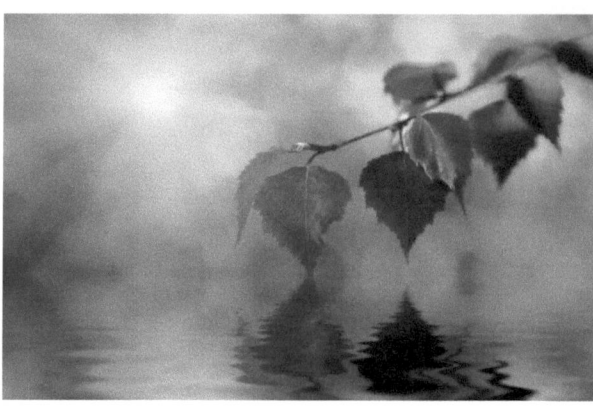

Common Names: River Birch, Black Birch

Scientific Name: Betula nigra

Family: Betulaceae

Origin: Widely diffused in the inland regions of Western United States and Canada, up to the east part of Alaska.

About Water Birch

This small tree can grow up to 35 feet tall, with many trunks from the single rootstalk. The trunks (covered by a red-brown and smooth bark), leave many branches populated by opposite, ovate leaves with serrated margins. Flowers are catkins: the male ones drooping down, the female erect. Seed have horizontal "leaflets" such as a helicopter (samara). This helps them fly for long distances when they detach from the tree.

Medicinal Parts:

- The leaves
- The bark

Habitat and Foraging:

- It can be found in swamps and floodplains.

Influence on the Body:

- Febrifuge
- Anti-inflammation

Traditional uses:

• Tea from the leaves and bark was used for its febrifuge properties.

• The tea was also used as a wash for mild skin ailments, such as pimples.

Possible Side Effects:

• Do not use during pregnancy.

Watercress

Common Names: Yellowcress

Scientific Name: Nasturtium Officinale

Family: Brassicaceae

Origin: This wild plant thrives in watery environments such as marshes and bogs, all over the United States and Canada.

About Watercress

This plant grows in floating mats with roots immersed into the water. It spreads in width rather than grow in height and can reach twenty inches at its best. The plant grows in an intricate entanglement of stems with alternate, ovate, three-lobed leaves. From May to July, small groups of three to five white flowers bloom at the top of the stems.

Medicinal Parts:

• The roots
• The leaves

Habitat and Foraging:

• It can be found in swamps, wetlands and close to streams of water.

• It can easily grow in your backyard, just by collecting it in the field and replanting it.

Influence on the Body:

• Detoxifying

• Carminative

Traditional uses:

• The leaves were used to spice food.

• The plant was consumed raw to treat coughs, colds, and indigestion.

• The plant also has strong diuretic characteristics and was recommended for cleansing and detoxifying.

Possible Side Effects:

• None

Wild Yam

Common Names: Rheumatism Root, Devil's Bones, Colic Root

Scientific Name: Dioscorea Villosa

Family: Dioscoreaceae

Origin: Native to North America (New England, Virginia, Texas, Minnesota)

About Wild Yam

The Wild Yam is a tuberous species native to the eastern part of North America. While the wild yam is edible, the root is also helpful in treating hormonal conditions like menopause, and it is also useful for treating arthritis.

Wild Yam is also helpful as an alternative to estrogen therapy, menstrual cramps, pre-menstrual syndrome, weak bones, and male sex drive. Wild Yam creams are also helpful for topical application and can reduce hot flashes, a symptom of menopause.

Medicinal Parts:

• The entire tuber

Habitat and Foraging:

• Wild Yam grows in moist thickets.

Influence on the Body:

• Vaginal dryness in older women

• Menstrual cramps

• Osteoporosis

Traditional uses:

• It was used to increase sexual drive and energy in men and to increase women's breast sizes.

Possible Side Effects:

• None

Willow

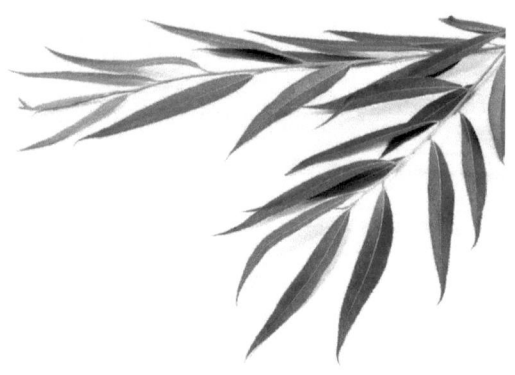

Common Names: Osiers, Sallows

Scientific Name: Salix Alba

Family: Salicaceae

Origin: Widely diffused in wet environments all over the North American Continent, both in the United States and Canada.

About Willow

The willow tree can grow up to 100 feet tall. From the wide central trunk spread many drooping branches widely populated by narrow and lance-shaped leaves with finely serrated margins. The drooping shape of its branches gives the tree its characteristic shape. Flowers, both male and female are in the shape of catkins: yellow for males, green for females.

Medicinal Parts:

• The bark

Habitat and Foraging:

• It grows in moist soil on riverbanks.

Influence on the Body:

• Diuretic

• Febrifuge

• Analgesic

Traditional uses:

• The bark decoction was used effectively for pain relief of tendinitis and arthritis.

Possible Side Effects:

• Due to its high salicin content, it can aggravate pre-existing conditions such as ulcers, and intestinal bleeding.

• The willow tree is full of cadmium, which it collects from the surrounding environment. Cadmium is a toxic chemical element.

Witch Hazel

Scientific Name: Hamamelis Virginiana

Family: Hamamelidaceae

Origin: Native to North America (Texas, Florida, Nova Scotia)

About Witch Hazel

Witch Hazel is a member of the witch hazel family. This shrub is native to North America and is used to produce ointments. The ointments are applied to the skin and scalp to help soothe sensitive skins as they prevent inflammation.

The Witch Hazel can be used as a natural treatment for inflammation and hemorrhoids. It is also used to fight acne and to sooth sore throats. This shrub is robust and is fit for use without any health consequences. You just need to make sure that you take it in regulated quantities and not all the time.

Medicinal Parts:

- The twig
- The bark

Habitat and Foraging:

- It tolerates different kinds of soils as long as there is adequate sunlight.

Influence on the Body:

- It alleviates scalp sensitivity.
- It helps treat hemorrhoids.
- It fights acne.
- It soothes sore throat.
- It reduces skin irritation.

Traditional uses:

- It was traditionally used for treating itchiness and skin inflammations.

Possible Side Effects:

- Stomach upsets

Yarrow

Common Names: Common Yarrow

Scientific Name: Achillea Millefolium

Family: Asteraceae

Origin: Widely diffused all over the North American continent in gardens and forests.

About Yarrow

This infesting plant is widely diffused all over North America. The plant produces several stems from the ground rhizome that can reach up to 3 feet in height. The hairy, bi-pinnate, cauline leaves widely populate the stems, and their size decreases towards the top where dense clusters of twenty to forty white flowers with five petals and yellow stamens are to be found.

Medicinal Parts:

- The leaves
- The flowers
- The stem

Habitat and Foraging:

- It can be found in a variety of environments, from plains to sub-alpine regions.

Influence on the Body:

- Astringent
- Diuretic
- Diaphoretic
- Analgesic

Traditional uses:

- Poultice from the leaves was used as a relief for common skin ailments such as eczemas, or burns and wounds.
- The Tea from the fresh plant was used to induce sweating and to treat fever.
- The whole plant decoction was used as a string diuretic and for its analgesic property as a topical wash in insect stings.
- Infusion from the leaves was used relaxation and sleep.
- Decoction from the roots was used as a wash for acne.

Possible Side Effects:

- It contains thujone, a carcinogenic substance, so it must be consumed in moderation.

Yellow Dock

Common Names: Curled Dock, Curly Dock

Scientific Name: Rumex Crispus

Family: Polygonaceae

Origin: Diffused all over the North American continent in gardens and yards.

About Yellow Dock

This small perennial plant is widely diffused all over North America. It can grow up to 40 inches from the taproot rhizome, which is brown on the outside and yellow on the inside. The taproot can sink to 30 inches deep in the ground. The basal leaves are long, narrow, and have curly edges. Flowers are red or white with vertical racemes. Seeds can be collected in winter at the top of the plant.

Medicinal Parts:

- The rhizome

Habitat and Foraging:

- It can be found in a variety of environments, ranging from cultivated grounds to tidal estuarine mud or on the coast.

Influence on the Body:

- Astringent
- Tonic
- Laxative
- Anti-inflammatory

Traditional uses:

- Poultice from the fresh rhizome was used to treat swollen joints and arthritis.
- The juice of the rhizome or the roasted seeds was used to treat diarrhea and dysentery.
- The powder obtained from dry rhizomes was used as an anti-hemorrhagic on wounds.
- The dried rhizome decoction was used as a powerful stimulant for the liver.

Possible Side Effects:

- Do not use in case of pre-existing kidney conditions.
- The high concentration of tannin can be dangerous if eaten in excess.

Yew

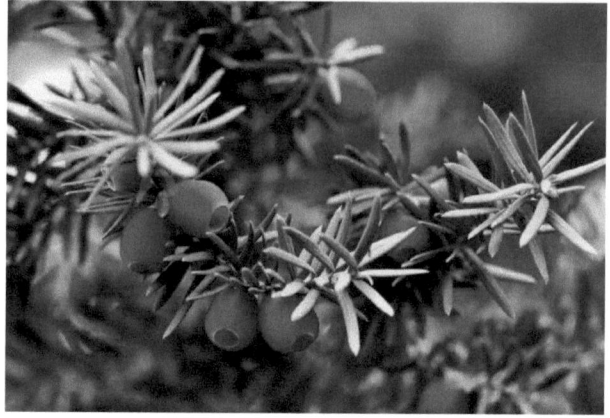

Common Names: Pacific Yew, Western Yew

Scientific Name: Taxus Brevifolia

Family: Taxaceae

Origin: Yew grows wild in the Pacific Coast States, from Northern California to Graham Island and in the North-Western part of Idaho.

About Yew

This evergreen tree can grow up to sixty feet in height. Leaves are lanceolate and small to avoid heat dispersion during the cold winter. It has small, red berries in the shape of a cup, with a black seed in the center.

Medicinal Parts:

- The fruit
- The leaves
- The barks

Habitat and Foraging:

- It can be found in a variety of environments, ranging from sides of stream to moist soils to ridge tops and slopes.

Influence on the Body:

- Astringent

- Tonic
- Laxative

Traditional uses:

- The decoction from the bark was used as an analgesic for stomachache.
- Poultice from fresh needles was used to treat burns and wounds.
- Yew berries were consumed raw to procure abortions, stimulate menstruation, or induce uterine contractions in difficult childbirths.

Possible Side Effects:

- Toxic to consume. Use only under medical supervision. It may cause abortions.

Yucca

Common Names: Adam's needle, Needle palm, Spoon Leaf Yucca

Scientific Name: Yucca Filamentosa

Family: Asparagaceae

Origin: Like other succulent plants, Yucca is mainly diffused in the hot, desert environments of the Southern United States and Mexico.

About Yucca

This perennial desert plant has no stem but only emerges from the ground in a whorl of basal, long, sword-like leaves. From this whorl of basal leaves pops up a straight single spike that can reach up to sixty inches, bearing a vertical cluster of white, bell-shaped flowers. The flowering period for this flower is from late spring to late summer.

Medicinal Parts:

- The roots
- The leaves

Habitat and Foraging:

- It blooms from May to September.
- It can be found in sandy soils and dunes, but also in rocky slopes and fields.

Influence on the Body:

- Analgesic
- Antiemetic
- Purgative

Traditional uses:

- The root extract was used as a natural soap to remove head lice.
- Decoction from the dried root was used to relieve gout and rheumatism.
- The water obtained by filtering the poultice of leaves was useful to calm uncontrolled vomit.

Possible Side Effects:

- None

Herbal Alphabetic Index

Honeysuckle; 106
Hops; 106
Horsetail; 107
Hyssop; 107
Ironwood; 108
Juniper; 108
Lady's Slipper; 109
Larch; 109
Lemon Balm; 110
Licorice (Wild American); 111
Mayapple; 111
Mexican Yew; 113
Milkweed; 112
Mint; 113
Mullein; 112
Nettle; 114
Oak; 115
Oregon Grape; 115
Oshà; 116
Partridge Berry; 116
Pasque Flower; 117
Passionflower; 118
Plantain; 118
Prickly Pear; 119
Queen of Meadow; 119
Red Clover; 120

Sagebrush; 121
Saint John's Wort; 122
Sarsaparilla; 123
Sassafras; 121
Saw Palmetto; 123
Skullcap; 124
Skunk Cabbage; 124
Slippery Elm; 125
Sumac; 126
Tobacco; 126
Toothwort; 127
Turtlehead; 127
Usnea; 128
Valerian; 129
Verbena; 129
Water Birch; 130
Watercress; 130
Wild Yam; 131
Willow; 131
Witch Hazel; 132
Yarrow; 132
Yellow Dock; 133
Yew; 134
Yucca; 134

Conclusion

We've now come to the end of this book.

Now, what next? Taking your time to apply all you've learned. Native American Herbs have long been used to cure many illnesses and conditions. They are still being studied for their hidden healing properties and will continue to be used in America and beyond to treat different conditions. So, take your chance with the remedies you've learnt in this book today and begin to live a freer, healthier and more fulfilled life.

BOOK 5: HERBAL APOTHECARY

Introduction

Most people want to know how medicinal plants were used by native North American populations. The most common belief was that in the early Native North American indigenous communities. The central figure was the medicine man.. However, more people may be involved including a priest, a sorcerer, a quack, and even a doctor.

The shaman was the priest's predecessor; the physician's predecessor was a lay healer, sometimes a woman. In some Native North American tribes, this division between the priest and healer was marked. Thus, the Ojibways had four shaman classes. The priests were highest in rank; then the "dawn men" who practiced a kind of medical magic; the seers and prophets were third; and finally were the herbalists, who, in the context of being healers, were the real medicine men. Any or all of these were merged into one entity in other tribes, a forerunner of today's holistic treatment aimed at concurrently curing body, mind and soul.

The knowledge and practice of medicine by the Native North Americans were not significantly different from their European counterparts when the European colonies were founded in North America in the 17th century. In both cases, the care of injuries caused externally was rational and always productive. Fractures, dislocations, burns, snake and insect bites, and so forth were included in this group. However, neither culture was able to treat most forms of prolonged internal illness where the trigger was not clear.

As European nations expanded throughout North America, as part of their subduing the tribes, they attempted to eliminate Native American culture. The shaman was the primary obstacle to this, both as a priest and as a tribal chief. He or she was seen by Christian missionaries and leaders alike as antagonistic to foreign ideas and societies.. Yet, despite this, among the early colonists, native North American medicine greatly influenced therapeutics.

Colonial health professionals were not always physicians, especially in frontier regions. Today, there are also concerns about insufficient care by physicians and hospitals in many rural parts of the United States. The colonists resorted to the native North American herbalists, the "medicine men" or "medicine women," where there were no colonial medical practitioners or where their prescribed remedies had failed. Some of their treatments were unsuccessful, as in Europe, but there are many others that worked.

They had been discovered through casual observation, sympathetic association and by trial and error. But there was barely a method for standardizing decoctions and identical preparations of course, and sometimes the specific batch had to be titrated against a patient's response. Nevertheless, many important remedies were first made by Native North Americans. About 170 preparations that were official in different editions of the United States Pharmacopeia or the National Formulary were used by the tribes in the present United States and Canada. Moreover, in the modern British Herbal Pharmacopoeia, the use of 25 percent of plants (more than fifty species) originated in North America, although they are now cultivated and used in Europe. Indian pinkroot (Spigelia marilandica), a Cherokee vermifuge, which was officially recognized in 1752 and included in the pharmacopeias of London, Dublin and Edinburgh, was one of the most important sources of early medicine.

At the beginning of the 17th century, sassafras bark was as commercially valuable as tobacco. Sassafras extract has been used in the treatment of rheumatism and gout as a febrifuge and carminative, whereas sassafras oil was used as a topical analgesic. At one time, wild cherry bark (Prunus virginiana and P serotina) was second only to home-medicated sassafras. The bark was applied directly as poultices and, as an injection, was used as an astringent in the treatment of coughs, colds, fever and cramps. As a sedative, narcotic, diaphoretic and emetic, Tobacco (Nicotiana tabacum) was legal in earlier editions of the USP. It has been used on crops as dust or an infusion, as an insecticide. Today, in reality, tobacco is cultivated mainly for smoking.

Cotton is indigenous to most of the subtropical countries. In the mid-16th century, Spanish explorers discovered that the North American species (G hirsutum) was grown by the Zui tribes in what is now western New Mexico; it is still the most commercially valuable species. Like tobacco, it is primarily cultivated for non-medicinal purposes. The fiber is still used for dressings. A decoction of the roots was used as an emmenagogue and oxytocic.

Indian (or American) cannabis (Apocynum cannabinum), which is native to North America, should not be mistaken for Indian hemp (Cannabis indica). The American hemp fiber was used to make bags, ropes ,quilts, etc. The root was used as a diuretic and a cathartic. The most commonly used (natural) cathartic on earth is said to be Cascara (Cascara sagrada). An anonymous Spanish priest found the native North Americans using it and was so struck by its mildness and effectiveness that he coined the botanical name "holy bark" (in Spanish).

As a demulcent and emollient, slippery elm (Ulmus fulva) is still being used. It was also used by native North Americans for the prevention of coughs, colds and dysentery. The bark was used as a poultice for the treatment of bullet wounds during 18th-century military interventions.

This book will explain in depth the different treatments and the different kinds of problems that can be managed using native American Herbal remedies.

Allergies

Native Americans have been using herbs for healing and spiritual purposes for centuries, and many of these herbs can be found in modern herbal stores. However, because the body's immune system is much more sensitive today than it was when Native Americans were using these herbs, people may now be allergic to them. Unfortunately, this often goes unnoticed until the person begins to feel symptoms such as asthma or hay fever.

It is important to always consult a doctor before taking any new medications or supplements, even if they are natural. And if you experience any negative reactions after taking an herb—whether it is an allergy or something else—stop taking it immediately and consult your physician right away; the negative effects could last much longer than just a few hours.

How to Know If You Are Allergic To Plants

Herbs are often used in combination either with other herbs or with other forms of medication. If you get an allergy from any of these herbs, you might also have an allergy to any medications that are used in combination with them since the pharmacology of the two substances is likely similar.

Check the ingredients on all over-the-counter medications or dietary supplements, including vitamins and pain relievers. If you think a product might contain an herb to which you are allergic, it is a good idea to avoid taking it until you have consulted a doctor.

If your allergies are severe or if you suffer from chronic allergies, it is important to know what unrelated medications could be the cause. In addition, if your allergy symptoms seem unusual for what is normally associated with that particular herb, contact your doctor right away.

Herbs to Watch Out For

Some herbs that have been known to cause allergic reactions include:

Cayenne pepper

Cayenne pepper has been used by Native Americans for hundreds of years as a natural pain reliever and as a way to stop minor bleeding. It has also been used to treat cold symptoms, heart disease, rheumatism, and arthritis. Cayenne pepper is now widely used as a spice in cooking.

In addition to anaphylaxis, cayenne pepper allergy can cause the throat to swell, itchiness and hives. In some cases, asthma attacks have also been associated with cayenne pepper allergy.

It is important to note that cayenne pepper sold in stores has been known to contain other substances that may produce an allergic reaction as well.

Chamomile

Chamomile is a healing herb used to treat indigestion, ulcers, insomnia, headaches, and heartburn. It can also treat inflammatory problems and can be used to relieve pain.

Most people more likely to be allergic to the flowers of the chamomile plant rather than its leaves. Some of the symptoms of an allergic reaction might include swelling in the mouth or throat that could cause breathing problems, as well as hives or anaphylaxis.

Ginseng

With its ability to boost energy levels and stimulate the immune system, ginseng has been widely used for both medicinal and spiritual purposes. It is also used to treat colds, asthma, heart disease, and many other conditions.

Because of the medicine's popularity, it is important to be aware of side effects such as allergies and toxicity. Some people are allergic to all parts of the ginseng plant, including the roots or the dried leaves. An allergy may develop to various ginseng products that contain only a tiny percentage of the herb itself.

According to Harvard Health Publications, ginseng can cause symptoms similar to those associated with an allergic reaction such as swelling in the throat and lips; breathing difficulties; itching; hives or welts on the body; or even fainting.

Cinnamon

You have probably heard that cinnamon helps sweeten things up, but you might not know that it also has been used for the care of digestive problems. Chronic users of cinnamon may develop an allergy to it, although the condition is uncommon.

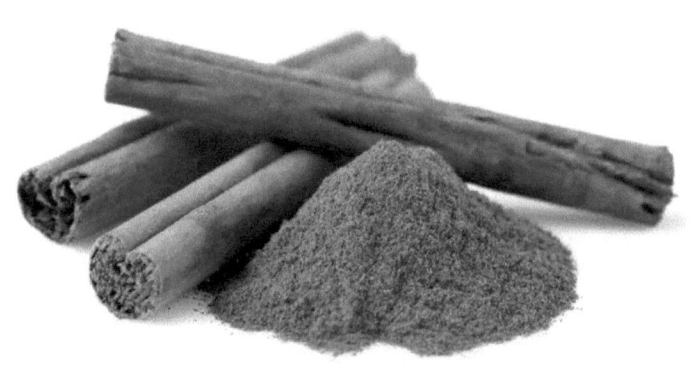

Those allergic to cinnamon may experience mild side effects such as a rash on their face and neck, while others may have more severe reactions such as breathing problems and difficulty in swallowing.

Always Try Small Quantities First

Since the body often responds positively to small amounts of highly potent herbs like black cohosh and ginseng, it is important to start with very small amounts of herbs before fully embarking on the herbal journey.

If you have allergies or other health problems, use the smallest quantities possible. Although this may not eliminate the negative effects of a new herb or supplement on your body, at least you will know what the supposed benefits are before taking an entire bottle.

It is also important to consider how long you have been taking a particular herb when you decide whether or not to continue using it.

Remember also that there are many herbs that have multiple uses, and some may not be safe for a person to use regularly. For example, some people have been known to develop a sensitivity to the aloe vera plant. Some who regularly use it on their skins or in their food may experience side effects such as burning, swelling, or itching.

Be Aware of the Herbs' Potential Side Effects

There is no doubt about it: herbs can help improve your health and make you feel better. However, you should consult with your doctor first so as to eliminate the risk of side effects.

Some herbs might be useful for curing an illness, but they could also cause other health issues. As mentioned above, regular use of aloe vera may have side effects. However, they may not experience any side effects until they start using it regularly. If you notice a rash on your skin after using aloe vera products, stop using them and contact a doctor right away.

Remedies to Treat the Most Common Illnesses and Pains (80-100 Recipes)

Digestive System

Bloating

Overeating, stomach gas, and the start of women's pre-menstrual cycles are just a few of the factors that can cause bloating. Herbs aid in evacuating toxins, excess gas, and accumulated fluid, allowing your body to recover to a more balanced state.

1. **Peppermint-Fennel Tea**

Makes 1 cup

If you think your bloating is caused by a buildup in your digestive tract, peppermint and fennel can help you feel better quickly. Strong anti-spasmodic compounds in these pleasant-tasting herbs relax the smooth muscle tissue in the digestive tract. If the flavor of this tea is too strong, add a teaspoon of honey.

Ingredients:

- 1 cup boiling water
- One teaspoon dried peppermint
- ¼ teaspoon fennel seeds, crushed

Directions:

1. Fill a large cup halfway with boiling water. Allow the tea to steep for 10 minutes after adding the peppermint and fennel.

2. Relax and sip your tea. This is a gentle cure that can be used as often as necessary.

2. **Dandelion Root Tincture**

Makes about 2 cups

Although dandelion root has a harsh flavor, it has powerful diuretic properties that help your body eliminate toxins and make you feel much better. If stored in a cool, dark place, this tincture will last for up to 7 years.

Ingredients:

- 8 ounces dandelion root, finely chopped
- 2 cups unflavored 80-proof vodka

Directions:

1. Place the dandelion root in a pint jar that has been sterilized. Fill the jar with vodka, filling it to the top and completely covering the roots.

2. Close the jar tightly and give it a good shake. For 6 to 8 weeks, keep in a cool, dark cabinet and shake it several times a week. If any of the alcohol evaporates, top up the jar with vodka until it's full again.

3. Soak a piece of cheesecloth in water and lay it over the funnel's mouth. Pour the tincture into another sterilized pint jar using the funnel. Squeeze the liquid out of the roots with the cheesecloth until there is no more liquid. Remove the roots and pour the tincture into dark-colored glass vials.

4. If feel bloated, take one teaspoon orally once or twice a day.

5. If the flavor is too strong for you, combine it with some water or juice and drink it.

Constipation

Constipation is unpleasant and may make life difficult. When you are feeling bloated and weighted down, you want immediate relief. You might be able to treat your constipation using natural solutions.

Having less than 3 bowel motions each week is considered constipation. It might be a recurring problem or something that just happens once in a while. Among the signs and symptoms are:

- Stool that is hard to pass.
- Straining to get a bowel movement.
- A sense of being "blocked" or unable to evacuate your bowels.
- Need assistance in emptying the rectum.
- Discomfort in the abdomen.
- Bloating and nausea.

Herbal treatments for constipation are quite simple to get. For one, herbal components are used in several laxatives. Then, anthraquinones, or chemicals that stimulate the intestines, are found in most laxative plants. These laxatives increase peristalsis (the spasm of the intestines that helps transfer food from the colon towards the rectum) by pulling fluid into the colon. Constipation necessitates the addition of fiber and water.

Below are some herbal treatments for constipation.

3. Bowel-Hydrating Infusion

Yields about 2 1/4 cups of herb mix, dried (enough for tea (14 - 18 quarts))

It is a bit sweeter than solo marshmallows and is a fantastic choice for those with dry, hard-to-pass, little "rabbit pellet" bowel function. Drink a quart or so every day.

Ingredients:

- ¼ cup of dried licorice root
- 1 cup of dried linden flower or leaf
- 1/4 cup of dried cinnamon bark
- 1 cup of dried marshmallow root

Directions:

1. Combine all of the herbs in a medium mixing bowl. Keep the container airtight.

2. Make a cold infusion by putting 2 to 4 tablespoons of herbs in every quart of water in a mason jar or a French press. Before filtering, add cold or room-temp water and soak for 4 to 8 hours.

4. Bowel-Motivating Tincture

Yields 4 fluid ounces approx. (30 - 60 doses)

Bitters and carminatives stimulate bile flow and intestinal peristalsis, inducing bowel movement.

Ingredients:

- 1 ½ fluid ounces dandelion root, tincture
- 1 and a half fluid ounces St. John's wort, tincture
- Half fluid ounce angelica root, tincture
- Half fluid ounce ginger, tincture

Directions:

1. Combine the tinctures in a small container. Cap and label the bottle.

2. Take 2–4 drops every twenty minutes until you feel better.

5. Bowel-Soothing Tea

Ingredients:

- Boneset flowers, one large handful
- Dandelion flowers, one large handful
- 4 ounces of cascara bark

- 2 quarts of water honey

Directions:

1. In a saucepan, mix the above herbs and two quarts of water. Bring to a boil and cook until the mixture is reduced to one quart; drain.

2. Drink a cup before breakfast and another before bed. To sweeten, you might use honey.

6. Purifying Digestive Tea

Ingredients:

- 2 cups of boiling water
- 2 tsps. of cascara sagrada
- 1 tsp. of Oregon grape root
- 3 to 4 slices of ginger root
- 1 tsp of cayenne

Directions:

1. In a saucepan, combine all herbs and two cups of boiling water;

2. Soak for 30 - 45 minutes, cool, and drain. Take two cups a day, one tbsp.. at a time.

Heartburn

Heartburn/Reflux/Gerd

Heartburn is a burning stomach pain that can spread up into the throat. It occurs when hydrochloric acid from the stomach backs up into the esophagus. It may occur if food is gulped or there is too much caffeine or alcohol in drinks. It can also occur if you eat while stressed or eat certain foods (such as spicy or fatty foods). Antacids are commonly taken for heartburn, but herbs can be just as effective.

Note: If you suffer from heartburn, avoid peppermint. Although it helps treat indigestion and other stomach problems, it can relax the esophageal sphincter and increase heartburn's tendency.

7. Marshmallow Infusion

Makes 1 quart.

If you have heartburn, you need a cold infusion of marshmallow root which heals the damaged tissue in the esophagus. When heartburn occurs, just sip on this slowly, and you will feel relief in no time.

Ingredients:

- 2–4 tbsps. dried marshmallow root

Directions:

1. In a quart-size mason jar, combine the marshmallow with enough cold or room-temperature water to fill the jar—cover and steep for 4–8 hours.

2. Keep refrigerated, where each batch will last for 2–3 days.

8. Preventive Bitter Tincture

Makes 3 ½ fl. oz. (30–60 doses)

To restore normal stomach acid levels and lessen the conditions for heartburn to develop, take these drops before every meal.

Ingredients:

- 1 fl. oz. tincture of dandelion root
- ½ fl. oz. tincture of catnip
- ½ fl. oz. tincture of chamomile
- ⅓ fl. oz. tincture of fennel
- ⅓ fl. oz. tincture of meadowsweet
- ⅓ fl. oz. tincture of self-heal
- ½ fl. oz. tincture of St. John's wort.

Directions:

1. In a mini bottle, combine the tinctures. Cap the bottle and label it.

2. Take ½–1 drop 10 minutes before eating.

9. Quick-Acting Heartburn Tea

Ingredients:

- 1 tsp. dried angelica root
- 1 tsp. crushed juniper berries
- 1 cup boiling water

Directions:

1. Combine the herbs in a nonmetallic container and cover with boiling water; steep for 20–30 minutes; strain.

- Take a tbsp. at a time, as needed.

10. Soothing Heartburn Tea

Ingredients:

- 1 tsp. catnip leaves
- 1 tsp. oxeye daisy herb
- 1 cup boiling water

Directions:

2. Combine the herbs in a non-metallic container and cover with boiling water; steep for 30 minutes; strain.

3. Take 1 tbsp. at a time, as needed.

Indigestion

Indigestion is characterized by bloating, belching, stomach ache, discomfort, etc. It often happens when the stomach reacts to something taken. The herbs below should offer the quick relief needed.

11. Pre-Emptive Bitter Tincture

Indigestion often refers to insufficient digestion. This solution stimulates all the digestive fluids, including saliva, stomach acid, bile, and pancreatic enzymes, to ensure thorough and complete digestion.

Ingredients:

- 1 fluid ounce tincture of dandelion root
- 1 fluid ounce tincture of sage
- 1 fluid ounce tincture of catnip
- 1 fluid ounce tincture of chamomile

Directions:

1. In a small bottle, combine the tinctures. Cap the bottle and label it.

2. Take 1 to 2 drops 10 minutes before eating.

12. Carminative Tincture

This combination warms the core of the body, activating the digestive organs and preventing the intestines from becoming sluggish; angelica can be used instead of peppermint if preferred.

Ingredients:

- 1½ fluid ounces tincture ginger
- 1 fluid ounce tincture fennel
- 1 fluid ounce tincture peppermint
- ½ fluid ounce tincture licorice

Instructions:

1. In a small bottle, combine the tinctures. Cap the bottle and label it.

2. Take 1 to 2 drops after each meal or whenever your guts feel uncomfortably stuck.

13. Strong Digestive tea

3. This is an excellent digestive aid, and it can provide fast relief for "flatus" or ringing in the ears, as well as indigestion.

Ingredients:

- 1 teaspoon angelica root
- 1 teaspoon grated ginger root
- 2 teaspoons chamomile flowers
- 2 teaspoons peppermint leaves
- 1 cup boiling water

Directions:

1. Combine the above ingredients in a vessel.

2. Take one tablespoon of the herb combination and place in boiling water; steep for 30 minutes; cool and strain.

3. Take as needed, up to two cups a day.

14. **Spicy Ginger Elixir**

Yield: 1 cup (235 ml)

This is a great digestive aid. It is also great for chest congestion.

Ingredients:

- 1/2 cup (50 g) hacked ginger
- 1 lemon, daintily cut
- 1 (4-inch, or 10 cm) cinnamon stick
- 2-star anise
- 2 cardamom units
- 1/2 cup (160 g) crude nearby honey
- 1 cup (235 ml) 100 proof vodka or liquor

Directions:

1. Add 1/2 tsp. of ginger root to 1 quart of boiling water.

2. Boil for 10 minutes, then allow to cool for approximately 20 minutes.

3. Strain out the ginger with a strainer or mesh cheesecloth, and drink the syrup warm or chilled in water.

4. NB: For stomach ailments, add 2 tbsp. of ground ginger with 1 cup of honey and cinnamon at night before bedtime to help soothe your stomach muscles and ease indigestion or gas pains in the morning.

Cardiovascular System

Anemia

Anemia is a disorder where the blood has low RBCs, hemoglobin, or a defective RBC. The term anemia comes from the Greek word 'mia,' which signifies blood and refers to a lack of sufficient red blood cells. A number of factors may cause anemia, but the most prevalent is a lack of iron in the blood.

The RBCs transport oxygen to all the critical organs of the body. A protein-bound iron in RBCs, hemoglobin, gives the blood cells their red color. It attaches oxygen, protects against infections, and prevents blood loss. According to the latest international health survey data, India has the greatest incidence of anemia at 39.9%, particularly among children and women of childbearing age.

In most situations, the symptoms of anemia are missed or misinterpreted; constantly look for signs and symptoms such as those listed below;

- General weakness and fatigue
- Hair loss
- Pale skin
- Increased heartbeat
- Lack of stamina
- Giddiness
- Shortness of breath (dyspnea)
- Poor appetite
- Swelling around eyes

Men's hemoglobin levels should be between 13.5 to 17.5 g/dl, while women's levels should be between 12.0 and 15.5 g/dl. Anemia is defined as a blood level of less than 12 g/dl for females and less than 12 g/dl for males. Anemia may be effectively controlled and treated by eating a nutritious diet rich in iron and using iron supplements.

Try these easy-to-use natural treatments to boost your iron levels as well as your strength and energy.

15. Moringa Leaves Paste

Vitamins C, A, magnesium, and iron are all abundant in moringa leaves. A serving of these extraordinary leaves has 28mg higher iron than spinach. Moringa leaves are very well known for improving hemoglobin levels.

Ingredients:

- Maringa leaves
- Jaggery powder

Directions:

1. To prepare a paste, finely chop about 20 to 25 moringa leaves, add a tsp. of jaggery powder, and mix well. To boost your iron levels, eat this at breakfast.

16. Beetroot Juice

Beets are high in copper, iron, magnesium, phosphorus, and vitamins B2, B1, B12, B6, and vitamin C. Beets' high nutritional content helps in the synthesis of RBCs in the body and improves hemoglobin levels.

Ingredients:

- Diced beetroot one cup
- Lemon juice

Directions:

1. Add about one cup of diced beetroot to a blender, mix well, filter the juice, add a tsp. of lemon juice, and enjoy this incredible juice every morning. Lemon juice boosts vitamin C absorption and improves iron absorption.

17. Sesamum Indicum (Sesame Seeds)

Copper, iron, selenium, zinc, folate, vitamin E, and vitamin B6 are abundant in sesame seeds. The inclusion of dark sesame seeds in the daily routine enhances hemoglobin levels and boosts iron absorption.

Ingredients:

- Black sesame seeds 1 tbsp.
- Honey 1 tbsp.

Directions:

1. 1 tbsp. black sesame seeds, dry roasted, combined with 1 tsp. honey; roll into a ball. Eat this healthy mixture daily.

2. Bed Sores

3. When bedridden people lie in the same position for long hours or days, the blood circulation to sensitive regions is disrupted. The reduced blood flow affects the skin and causes bedsores.

4. The initial red color fades and starts to become purple as the bedsores progress. Once a bedsore develops and matures, it will take a long time to cure entirely.

18. Aloe Vera Gel

Aloe Vera is a plant that works wonders. It has anti-inflammatory, antibacterial, therapeutic, and relaxing qualities. Alpe vera prevents and cures bedsores. Put aloe vera gel directly onto the bedsores. The natural cooling qualities of aloe vera help to avoid burning and irritation. This plant is among the most powerful natural remedies for curing bedsores and providing immediate relief.

Steps to make aloe vera gel"

Ingredients:

- Aloe vera leaf
- Vitamin E and C (preservatives)

Directions:

1. Slice off one of the plant's outer leaves from the base.

2. You may also use a leaf from the market.

3. Wash and remove any dirt; then set it upright in a jar or basin for 10 to15 minutes. This allows the yellow-tinted resin in the leaf to seep out.

4. Because the resin includes latex, which might irritate the skin, finishing this step is essential.

5. Wash off the remaining resin on the leaf, then peel off the thick skin with a sharp vegetable peeler when the resin has entirely drained.

6. The organic aloe vera gel may be seen once the leaf has been peeled.

7. Scrape it into the blender with a little spoon. Make sure there are no fragments of aloe vera skin in the mix.

8. It should just take a few seconds to blend the gel till it's foamy and dissolved.

9. It is now be ready to use. If you wish to preserve it for more than one week, you need to add preservatives.

10. Vitamins E and C are powerful preservatives that may help your aloe vera gel last for a long time. While the gel itself has some of these nutrients naturally, they are not enough to keep it fresh for more than a week. So. If you want

11. to increase the shelf life of the gel, add additional vitamins.

19. Golden Paste

Turmeric on its own is an excellent treatment for bed sores.. Its antimicrobial properties guard against any infection that may result from the sores. It rapidly offers comfort and relieves pain.

Steps to make this golden paste:

Ingredients:

- 1 cup water (purified)
- 1 teaspoon black pepper (finely ground)
- 1/4 cup coconut oil or any other fat like olive oil or ghee
- 1/2 cup turmeric powder (organic)

Directions:

1. Mix the water and turmeric in a skillet over medium-low heat till it forms a thick paste.

2. Mix in the black pepper and oil of choice, modifying the turmeric and water quality as required.

3. If desired, you might even add 1 to 2 tbsp. raw honey.

4. Once the paste has reached the desired consistency, store in the refrigerator for about 1 to 2 months in a glass jar covered with a lid.

5. This paste reduces inflammation whether taken orally or applied topically.

Bruise

Deep, severe bruises may indicate the presence of underlying injuries or health issues. Something as easy as bumping against a piece of furniture can result in minor bruises. Consult your doctor if you notice you are bruising more easily than normal, as this could indicate an underlying health problem.

20.   Fresh Hyssop Poultice

Makes one treatment Hyssop, offers pain relief and stimulates circulation, helping your bruise heal faster. If you have not yet planted hyssop in your garden, use a drop or two of hyssop essential oil to treat a bruise. Rehydrate a teaspoon of dried hyssop with a tablespoon of warm water and use it to make a poultice.

Ingredients:

- One tablespoon finely chopped fresh hyssop leaves

Directions:

1. Cover the injured area with the chopped leaves and a soft cloth. Allow 10 to 15 minutes for the poultice to dry. Repeat this process two or three times per day until your bruise is gone.

2. Precautions: If you have epilepsy or are pregnant, avoid using hyssop because it might cause involuntary muscle contractions.

21.   Arnica Salve

Makes about 1 cup.

Arnica is a strong anti-inflammatory agent, and its ability to relieve pain makes this simple salve an excellent choice for bumps and bruises.

Ingredients:

- 1 cup light olive oil
- 2 ounces dried arnica flowers
- 1-ounce beeswax

Directions:

1. Combine the olive oil and arnica flowers in a slow cooker. Set the slow cooker to the lowest heat setting, cover it, and let the herbs steep in the oil for 3 to 5 hours. Allow the infused oil to cool after turning off the heat. In the base of a double boiler, bring about an inch of water to a simmer. Reduce the heat to a low setting.

2. Over the top part of the double boiler, drape a piece of cheesecloth. Pour the infused oil into the cheesecloth, then wring and twist it until no more oil comes out. Remove the cheesecloth and the herbs used.

3. Place the double boiler on the base and add the beeswax to the infused oil. Warm gently over low heat. Remove the pan from the heat once the beeswax has completely melted. Pour into clean, dry jars or tins as soon as possible and allow it to cool fully before capping.

4. Apply a pea-size amount to the bruised region with your fingertips or a cotton cosmetic pad. Repeat twice a day until your bruise fades, adding a bit more or less as needed.

Precautions: Do not use on skin that has been broken. Long-term use can cause skin irritation; if signs of skin irritation arise, stop using it.

Respiratory System
Asthma

Inflammation in the airways throughout the lungs and restricted bronchial tubes characterize this chronic disease. Asthma attacks can be terrifying and can cause panic attacks.

22.   Ginkgo-Thyme Tea

Makes 1 cup

Ginkgo biloba and thyme widen the airways and relax chest muscles, allowing for easier breathing. Add a teaspoon of honey or dried peppermint to the mix to sweeten it if you prefer.

Ingredients:

- 1 cup boiling water

- One teaspoon dried Ginkgo Biloba
- One teaspoon dried thyme

Directions:

1. Fill a large cup halfway with boiling water. Allow the tea to steep for 10 minutes after adding the dry herbs and covering the mug.

2. Relax and inhale the steam while slowly drinking the tea. Repeat this process up to four times a day.

Precautions: If you are taking a monoamine oxidase inhibitor (MAOI) for depression, don't take it. Ginkgo biloba can take blood thinners to work better, so consult your doctor before taking it.

23. **Peppermint-Rosemary Vapor Treatment**

Makes one treatment

Rosemary leaves contain important histamine-blocking oil, while peppermint helps expand your airways and aid breathing. If you don't have fresh herbs on hand, substitute two drops of peppermint essential oil and four drops of rosemary essential oil for this therapy.

Ingredients:

- 4 cups steaming-hot water (not boiling)
- ½ cup crushed fresh peppermint leaves
- ½ cup finely chopped fresh rosemary leaves

Directions:

1. Combine all of the ingredients in a large, shallow bowl. Place the bowl on a table and take a seat in front of it comfortably.

2. Cover your head and the bowl with a big towel. Inhale the fumes released by the herbs. As needed, get some fresh air and close your eyes if the vapours are too powerful. Continue to treat the water until it has cooled.

3. If asthma symptoms begin, repeat as required. This therapy is mild enough t to use as often as you want.

Precautions: If you have epilepsy, avoid using rosemary. While some relaxing oils, such as jasmine, ylang-ylang, chamomile, and lavender, have been proven to help prevent seizures, more aromatic oils, such as rosemary, fennel, sage, eucalyptus, hyssop, camphor, and spike lavender, have been known to cause seizures.

Bronchitis

Bronchitis occurs when the bronchial linings become inflamed as a result of irritation, infection, or allergies. A heavy, rasping cough is also a common symptom of the illness. When paired with increased fluid intake and lots of rest, herbal therapies have been shown to help reduce and eliminate bronchitis symptoms.

24. **Rosemary–Licorice Root Vapor Treatment**

Makes one treatment

Rosemary and licorice roots expand the airways, increase circulation, and relieve the pain and inflammation associated with bronchitis.

Ingredients:

- 5 cups water
- ¼ cup chopped dried licorice root
- ½ cup finely chopped fresh rosemary leaves

Directions:

1. Combine the water and the dried licorice root in a saucepan. Bring the mixture to a boil, then lower the heat to a low setting. Cook for 10 minutes on low heat.

2. In a shallow dish, combine the water, licorice root, and rosemary leaves.

3. Cover your head and the bowl with a big towel. Inhale the fumes released by the herbs. As needed, get some fresh air and close your eyes if the vapours are too powerful. Continue to treat the water until it has cooled.

4. As needed, repeat the process. This therapy is mild enough to use as often as you want.

Precautions: If you have epilepsy, high blood pressure, diabetes, kidney difficulties, or heart disease, you should not use this therapy.

25. Goldenseal-Hyssop Syrup
Makes about 2 cups

Hydrastine and berberine are two powerful antiviral and antibacterial compounds found in goldenseal. Hyssop relieves bronchial spasms and helps eliminate lung congestion while also providing a relaxing, soothing effect. This syrup can also be used to treat common colds. When refrigerated, it will last up to 6 months.

Ingredients:

- ½ ounce dried goldenseal root, chopped
- 1 ounce dried hyssop
- 2 cups water 1 cup honey

Directions:

1. Combine the goldenseal and hyssop with the 2 cups of water in a saucepan. Reduce the liquid by half by bringing it to a low simmer and partially covering it with a lid.

2. Fill a glass measuring cup halfway with the contents of the saucepan, then strain the mixture through a soaked piece of cheesecloth into the saucepan, wringing the fabric until no more liquid comes out.

3. Warm the mixture over low heat with the honey, stirring regularly until the temperature reaches 105°F to 110°F.

4. Fill a sterilized jar or bottle with the syrup and keep it in the refrigerator.

5. Orally take one tablespoon three to five times a day, until your symptoms go away.

Precautions: If you are pregnant or breastfeeding, if you have high blood pressure or epilepsy, don't use it. In addition, diarrhea and heartburn can be aggravated by goldenseal. Children under the age of 12 should take one teaspoon twice a day, two to three times a day.

Cough and Cold

The common cold is an inflammation of the upper respiratory tract caused by more than 100 viruses. Watery eyes, a runny or stuffy nose, head congestion, fatigue, sneezing, and coughing are typical common cold symptoms. The cough that often accompanies a cold is the body's effort to rid the air passage of mucus, dust, or other irritants.

Other symptoms of the common cold include impaired taste and smell, fever or chills, a general aching sensation of pain and listlessness and as the cold progresses, a sore throat, ranging from mild to extreme. Any or all of these symptoms may be experienced.

26. Antitussive Oxymel
Makes 20 to 60 doses.

An oxymel is essentially a vinegar and honey mixture that combines the astringent and stimulating properties of vinegar with the moistening and calming properties of honey. With the addition of lung-specific herbs, this is a go-to for coughs of all types.

Ingredients:

- 1/3 cup dried pine needles
- 1/3 cup dried sage leaf
- 1/3 cup dried thyme leaf
- ¼ cup dried ginger
- 1-quart of apple cider vinegar
- Honey as needed to fill the container

Directions:

1. Fill the jar four-fifths of the way with vinegar, then with honey.

2. Cover the pot and let macerate for four weeks.

3. Strain and bottle the oxymel. Cap the bottle and label it.

4. Take 1 to 3 tablespoons as needed.

27. **Cough Syrup**

This cough syrup is a great way to relieve a nasty cold or flu.

Ingredients:

- 2 teaspoons coltsfoot leaves
- 1 tablespoon wild plum root
- 2 teaspoons mullein leaves
- 2 cups boiling water
- 1 pound honey

Directions:

1. Combine the herbs in boiling water, steep for 30 minutes, and strain in non-metallic containers.

2. Add one pound of honey, heating, and stirring until the honey is dissolved; cool and store in a glass container.

28. **Soothing Cough and Cold Formula**

The components in this formula may aid in promoting much-needed relief for any respiratory infections.

Ingredients:

- 30 drops echinacea tincture
- 20 drops wild indigo root tincture
- 2 cups white cedar leaf tips tea

Directions:

1. Combine the above ingredients and take half a cup at a time, hot.

2. Take up to three times a day.

29. **Lakota Cough and Cold Formula**

Also known as plantain, dandelion, or yucca root, this is a great herbal remedy for sore or dry throats caused by the common cold.

Ingredients:

- 1 teaspoon goldenseal root
- 1 teaspoon mullein leaves
- 1 teaspoon Osha root
- 1 teaspoon pleurisy root
- 1 teaspoon yerba mansa root
- 2 teaspoons yerba santa leaves
- 2 cups boiling water

Directions:

1. Combine the above herbs and cover with boiling water; steep for 30 minutes, calm, and strain.

2. As required, take two teaspoons at a time, up to two cups a day.

30. **Lumbee Cough And Cold Formula**

This formula is formulated with natural ingredients that help to relieve the discomfort of colds and flu.

Ingredients:

- 3 teaspoons goldenrod leaves,
- 4 teaspoons horehound leaves
- 2 teaspoons white pine inner bark
- 4 cups boiling water

Directions:

1. Combine the above herbs in cheesecloth; tie closed with a string.

2. Place the bag in the boiling water; simmer for 15 minutes; cool; remove the bundle.

3. Take half a cup of the hot mixture at a time, as needed, up to two cups a day.

31. Quick-Acting Cough and Cold Formula

This tea can quickly relieve cold and flu symptoms.

Ingredients:

- 4 teaspoons agrimony leaves
- 2 teaspoons mullein leaves
- 2 teaspoons blue vervain leaves
- 1 teaspoon oxeye daisy
- 3 teaspoons horehound leaves
- 2 teaspoons speedwell
- 2 cups boiling water

Directions:

1. Combine the herbs with water, steep for 30 minutes, calm, and strain.

2. Take up to two cups each day.

32. Expectorating Cough and Cold Tea

This formula contains known expectorant herbs that can help to relieve cough and sore throat.

Ingredients:

- 2 teaspoons boneset herb
- 2 teaspoons licorice root
- 2 to 3 slices ginger root
- 2 teaspoons wild cherry bark
- 2 cups boiling water

Directions:

3. Combine the herbs with water, steep for 30 minutes, calm, and strain.

4. Take up to two cups each day.

33. Quick-Acting Mullein Cough Syrup

This syrup helps relieve cough

Ingredients:

- 1 cup mullein tea
- 1 pound honey

Directions:

1. Heat until the honey is liquid.

2. Remove from heat, calm, and pour into a glass container. Take a tablespoon at a time, as needed.

Nervous System
Headache

Headaches are widespread and can be dull and steady, stabbing, gnawing, or throbbing. There are many kinds of headaches with many different causes. Sometimes tension, fatigue, or stress can cause a headache. Problems with the eyes, ears, nose, throat, or teeth such as allergies, injuries, infections, tumors, and many diseases can bring on headaches. Headaches are also big business; most people take non-steroidal anti-inflammatory drugs (NSAIDs) such as aspirin, ibuprofen, or indomethacin, or even more potent painkillers for relief. But these drugs have unwanted and sometimes severe side effects, including ulcers and an increased tendency to bleed. Herbs can offer a safer alternative.

Headaches also arise from a variety of imbalances. Some are simple one-off causes such as dehydration, sleep debt, dietary excesses, alcohol, caffeine and medications. Following are recipes for quick pain relief while y supplying what's missing or while simply waiting for the body to recover.

34. Cooling Tea for Headache

This is for a headache that causes flushes and the pain feels hot, intense, and highly sensitive to the touch. Front strain, stress or worry, nasal congestion, or acute nerve pain are all common causes of this kind of headache. These herbs relax, cool, and drain (but the wild lettuce might cause sleepiness).

Ingredients:

- 1 cup meadowsweet flower, dried
- 1 cup betony flower and leaf, dried
- 1/2 cup linden flower and leaf, dried
- 1/4 cup wild lettuce stalk and leaf, dried
- 1/2 cup marshmallow leaf, dried

Directions:

1. Combine all the herbs in a medium mixing dish. Keep the container sealed.

2. Prepare a steaming infusion: bring a pot of water to a boil. In a French press or mason jar, measure 2–3 tbsp. of herbs in every quart of water.

3. Fill the pot halfway with boiling water, cover, and steep for 30–40 minutes. Drink hot or cold. A cup of this tea will help you feel better.

35. Warming Tea for Headache

Yields about 3 1/4 cups of herb mix, dry (enough for 22 - 28 quarts of tea)

Try this combination if your headaches leave you with a pale face and the pain feels chilly, dull, and broad. Hypothyroidism, Sin, hepatic congestion, and circulation stasis are all common causes of this form of headache. These herbs are warming, astringent, and circulatory. (If you regularly use coffee to relieve headaches, try this.) Drink a quart or so every day as a preventative if you suffer frequent headaches.

Ingredients:

- 1 cup tulsi leaf, dried
- 1 cup betony flower and leaf, dried
- ½ cup chamomile flower, dried
- ¼ cup ginger, dried
- ½ cup sage leaf, dried

Directions:

1. Combine all the herbs in a medium mixing dish. Keep the container sealed.

2. Make a hot infusion: boil some water in a pot. In a French press or mason jar, measure 2 to 3 tbsp. of herbs every quart of water.

3. Fill the container halfway with boiling water, cover, and steep for 30 - 40 mins. Have it warm to hot. A cup of this tea will help you feel better.

36. Peppery Tea for Headache

Ingredients:

- 1 cup of boiling water
- 1 tsp. of feverfew leaves
- 1 tsp. of peppermint leaves
- Honey, to taste

Directions:

1. In a nonmetallic container, combine the herbs mentioned above and cover with boiling water.

2. Soak for 30 minutes; strain.

3. Taste and add honey as needed. Take one tbsp. at a time, about one cup per day.

37. Soothing Tea for Headache
Ingredients:

- 1 to 2 cups of boiling water
- 1 tsp. of catnip leaves
- 2 tsp. of feverfew leaves

Directions:

1. In a glass jar, combine the catnip and feverfew.

2. Cover the herbs with one to two cups of boiling water and soak for 30 minutes before straining.

3. Start with one tbsp. at a time increasing to up to a cup per day.

Insomnia

Insomnia is a sleep disorder that makes it difficult to fall asleep, or causes people to wake up in the night and be unable to sleep again. Insomnia may deplete energy and attitude because of exhaustion, as well as impact health, job performance, and overall quality of life.

The amount of sleep required varies for everyone, although most individuals need 7 to 8 hours each night.

38. Good Dreams Tea
Ingredients:

- 2 tsp. catnip leaves
- 2 tsp. chamomile flower
- 1 tsp. hops
- 1 cup of boiling water
- 2 tsp. passionflower

Directions:

1. In a glass container, mix all the herbs.

2. Add boiling water and let it steep for thirty minutes.

3. Cool and strain.

4. Take it an hour before going to bed.

39. Anti-Insomniac Elixir

This combination of relaxants and mild sedatives does not force sleep, but it does assist to ease the tension, nervousness, and distractions that make it hard to fall asleep. This combination (as well as other herbs used to assist in sleeping) is better taken in 'pulse doses,' which are much more beneficial than taking the whole amount shortly before bedtime. It allows the herbs to begin operating in the system and signals to the body that it is time to sleep.

Ingredients:

- 1 fluid oz. chamomile tincture
- ¾ fluid oz. ashwagandha
- 1 fluid oz. betony tincture
- ½ fluid oz. catnip tincture
- ¼ fluid oz. honey
- ½ fluid oz. linden tincture

Directions:

1. Combine honey and tinctures in a medium size bottle. Cover the bottle and label it.

2. Take one to two drops, 1 hour before going to bed.

3. Take another one to two drops, 30 minutes before going to bed.

4. Then take the final one to drops before going to bed.

40. Insomnia Relieving Tea
Ingredients:

- 1 tsp. chamomile flowers

- 1 tsp. valerian root
- 1 tsp. hops
- 1 cup of boiling water

Directions:

1. Mix all the herbs.

2. Add 1 tbsp. of mixture in boiling water.

3. Let it steep for at least thirty minutes; strain.

4. Drink half cup when needed.

Stress

Any mental or physical discomfort is referred to as stress. Anything that makes one angry, upset, or anxious may cause it. The response of the body to a threat or a demand is called stress. Stress causes the body to release hormones which increase the pulse and make the brain more alert. They also cause muscles to tense up. These responses are beneficial in the short term because they assist in dealing with stressful situations. They are the body's attempt to defend itself.

41. Soothing Tea

This is the ideal combination for those days when everything seems to be coming apart.: take a minute, brew a cup, sip it slowly, and let the warmth and tranquility wash over you.

Include quarter cup dried goldenrod and sage if your stress appears as a sensation of heaviness and dismal weariness.

If you're experiencing stomach issues, add 1/4 cup dried chamomile and catnip to the mix.

Drink a quart or so every day.

Ingredients:

- 1 cup tulsi leaf, dried
- 1 cup betony flower and leaf, dried
- 1/2 cup linden flower and leaf, dried
- 1/2 cup rose petals, dried
- 1/4 cup St. John's wort flower and leaf, dried
- 1/2 cup elderflower, dried

Directions:

1. Combine all the herbs in a medium dish. Keep the container sealed.

2. Make a hot infusion: boil some water in a pot. In a French press or mason jar, measure 2–3 tbsp. of herbs in every quart of water.

3. Pour in boiling water then cover and soak for 20 minutes, or until cold enough to drink.

42. Elixir to the Rescue

This is your best buddy when you need a little break after a stressful day. If you can go away to a quiet place for a few moments, this cure will work best. Take a few deep breaths to center yourself, then take your tincture and breathe several more times before returning to the world. A little ritual may go a long way.

Ingredients:

- ½ fluid ounce of honey
- 1 fluid ounce tulsi, tincture
- 1 fluid ounce betony, tincture
- 1/2 fluid ounce catnip, tincture
- 1/2 fluid ounce chamomile, tincture
- 1/2 fluid ounce elderflower, tincture
- 1/2 fluid ounce rose, tincture
- ¼ fluid ounce goldenrod, tincture
- ¼ fluid ounce sage, tincture

Directions:

1. Mix the tinctures and honey in a tiny container. Cap and label the bottle.

2. When required, take 2 to 4 drops.

43. Shaking-It-Off Tea

Ingredients:

- 1 cup of boiling water
- 1 tsp. of valerian root
- 1 to 2 tsp. of peppermint leaves

Directions:

1. Combine the following ingredients in a large mixing bowl, cover with boiling water.

2. Soak for 20 - 30 minutes and drain.

3. As required, drink one cup per day.

44. Nerve-Relaxing Tea

Ingredients:

- 1 tsp. of kava root
- 1 tsp. of betony leaves
- 1 tsp. of hops
- 1 cup of boiling water
- 1 tsp. of skullcap, dried

Directions:

1. In a nonmetallic container, combine all the herbs.

2. Place 2 tsp of the mixture in a similar container and cover with boiling water.

3. Soak for 30 min; cool and drain.

4. As required, take one tbsp. at a time.

45. Calming Tea

Ingredients:

- 1 tsp. of powdered valerian root
- 1 tsp. of powdered ginger
- 2 cups of boiling water
- 1 tsp. of powdered pleurisy root

Directions:

1. In a nonmetallic container, combine all the herbs and cover with boiling water.

2. Soak for 30 minutes; cool and drain.

3. Take 1 tbsp. at a time, up to 2 cups each day, as required.

Excretory System

Uremia

Uremia is when there are high levels of urea in the blood. It can be described as the terminal clinical manifestation of kidney failure.

The most common signs of uremia are: progressive weakness and easy fatigue, tremors, loss of appetite due to nausea and vomiting, muscle atrophy, abnormal mental function, and frequent shallow respiration.

46. Corn Infusion

Recommended Dosage: One Cup three times daily; Take before your meals

Ingredients:

- 250 ml water
- Two to four tablespoons of corn

Directions:

1. Bring the water to a boil.

2. Place the corn in a bowl.

3. Ladle hot water over it.

4. Allow the tea to steep for ten to fifteen minutes.

5. Remove the tea strainer and serve hot.

Kidney Stones

A kidney stone is a hard object formed by chemicals found in urine. Kidney stones are classified into four types: uric acid, calcium oxalate, struvite, and cystine.

Common symptoms are extreme lower back pain, blood in the urine, nausea, vomiting, fever, and chills, or urine that smells bad or appears cloudy.

47. Agrimony Tincture

Recommended Dosage: one cup daily; Take it 30 minutes before eating or two hours after eating.

- Ingredients:
- Filtered water
- Tincture or fluid extract

Directions:

1. Bring 200ml of filtered water to a boil in a saucepan.

2. Turn off the heat and apply the tinctures directly.

Oedema

Oedema is described as fluid retention. It was previously known as dropsy. Oedema is most visible around the ankles after standing for a while. Eyes can also appear puffy and swollen after lying down for a while. Oedema can also collect in the lungs and leave one out of breath in extreme cases.

48. Hawthorn Berry Tea

Recommended Dosage: 250–500 mg three times daily; can be taken any time of the day

Ingredients:

- ¼ tsp. dried heartsease
- Honey
- ½ tsp. dried wood betony
- ½ tsp. dried albizia bark
- One tsp. dried hawthorn berries
- ¼ tsp. dried rosebuds or petals
- 1¼ cups filtered water
- One tsp. dried or fresh lemon balm

Directions:

1. Place hawthorn berries and albizia bark in a small saucepan with measured water.

2. Bring to a boil, then reduce to low heat and simmer for five minutes

3. Take the pan off the heat and quickly add the remaining herbs.

4. Allow to steep for 10 minutes, covered with a lid.

5. Pour into a big mug and top with honey, if desired

Skeletal System
Abscess

An abscess is a pus-filled inflamed, or diseased area that is painful and hot to the touch. An abscess becomes more painful as it grows larger. If herbal therapies don't work, get medical help since an infection inside a large abscess can spread to adjacent tissue and into the circulation.

49. Fresh Yarrow Poultice

Makes one poultice

Anti-inflammatory and antibacterial substances are found in yarrow. It disinfects the abscess, reduces swelling, and speeds up the healing process.

Ingredients:

- One tablespoon finely chopped fresh yarrow leaves

Directions:

1. Apply the chopped leaves to the abscess, then cover with a soft cloth. Leave the poultice in place for 10 to 15 minutes.

2. Repeat two or three times per day until the abscess is healed.

3. Precautions: Do not use if you are pregnant. People who are allergic to plants in the Asteraceae family may get cutaneous responses from yarrow.

50. Echinacea and Goldenseal Tincture

Makes about 2 cups

Echinacea and goldenseal have powerful antibacterial properties, as well as boosting the natural immune response. Make this tincture ahead of time so you will always have it at hand. It can last up to 7 years if kept in a cool, dark place. It can be used whenever you have an infection.

Ingredients:

- 5 ounces dried echinacea root, finely chopped
- 3 ounces dried goldenseal root, finely chopped
- 2 cups unflavored 80-proof vodka

Directions:

1. Combine the echinacea and goldenseal in a sterilized pint jar. Fill the jar with vodka, filling it to the top and completely covering the herbs.

2. Close the jar tightly and give it a good shake. For 6 to 8 weeks, keep it in a cool, dark cabinet and shake it several times a week. If any of the alcohol evaporates, top up the jar with vodka until it's full.

3. Soak a piece of cheesecloth in water and lay it over the funnel's mouth. Pour the tincture into another sterilized pint jar using the funnel. Squeeze the liquid out of the roots with the cheesecloth until there is no more liquid. Remove the roots and pour the tincture into dark-coloured glass vials.

4. Take ten drops orally two or three times a day for 7 to 10 days to treat an abscess.

Precautions: Do not use if you are pregnant. If you have diabetes, be cautious because goldenseal might reduce blood sugar.

Backache

While overwork or injury is the most common cause of back pain, it can also be caused by inactivity, muscle spasms, or inflammation. Rest as much as possible to help your body heal, and visit your doctor if the pain is severe or is accompanied by numbness, tingling, or incontinence.

51. Passionflower–Blue Vervain Tea

Makes 1 cup

Passionflower and blue vervain both calm the nervous system and relieve muscle pain. This is a wonderfully calming combination, so use it when you have a chance to unwind.

Ingredients:

- 1 cup boiling water
- One teaspoon dried passionflower
- One teaspoon dried blue vervain

Directions:

1. Fill a large cup halfway with boiling water. Allow the tea to steep for 10 minutes after adding the dry herbs and covering the mug.

2. Slowly sip the tea as you relax for up to two times each day.

Precautions: Passionflower and blue vervain should not be used during pregnancy. If you have prostate issues or baldness, stay away from passionflower.

52. Ginger-Peppermint Salve

Makes about 1 cup

Potent elements in ginger and peppermint permeate the skin, causing a warming sensation that aids muscle relaxation. When stored in a cold, dark place, this salve will last for up to a year.

Ingredients:

- 1 cup light olive oil
- 1 ounce dried ginger root, chopped
- 1 ounce dried peppermint, crushed
- 1-ounce beeswax

Directions:

1. Combine the olive oil, ginger, and peppermint in a slow cooker. Set the slow cooker to the lowest heat setting, cover it, and let the herbs steep in the oil for 3 to 5 hours. Allow the infused oil to cool after turning off the heat.

2. In the base of a double boiler, bring about an inch of water to a simmer. Reduce the heat to a low setting.

3. Over the top part of the double boiler, drape a piece of cheesecloth. Pour the infused oil into the cheesecloth, then wring and twist it until no more oil comes out. Remove the cheesecloth and herbs used.

4. Place the double boiler on the base and add the beeswax to the infused oil. Warm gently over low heat. Remove the pan from the heat once the beeswax has completely melted. Pour the contents into clean, dry jars or tins as soon as possible, and set aside to cool fully before capping.

5. Using your fingers or a cotton cosmetic pad, apply one teaspoon to the affected area, massaging well. Use a little more or less as needed. Repeat the treatment up to four times per day.

Precautions: If you're on blood thinners, have gallbladder illness, or have a bleeding issue, don't use ginger.

Muscular System
Sprains and Strains

A sprain occurs when a ligament is severely wrenched, while a strain is a tearing and overstretching of muscle fibers. The same injuries that can cause a sprain can cause a strain as well. The difference is that a sprain involves ligaments and tendons, while a strain involves muscles. Movement in the affected area is often limited because of the pain and swelling.

53. Soft Tissue Injury Liniment

It makes about eight fluid ounces

Ingredients:

- 3 fluid ounces ginger-infused oil
- 2 fluid ounces Solomon's seal-infused oil or tincture of Solomon's seal
- 1 fluid ounce tincture of St. John's wort
- 1 fluid ounce tincture of self-heal
- 1 fluid ounce tincture of meadowsweet
- 40 drops peppermint essential oil
- 40 drops cinnamon essential oil

Directions:

1. In a small bottle, combine the infused oils, tinctures, and essential oils. Cap the bottle and label it, including 'Shake well before each use.'

2. Hold your palm over the bottle's mouth and tilt to deposit a small amount in your palm. 3. Rub between your hands to warm the treatment, then apply to the painful joints.

3. Massage the oil into the joints until your hands no longer feel oily. Work the cream into the tissue.

4. Repeat the application 3 to 5 times per day. More is better!

54. Sweet Relief Tea
Ingredients:

- 1 tablespoon raspberry leaf
- 1 teaspoon white willow bark
- 2 cups boiling water

Directions:

1. Combine the above herbs and cover with boiling water; steep for 30 minutes; strain.

2. Take as needed.

Endocrine System
Body Odor

Body odor is the odor that our bodies emit as bacteria that live on our skin break down sweat into acids. Some attribute it to the odor of bacteria developing in the body, but bacteria break down protein into specific acids.

55. Witch Hazel Spray

Recommended Dosage: Spray as needed

Use in the morning and before you go to bed

Recommended Dosage Time: Till your body smells nice

Ingredients:

- One part of aloe juice
- Three parts of Witch Hazel
- A couple of drops of essential oil for your skin type

Directions:

1. Combine the ingredients in a 4-ounce spray bottle

2. Store in a cool, dry, dark place

Chapped Lips

Chapped Lips are a common disorder that affects the majority of people. However, some people can develop cheilitis, a more severe type of chapped lips. Cheilitis is caused by an infection and is distinguished by broken skin at the corners of the lips.

56. Chamomile Lip Scrub

Recommended Dosage: As needed

How to Use:

This recipe yields enough for one use. Kindly rub a tiny amount all over your lips with your fingertips/massage for a minute or two in circular movements. Pat dry after rinsing with warm water /apply a natural moisturizing lip balm afterward.

Best time of the day to apply it: In the afternoon

Ingredients:

- One tsp. coconut sugar
- One tbsp. dried chamomile flowers
- One tbsp.. raw sugar
- One drop of pure orange essential oil
- One tsp. raw honey
- One tbsp.. apricot kernel oil

Directions:

1. Soak the dried chamomile flowers in apricot kernel oil for 48 hours. Make sure the flowers are fully submerged

2. Shake the container occasionally.

3. When the flowers have finished infusing, strain the liquid through a fine sieve or hemp coffee filter. Set the oil aside.

4. Stir the raw sugar and the coconut sugar together in a small cup.

5. If using, add the infused apricot oil, honey, and essential oil. Mix all with a whisk. If necessary, add a little more apricot oil.

Menopause

Menopause marks the end of a woman's menstrual cycle. The word can refer to all of the changes you go through just before or after your cycle stops, signaling the end of your reproductive years.

Ovaries produce the hormones estrogen and progesterone, which regulate the menstrual cycle and egg release (ovulation). Menopause occurs when the ovaries no longer produce an egg each month and menstruation ceases.

57. Hot Infusion Tea

Take two cups per day of an infusion for someone weighing 130 to 160 pounds

Ingredients:

- One pound of dried alfalfa
- One pound of dried horsetail
- One pound of dried nettles
- One pound of dried spearmint
- One pound of dried nettles
- One pound of dried oat-straw

Directions:

1. Combine one pound of dried, sliced, and sifted nettles, oat-straw, red clover, alfalfa, horsetail, and spearmint.

2. Place one cup of the mixture in a quart bottle, cover with hot water, and leave overnight.

3. Strain the mixture in the morning to extract all of the spices, and drink it for the next two days.

4. Do not hold infusions for more than two days, as they will spoil.

Irregular Menstrual Cycle

Menstruation is the period of the menstrual cycle during which the endometrium, or uterine lining, is shed. This manifests as womb bleeding that is expelled through the vagina. Monthly periods typically begin during puberty, between the ages of 10 and 16, and last until menopause, when a woman is 45 to 55.

Irregular cycles, also known as oligomenorrhea, may occur due to a shift in the contraceptive process, a hormone imbalance, hormonal changes during menopause, and endurance exercise.

58. Daily Soothing Menstrual Tea

Recommended Dosage: Half a cup four times daily.

Take every 4 hours during menstruation.

Ingredients:

- Two cups cold water
- Two teaspoons black haw root or bark
- Two teaspoons passionflower

Directions:

1. Combine the herbs mentioned above in a pan and cover with cold water; soak overnight; strain.

2. Take half a cup up to four times per day.

Immune System

Cold Sores

Cold sores are small, painful, fluid-filled blisters on the mouth caused by the herpes simplex virus. Tingling, itching, and burning may give you a warning that a cold sore is about to erupt. The blisters may appear a few hours or days after the initial warning signs. After a few days, they eventually dry and form a crust. They usually completely heal within a week or two.

59. Cold Sore Compress

Makes 5 cups dried herb mix

Ingredients:

- 1 cup dried calendula flower
- 1 cup dried plantain leaf
- 1 cup dried chamomile flower, dried self-heal leaf, and flower
- ½ cup dried St. John's wort leaf and flower

Directions:

1. Mix all the herbs.

2. Store in an airtight container.

3. Relax and place a wet cloth over the affected area. Cover with a dry cloth and lay the hot water bottle on top. Let it sit and soak in for 10 to 20 minutes.

4. Repeat 2 to 3 times each day.

60. Cold Sore Balm

Makes 5 ounces

Ingredients:

- 1 fluid ounce calendula-infused oil
- 1 fluid ounce plantain-infused oil
- ½ fluid ounce self-heal–infused oil
- ½ fluid ounce chamomile-infused oil
- ½ fluid ounce St. John's wort–infused oil
- ½ fluid ounce thyme-infused oil
- 1-ounce beeswax, plus more as needed

Directions:

1. Make a nice and soft salve if you'll keep it in little jars; make it slightly firmer if you're using lip balm tubes.

61. Cold Sore Tea

Ingredients:

- 1 teaspoon burdock root
- 1 teaspoon dried and powdered goldenseal root
- 1 cup boiling water
1. Honey, to taste

Directions:

2. Combine all the herbs in a glass container.

3. Steep for 30 minutes, calm, and strain.

4. You may want to sweeten with honey.

5. Take up to one cup a day.

62. Cold Sore Mouthwash

Ingredients:

- 1 teaspoon echinacea root
- 1 teaspoon yerba mansa root
- 1 tablespoon white oak bark
- 1 cup boiling water

Directions:

1. Combine the herbs in a glass container.

2. Steep 30 minutes, calm, and strain. Use the solution as a wash to treat cold sores.

Fever

The "normal" body temperature is 98.6°F, but this can vary between individuals and even within the same person at various times of the day. Our body temperature, for example, is lowest in the early morning and highest in the late afternoon. A fever, is described as any temperature above 100°F.

A fever is usually an indication that the body is battling an infection. The decision on whether or not to treat a fever is a contentious one. Fever, in my view, is the body's way of healing itself and should not be silenced. Fever in children and adults with heart disease or other illnesses can be dangerous and should be handled.

63. Honey-Ginger Tea

Ginger's antioxidant, analgesic, and anti-inflammatory qualities have the incredible potential to provide comfort and lessen the sensations of viral fever. Honey's antibacterial qualities help to fight infections and relieve coughs.

Ingredients:

- Ginger 1 tsp.
- Honey

Directions:

1. Boil 1 tsp. grated ginger in a hot water cup for approximately two to five minutes to relieve viral fever.

2. Filter the mixture and add a tsp. of honey.

3. Take this tea two times a day.

64. Fever Relieving Tea #1

Yields 1 3/4 cups of herb mix, dry (enough for 14 - 24 pints of tea)

These soothing diaphoretics and refrigerants will reduce tension and discharge heat without igniting other fire if the fever is too intense to bear. The wild lettuce inside the mix can make you feel tired, which is a good thing since sleep is your body's finest healer. Go to sleep.

Ingredients:

- ½ cup catnip flower and leaf, dried
- ½ cup elderflower, dried
- ½ cup peppermint leaf, dried
- 1 pint of boiling water
- ¼ cup wild lettuce leaf and stalk, dried

Directions:

1. Combine all the herbs in a medium size mixing dish. Keep the container sealed.

2. Prepare a hot infusion: measure 1–2 tbsps. of herbs in a miniature glass jar.

3. Fill the pot halfway with boiling water, cover, and steep for 20 minutes, or until cool. Drink this tea at a little lower temperature than normal.

4. If you have a fever, drink a mugful of it.

65. Fever Relieving Tea #2

Ingredients:

- 1 tsp. of ground ivy leaves
- 1 tsp. of angelica root
- 1 tsp. of barberries
- 1 tbsp. of yarrow, dried
- 2 tsp. of peppermint leaves
- 2 tsp. of blue vervain leaves
- 1 cup of boiling water
- 1 tsp. of catnip leaves

Directions:

1. Combine all the listed herbs.

2. Put one tablespoon of the mixture in a cup; pour boiling water over the herbs.

3. Soak for 30 minutes; drain.

4. Take one cup every day.

66. Rapid-Acting Fever Tea

Ingredients:

- 1 tsp. of echinacea root
- 1 cup of water
- 1 tsp. of white willow root

Directions:

1. Combine the roots and cover them with water in a pan.

2. Bring to a boil, reduce to low heat, and cook for 30 minutes, straining afterward.

3. Take half a cup, 4 times a day.

Gingivitis

Gingivitis, also known as periodontal disease, is a mild and early type of gum disease. It occurs when bacteria invades the gums, causing them to swell, redden, and bleed easily.

Gingivitis may be treated using herbal remedies, which are both inexpensive and effective. Gingivitis may typically be cleared up with home treatments if started early enough.

It is important to cure plaque before it hardens into tartar. Flossing and brushing should be done more often and for longer periods.

The herbal medicines listed below are usually considered safe for use. Get medical counsel before using if you are pregnant, breast feeding, or have any medical problem.

Visit your physician or dentist if you're suffering severe symptoms, including intense pain or bleeding. Gingivitis, if left untreated, may lead to more severe health issues.

Continue reading to understand how several herbal treatments may help you get rid of your symptoms and how to avoid gingivitis in the future.

67. Mouthwash from Lemongrass Oil

Lemongrass Oil was found to be significantly effective in reducing plaque accumulation than standard chlorhexidine mouthwash.

Ingredients:

- Water
- Lemongrass
- Essential oil

Directions: For using this mouthwash, follow these steps:

1. In a cup of water, dilute 2 to 3 droplets of lemongrass essential oil.

2. For 30 to 40 seconds, swish the liquid in your mouth.

3. Spit it out..

4. Do this 2 to 3 times a day.

Lemongrass oil is typically safe to use, although it is quite powerful. To avoid causing more discomfort, always start with an extremely diluted combination.

68. Mouthwash from Aloe Vera

Aloe vera was proven to be just as efficient as chlorhexidine in eliminating gingivitis and plaque in studies. Both methods resulted in considerable reduction in symptoms.

Aloe vera juice, unlike other mouthwashes, does not have to be diluted. Assure the juice is 100% pure before using it.

Ingredients:

- Aloe vera juice

Directions:

1. For thirty seconds, swish the liquid around in your mouth.

2. Spit it out.

3. Do this 2 to 3 times a day.

4. Always get aloe vera from a reliable supplier then follow all label directions.

5. Don't use it if you have had an allergic response to aloe vera.

69. Mouthwash from Tea Tree Oil

Tea tree oil rinsing seems promising for the healing of gingivitis, as per 2020 research.

Ingredients:

- 1 cup hot water
- 3 drops tea tree oil

Directions:

1. In a cup of hot water, add up to 3 drops of the oil.

2. Swish the liquid in your mouth for 30 seconds..

3. Spit it out.

4. Do this 2 to 3 times a day.

You can also put a drop of this oil in your toothpaste when brushing your teeth.

Apply an extremely diluted dose of tea tree oil when using for the first time. High concentrations may lead to the following effects:

- Mild burning
- Rash
- Allergic reaction

70. Mouthwash from Sage

In a 2015 survey, researchers discovered that sage mouthwash reduced the amount of germs that create tooth plaque. The solution could be rinsed for up to 1 min without causing irritation.

Ingredients:

- 1-2 cups water
- 1 tbsp. dried sage or 2 tbsp. fresh sage

Directions:

1. Bring 1–2 cups of water to a boil.

2. Mix in 1 tbsp. dried sage or 2 tbsp. fresh sage in water.

3. Simmer for 5 - 10 minutes.

4. Drain the water and set it aside to cool.

5. Rinse with the solution 2 to 3 times each day.

Sage possesses anti-inflammatory and anti-bacterial qualities that may aid in the healing and treating of sore gums.

71. Mouthwash from Guava Leaves

Guava leaves have long been used as an efficient oral hygiene treatment. Their anti-microbial and anti-bacterial characteristics gargle decrease plaque. It can also:

- Freshen breath
- Relieve pain
- Reduce gum inflammation

Ingredients:

- 5 to 6 guava leaves
- 1 cup hot water
- A pinch of salt

Directions:

1. Using a pestle and mortar, crush 5 to 6 tender guava leaves.

2. Pour 1 cup of hot water over the crushed leaves.

3. Cook for fifteen minutes on low heat.

4. Allow the fluid to cool before adding a pinch of salt.

5. Swish the mouthwash in the mouth for up to 30 seconds.

6. Spit it out.

7. Do this two or three times a day.

Topical Treatments

If mouthwashes are not really working, a topical lotion or gel applied to your gums may be therapeutic.

72. Clove Application

Studies suggest that cloves can prevent plaque and decrease inflammation, but more research is required in the subject. Cloves contain antioxidant and antiviral effects, so they're a good choice. They might also aid in pain relief.

Ingredients:

- Chopped cloves
- Cotton balls
- Water

Directions:

1. Cloves may be used topically in the following ways:

2. Chop 1 tsp. cloves finely.

3. Dip a moist cotton ball into the chopped cloves, squeezing out as much as possible.

4. Gently massage your gums with the clove-covered ball.

5. Leave the cloves on the gums for a minute or more.

6. To gather all the cloves, swish water in your mouth.

7. Spit out the clove water.

8. Do not use cloves for a long time or in large quantities.

73. Turmeric or Curcuma Gel Application

According to a 2015 research, turmeric gel may effectively reduce plaque and gingivitis most probably because of its anti-inflammatory characteristics.

Turmeric has anti-fungal and anti-bacterial properties. It may aid in the healing of gum reddening and bleeding.

Curcuma or turmeric gel may be used as a therapy. Turmeric's active component is curcumin; therefore, it may be labeled as either.

Ingredients:

- Curcuma

Directions:

1. Brush your teeth before applying the turmeric gel.

2. Thoroughly rinse.

3. Gently massage the gel into your gums.

4. Set aside the gel for ten minutes.

5. To gather all of the gel, swish water in your mouth.

6. Spit out the water

7. Do this twice a day.

Hangover

In this section, we will look at what a hangover is and offer several best treatments.

What Are the Causes of a Hangover?

The liver is in charge of breaking down alcohol. As alcohol is degraded, it creates acetaldehyde is which is a harmful chemical that results from ethanol metabolism. This may be found in less expensive wines and other alcoholic drinks

Not drinking alcohols with high amounts of acetaldehyde, such as cheap whiskey, red wines, black spirits, and fruit brandy, is the first way of avoiding a hangover. If you must drink, drink pure spirits and top-quality red wines that has not been sulfated.

If you choose organic, you'll get fewer sulfites and a higher-quality and a more organic product that's simpler for your liver to digest.

Dehydration, weariness, blood-sugar fluctuation, nausea, and reduced immunity are some of the most common symptoms of a hangover.

The best way to cure a hangover is to enhance the detoxification processes that occur during stages one and two while simultaneously delivering a high dosage of anti-oxidants. Herbs which strengthen and tonify the liver's processes are also available.

Keep the following herbal remedies in your hangover treatment kit.

74. Hangover Infusion

Yields three and a half cups of herb mix, dry (enough for 20 - 28 quarts of tea).

This soothing tea relieves the most frequent hangover symptoms and aids in dehydration. It is is best to make it beforehand so that it is ready when required. Drink a quart or so steadily throughout the day.

Ingredients:

- 1/2 cup plantain leaf, dried
- ½ cup betony flower and leaf, dried
- 1/2 cup calendula flower, dried
- 1/2 cup chamomile flower, dried
- 1/3 cup linden leaf and flower, dried
- 1/3 cup marshmallow leaf, dried
- 1/3 cup self-heal flower and leaf, dried
- 1 tbsp licorice mat, dried
- ¼ cup St. John's wort flower and leaf, dried
- 1 tbsp ginger, dried

Directions:

1. Combine all of the herbs in a medium size mixing dish. Keep the container sealed.

2. Prepare a steaming infusion: bring a pot of water to a boil. In a French press or mason jar, measure 2–3 tbsp. of herbs in every quart of water.

3. Pour in boiling water, cover and soak for 20 minutes, or until cold enough to drink..

P.S: If you are taking medicines simultaneously, skip the St. John's wort.

75. Hangover Tea

Ingredients

- 1 tsp. of ripe barberry berries
- 2 cups of boiling water
- 1 tsp. of Oregon grape root

Directions:

1. In a non-metallic container, combine the herbs and cover with boiling water.

2. Soak for 30 minutes; cool, and filter.

3. Drink about one cup of it every day, diluted with lots of cool water.

76. Rapid-Acting Hangover Tea

Ingredients:

- 1 tsp. of goldenseal root, dried
- 1 tsp. of bayberry root
- 2 cups of boiling water
- 1 tsp. of Oregon grape root

Directions:

1. In a non-metallic container, combine the herbs and cover with boiling water.

2. Soak for 30 minutes; drain.

3. In a glass with 8-ounces of water, put a tbsp. of the mixture.

4. Drink a few glasses throughout the day.

77. Spicy Tea

Ingredients:

- 1 tsp of peppermint leaves
- 1 tsp of chaparral leaves, dried
- 2 cups of boiling water
- 1 tsp of catnip leaves

Directions:

1. In a non-metallic container, combine the herbs and cover with boiling water.

2. Soak for 20 to 30 minutes; drain.

3. Start with half a cup and work your way up to two cups each day.

Immune System Boosters

78. Vitamin C Pills

These are great for boosting the immune system and fighting off colds and flu-like symptoms.

Ingredients:

- 1 tablespoon rose hip powder (the fruit of a rose plant, which has a high vitamin c content)
- 1 tablespoon amla powder (an Indian gooseberry, which has strong antibacterial properties)
- 1 tablespoon acerola powder (a Barbados cherry, which is great for stomach discomfort)
- Honey
- Orange peel powder (optional) (orange is a citrus fruit, and its peel is often used for flavor)

Directions:

1. Blend the powdered herbs, smoothing out any clumped powder. Pour a few droplets of slightly warmed honey into the powdered mix.

2. Stir, add a few more droplets, and stir again. Mix until the combination holds together without being too sticky or moist.

3. Shape the mix into pea-size balls. Roll these around in the orange powder if want. The mixture should make 45 balls. Store these in an air-tight container to give them an extended shelf life. Take 1-3 daily.

79. Elderberry Gummy Bears

This is great for boosting the immune system.

Ingredients:

- 50 g elderberries, dried
- 30 g rosehips, dried
- 15 g cinnamon chips
- 7 g licorice root
- 0.5 g pepper, freshly ground (a flowering vine, which is often used for seasoning)
- 3 cups apple cider
- 3 tablespoons gelatin (derived from collagen and used as a gelling agent in food)

Directions:

1. Place all ingredients (minus the gelatin) into a medium-size saucepan. Bring the mixture to

simmer and continue to simmer for 20 minutes. Strain, squeeze well to extract the juice.

2. Measure 2 cups juice (you can add more apple cider to make the mixture fill 2 cups). Put 1/2 cup into the fridge, then after it's chilled, dust the gelatin on top of it. Allow this to sit for one minute.

3. Bring the rest of the mixture to a simmer. Combine the hot juice with the cooled gelatin mixture. Stir quickly with a whisk. If you want to sweeten this up more, add sugar or honey.

4. Pour the mixture into molds and refrigerate. Eat 1–3 gummies per day. Store in a sealed container in the fridge.

Integumentary System

Acne

Infected sebaceous glands produce painful pimples that are red and inflamed. While this mostly affects teenagers, it can also impact adults. Herbal medicines can help you look and feel better whether your acne is limited to your face or has spread to your chest, back, or other body regions.

80. Calendula Toner

Makes about ½ cup

This basic toner contains witch hazel, which targets bacteria while relaxing your skin, as well as calming calendula, which reduces irritation. This toner will last for at least a year if maintained in a cold, dark place.

Ingredients:

- Two tablespoons calendula oil
- ⅓ cup witch hazel

Directions:

1. Combine the ingredients in a dark-colored glass bottle and shake gently.

2. Apply 5 or 6 drops to your freshly cleaned face or any areas of concern with a cotton cosmetic pad. Add or remove as needed.

3. Repeat twice a day as long as the acne persists. If you want a chilly sensation, keep the bottle in the refrigerator.

81. Agrimony-Chamomile Gel

Makes about ⅔ cup

Redness and irritation are reduced when agrimony and chamomile are mixed with aloe vera gel. The gel should be kept in the refrigerator. It will stay fresh for up to two weeks if kept in an airtight container.

Ingredients:

- Two teaspoons dried agrimony
- Two teaspoons dried chamomile
- ½ cup water
- ¼ cup aloe vera gel

Directions:

1. Combine the agrimony and chamomile with the water in a saucepan. Over high heat, bring the mixture to a boil, then reduce the heat to low. Reduce the mixture by half, remove it from the heat and set it aside to cool completely.

2. Soak a piece of cheesecloth in water and lay it over the funnel mouth. Pour the contents into a glass bowl using the funnel. Squeeze the liquid out of the herbs with the cheesecloth until there is no more left.

3. Blend the aloe vera gel into the liquid using a whisk. Fill a sterile glass jar halfway with the final gel. Refrigerate with the container tightly closed.

4. Apply a tiny coating to all affected areas twice a day with a cotton cosmetic pad.

Precautions: If you take blood thinners or are allergic to plants in the ragweed family, leave out the chamomile.

Allergies

Allergies are immunological reactions to common substances like cat dander, pollen, or dust. Food, drinks, and the environment all contain allergens, making it impossible to avoid them entirely. Herbal medicines are significantly milder than conventional treatments, which block the body's immune reaction to allergens that impact you.

82. Feverfew-Peppermint Tincture

Makes about 2 cups

During an allergic attack, feverfew and peppermint open up the airways. Peppermint csn be used on its own. In a cool, dark spot, the tincture will last up to 7 years.

Ingredients:

- 2 ounces dried feverfew
- 6 ounces dried peppermint
- 2 cups unflavored 80-proof vodka

Directions:

1. Combine the feverfew and peppermint in a sterilized pint jar. Fill the jar to the top with vodka.

2. Close the jar tightly and give it a good shake. Keep it in a cool, dark cabinet for 6 to 8 weeks and shake it several times a week.

3. Soak a piece of cheesecloth in water and lay it over a funnel mouth. Pour the tincture into another sterilized pint jar using the funnel. Remove the moisture from the herbs by wringing it out. Transfer the final tincture to dark-colored glass bottles after discarding the spent herbs.

4. When allergy symptoms flare up, take five drops orally. If the flavor is too strong, combine it with some water or juice.

Precautions: If you are allergic to ragweed, do not take feverfew. Feverfew should not be used during pregnancy.

83. Garlic-Ginkgo Syrup

Makes about 2 cups

Ginkgo biloba is a natural antihistamine with over a dozen anti-inflammatory ingredients, while garlic helps to boost your immune system. If feasible, use local honey to help build resistance to allergies common in your area. When refrigerated, this syrup will last up to 6 months.

Ingredients:

- 2 ounces fresh or freeze-dried garlic, chopped
- 2 ounces ginkgo Biloba, crushed or chopped
- 2 cups water
- 1 cup local honey

Directions:

1. Combine the garlic, Ginkgo Biloba, and water in a saucepan. Reduce the liquid by half by bringing it to a low simmer and partially covering it with a lid.

2. Fill a glass measuring cup halfway with the contents of the saucepan, then strain the mixture through a soaked piece of cheesecloth into the saucepan, wringing the fabric until no more liquid comes out.

3. Warm the mixture over low heat with the honey, stirring regularly until the temperature reaches 105°F to 110°F.

4. Fill a sterilized jar or bottle with the syrup and keep it in the refrigerator.

5. Take one tablespoon orally three times a day until your allergy symptoms go away.

Precaution: If you are taking a monoamine oxidase inhibitor (MAOI) for depression, don't take it. Ginkgo biloba can take blood thinners to work better, so consult your doctor before taking it. Take one teaspoon three times a day for children under the age of 12.

Athlete's Foot

A fungus that thrives in moist, warm, dark environments causes this itchy, often severe infection. Make sure you get rid of it before it reaches beneath your toenails, where it can cause discoloration that is difficult to remove.

84. Fresh Garlic Poultice

Makes one treatment

Garlic is a powerful anti-fungal agent that can help get rid of athlete's foot. Raw honey aids in the binding of garlic to your foot while also acting as an anti-fungal agent. While you can prepare a double or triple batch of this remedy and use it over two to three days, you will get better results if you produce a fresh batch for each treatment.

Ingredients:

- One garlic clove, pressed
- One teaspoon raw honey

Directions:

1. Combine the garlic and honey in a small bowl. Apply the blend to the afflicted region using a cotton cosmetic pad.

2. Put on a clean pair of socks and lie down with your feet elevated for 15 minutes to an hour, with the poultice in place. After that, wash and dry your feet. Repeat the procedure once or twice a day, and then apply Goldenseal Ointment to the affected area. Continue for three days after the symptoms have subsided.

Precautions: Garlic can induce a rash in people who are allergic to it.

85. Goldenseal Ointment

Makes about 1 cup

Goldenseal is an anti-bacterial substance that aids in the treatment of athlete's foot. You can use this ointment on its own or combined with a Fresh Garlic Poultice to speed up healing. When stored in a cold, dark place, it will last for up to a year.

Ingredients:

- 1 cup light olive oil
- 2 ounces dried goldenseal root, chopped
- 1-ounce beeswax

Directions:

1. Combine the olive oil and goldenseal in a slow cooker. Set the slow cooker on the lowest heat setting, cover it, and steep the roots in the oil for 3 to 5 hours. Allow the infused oil to cool after turning off the heat.

2. In the base of a double boiler, bring about an inch of water to a simmer. Reduce the heat to a low setting.

3. Over the top part of the double boiler, drape a piece of cheesecloth. Pour the infused oil into the cheesecloth, then wring and twist it until no more oil comes out. Remove the cheesecloth and herbs that have been used.

4. Place the double boiler on the base and add the beeswax to the infused oil. Warm gently over low heat. Remove the pan from the heat once the

beeswax has completely melted. Pour the contents into clean, dry jars or tins as soon as possible, and set aside to cool fully before capping.

5. Apply 14 teaspoons to each affected region with a cotton cosmetic pad. Apply a bit more or less as needed, and do so up to three times per day, the last time being before bed. To avoid slippage, put on a pair of clean socks over the ointment.

Precautions: If you are pregnant, breastfeeding or have high blood pressure, don't use it.

Bee Sting

A bee sting is generally accompanied by pain, redness, and swelling, and the discomfort can persist for days. Herbs can help with pain relief. If you're allergic to bee venom, keep in mind that herbal remedies are not meant to take the place of emergency EpiPens.

86. Fresh Plantain Poultice

Makes one treatment

The modest plantain plant—not to be confused with its banana-like namesake—is a weedy green plant that contains aucubin, a powerful antitoxin glucoside. Anti-septic and anti-inflammatory properties are provided by other components, making this simple treatment quite effective. If fresh plantain leaves are unavailable, rehydrate a teaspoon of dried, crushed plantain in a tablespoon of water for use as a poultice.

Ingredients:

• One tablespoon finely chopped fresh plantain leaves

Directions:

1. Cover the injured area with the chopped leaves and a soft cloth. Allow 10 to 15 minutes for the poultice to dry.

2. Repeat as necessary until the pain is gone.

87. Comfrey-Aloe Gel

Makes about ¼ cup

Because of its anti-inflammatory and analgesic characteristics, comfrey can help relieve the pain and swelling associated with bee stings. Aloe vera soothes and speeds up the healing process. If you like this balm, you will find it useful for a variety of little cuts and scrapes. When kept in the refrigerator, it stays fresh for about two weeks.

Ingredients:

• Two teaspoons dried comfrey
• ¼ cup water
• Two tablespoons aloe vera gel

Directions:

1. Combine the comfrey and water in a saucepan. Over high heat, bring the mixture to a boil, then reduce the heat to low. Reduce the mixture by half, remove it from the heat and set it aside to cool completely.

2. Soak a piece of cheesecloth in water and lay it over the funnel's mouth. Pour the contents into a glass bowl using the funnel. Squeeze the comfrey liquid out of the cheesecloth until no more liquid comes out.

3. Blend the aloe vera gel into the liquid using a whisk. Fill a sterile glass jar halfway with the final gel. Refrigerate with the lid of the container tightly closed.

4. Apply a tiny coating to the affected region with a cotton cosmetic pad as needed until the discomfort and swelling go away.

Burns

Skin burns may be caused by heat (either from a blaze or boiling liquids), corrosive chemicals, electricity, or radiations like UV or radiation treatments. Burns are classed as follows depending on the degree of tissue damage:

- 1st-degree burns: The epidermis which is the skin's outer layer, is affected by 1st-degree burns that cause redness and pain. That prototype is a minor sunburn.
- 2nd-degree burns: These reach the dermis the skin's second layer, producing redness, oozing blisters, and pain. Deep 2nd-degree burns might become 3rd-degree burns over time
- 3rd-degree burns: These affect both the bottom and top layers of the skin and the underlying muscles, tendons, and bones. The burned area looks leathery or pale in appearance. Since the nerve endings in the region have been damaged, there is usually no pain within the area.
- 4th-degree burns: These penetrate the subcutaneous fat and skin into the bone and muscle underneath it. These burns are scorched and rigid.

If not treated appropriately, any burns, even mild ones, may lead to dire consequences. The body's natural barrier against any infection is the skin, and burns obliterate that barrier. As a result, most treatments seek to prevent or cure infections.

88. Honey for Burn Recovery

Yields 1 pint approx.

Honey is the most effective treatment for burns: Raw honey is excellent and is even better when infused with these medicinal herbs.

Ingredients:

- ½ cup calendula flower, fresh
- ½ cup rose petals, fresh
- 1 pint gently warmed honey

Directions:

1. In a pint-size glass jar, combine the calendula and rose petals.

2. Pour the warm honey into the container. Seal the jar and let it infuse for a month in a warm location.

3. Gently reheat the closed jar in a double boiler till the honey has a fluid consistency. In a fresh jar, extract as much honey as possible.

4. Apply a small amount of the infused honey to a burn spot once it is cooled and cleaned, and cover gently with a gauze bandage. Refresh at least twice a day

89. Spray for Sunburns

Yields 8 fluid ounces approx.

A few spritzes can help to calm the skin and minimize irritation.

Ingredients:

- 1 tbsp. of dried peppermint leaf
- 4 fluid ounces of rose water
- 1 tbsp. of dried plantain leaf
- 1 tbsp. of dried self-heal flower or leaf
- 1-quart of boiling water
- 1 tbsp. of dried linden flower or leaf

Directions:

1. Make a hot infusion by combining the peppermint, self-heal, plantain, and linden in a mason jar. Fill the container halfway with boiling water, cover, and steep for twenty minutes.

2. Place the container in the refrigerator until it is completely cold.

3. Strain 4 fluid ounces of infusion into an 8-ounce bottle and top with a fine-mist sprayer. Use the rest of the infusion to make compresses or a refreshing drink. It will last 3 days in the refrigerator.

4. Fill the spray container with rose water. Cap and label the bottle.

5. Use a lot of it and do it often. When not in use, keep the spray refrigerated.

90. Topical Ointment for Burn
Ingredients:

- 1 tbsp. of coneflower flowers, dried
- 1 tbsp. of hyssop flowers, dried
- 1 tbsp. of goldenrod flowers, dried
- 1 tbsp. of sunflower petals, dried

Directions:

1. Mix the above ingredients; moisten with boiling water and place between 2 layers of cheesecloth; cool before applying to the affected area.

2. Remoisten when it has dried. Use as frequently as you need.

91. Immunity Booster Tincture
Burns weaken the body, making it more susceptible to illness and infection. To boost your immunity, drink this tea.

Ingredients:

- 30 chaps of echinacea tincture
- 1 cup of warm water
- 20 drops of root tincture wild indigo

Directions:

1. In a bowl of warm water, combine the herbs listed above.

2. Take up to 5 times per day.

Rashes

A rash can be excruciatingly irritating regardless of what caused it and there are many lotions, creams, or antihistamines for relief. Scratching aggravates the situation and increases the risk of infection. Here are several options for pain relief and reasons of why they could help.

92. Salve for Dry Rash
Because of their oil and wax composition, salves are emollient, particularly when a moisturizing oil, such as olive oil, is used as the basis. The soothing and anti-inflammatory properties of the herbs improve its emollient effect.

Ingredients:

One moue beeswax

- Three fluid ounces of calendula-infused oil
- Two fluid ounces of licorice-infused oil
- Three fluid ounces of plantain-infused oil

Directions:

1. Make a salve as usual.

2. At least twice a day, gently apply a layer to the afflicted region.

93. Poultice for Weepy Rash
Poison ivy and other related plants may cause fluid-filled blisters. Astringents are needed for treatment and they are best supplied in the form of water extracts, such as poultice or compress.

Learn how to recognize the plants in your vicinity that cause contact rash! Poison ivy, poison oak, and poison sumac all thrive in the United States.

Ingredients:

- 1 cup rose petals, dried
- 1 cup calendula flower, dried
- 1 cup leaf wadi-lower (self-heal), dried
- 1/2 cup. St. John's wort flower and leaf, dried
- 1/2 cup uva-ursi leaf, dried
- Boiling water
- 1/2 cup yarrow flower and leaf, dried

Directions:

1. Combine all the herbs in a large mixing bowl. Store in a sealed container.

2. Place 4 to 6 tablespoons of the herb mixture in a heat-proof dish.

3. Pour adequate boiling water over the herbs to completely submerge them, but not so much that they float. Allow 5 minutes for the herbs to soak.

4. Apply a warm, moist mound of herbs to the afflicted body part. Cover the dish with a towel. Allow for a 5 to 10 minutes cooling period before gently patting dry.

5. Do this one to three times each day.

TIP: If you don't have access to these herbs, simple black or green tea bags will suffice! Simply get them warm and moist, put them on the rash for 20 minutes.

94. Skin-Healing Tea

Ingredients:

- 1 tsp. of Oregon grape root
- 1 tsp. of burdock root
- 1 tsp. of echinacea root
- 2 cups of water
- 1 tsp. of yellow dock root

Directions:

1. In a pan, combine the herbs and cover them with water.

2. Bring to a boil, lower the heat and cook for 10 to 15 minutes, until cool enough to drain.

3. Start with a tbsp. and work your way up to 1/2 cup every day.

95. Rash Wash

Ingredients:

- 1 tsp. of white pair bark or leaves
- 1 tsp. of comfrey root
- 2 cups of water
- 1 tsp. of slippery elm bark

Directions:

1. Fill a container halfway with water and add the herbs.

2. Bring to a boil and cook for 20 - 30 min; cool and drain.

3. Use as a topical wash as required.

Lymphatic System
Fibrocystic Breasts

Fibrocystic breasts are sore and lumpy. This widespread disorder, formerly known as fibrocystic breast disease, is not a disease. Many women go through these natural breast changes, which typically occur about the time of their period. The female breast is one of two mammary glands (milk secretion organs) on the abdomen.

96. Violet Leaf Balm

Recommended Dosage: Twice a day;

Can apply anytime of the day for up to two months

Ingredients:

- 3 1/2 ounces of violet leaf infused oil
- A bit under 1/2 ounce of beeswax

Directions:

1. Melt the two ingredients together in a heat-proof jar placed in a pan of simmering water, then carefully pour into cooling containers.

Swelling

Swelling happens when the muscles, skin, or other body parts swell. It is usually caused by inflammation or fluid accumulation. Swelling can occur internally or externally, affecting the skin and muscles. A variety of conditions can cause swelling.

97. Swellings Tea

Recommended Dosage: Half a cup a day; take everyday (every morning)

Ingredients:

- Two cups boiling water
- One teaspoon echinacea root
- One teaspoon granulated Oregon grape root
- One tablespoon white oak bark
- One teaspoons barberries

Directions:

1. Place the herbs in a glass container and mix well.

2. Soak the herbs in boiling water for three hours before straining.

Reproductive System

Erectile Dysfunction

Erectile dysfunction (ED) is the failure to obtain or maintain a solid enough erection for sexual intercourse. It is often referred to as impotence, though this term is becoming less common. It is frequent in men during periods of stress.

98. Horny Goat Weed Tea

Recommended Dosage: Two cups daily; consume on an empty stomach

Ingredients:

- A handful of horny goat weed leaves
- A handful of damiana

Directions:

1. Mix together equal parts of each herb.

2. Use one tablespoon of dried herb to two cups of hot water.

3. Bring to a slow boil and simmer for 20 minutes.

Menstrual Cramps

A menstruating woman is likely to have pain in the lower back, thighs, and abdomen. The womb muscles relax and contract throughout the period to remove constructed lining. Cramping occurs from time to time, indicating that the muscles are working. Some women may also have the following symptoms:

- Vomiting
- Nausea
- Diarrhea
- Headaches

Experts are baffled as to why some women have terrible symptoms while others do not. Some of the reasons linked to more acute discomfort include:

- The birth of the first child
- Heavy menstrual flow

- When she is under the age of twenty or about to start her cycle
- Having an excess susceptibility to prostaglandins, a kind of chemical in the body that has an effect on the womb.

Other considerations include:

- The use of contraception
- Endometriosis
- Tumors in the uterus

Some natural treatments might offer some relief from mild to temporary cramping. The following are quick relief suggestions and information on minimizing the discomfort during the period.

99. Tea for a Steady Cycle

Yields about 3 and a half cups of herb mix, dry (enough for 20 - 28 quarts of tea)

These herbs feed the body while stimulating the kidneys and the lymphatic and endocrine systems. For women with menstrual problems, long-term usage of a mixture like this will be the key to improvement. If you have a cold, add ginger, betony if you are regularly worried, and peppermint for flavor (if you like it). Drink a quart or so daily.

Ingredients:

- 1 cup dandelion leaf, dried
- 1 cup nettle leaf, dried
- 1/2 cup goldenrod flower and leaf, dried
- 1/2 cup self-heal flower and leaf, dried
- 1/4 cup kelp, dried
- 1/4 cup tulsi leaf, dried

Directions:

1. Combine all the herbs in a small dish. Keep the container sealed.

2. Make a lengthy infusion: boil some water in a pot. In a French press or mason jar, measure 2–3 tbsp. of herbs in every quart of water.

3. Fill the pot halfway with boiling water, cover, and steep overnight.

100. Say No to Pain Tea

Makes 3 naps of herb mix, dry (enough for 20 - 26 quarts of tea)

This tea should be drunk 3 to 7 days before the next period is due to start to induce menstruation. To get the greatest benefits, the tea should be drunk when extremely hot. Reheat as needed, then serve or drink a quart or so throughout the day. Drop a bit of angelica tincture with each cup of tea for a greater impact.

Ingredients:

- 1 cup tulsi leaf, dried
- 1 cup chamomile flower, dried
- 1/2 cup goldenrod flower and leaf, dried
- 1/3 cup angelica root, dried
- 1/3 cup ginger, dried

Directions:

1. In a small bowl, mix all the herbs. Store in an airtight container.

2. Combine all the herbs in a small dish. Keep the container sealed.

3. Make a hot infusion: boil some water in a kettle, then measure 2–3 tbsp. of herbs every quart of water in a French press or mason jar.

4. Fill the cup halfway with boiling water, cover, and steep for 20 minutes, or until cold enough to consume.

101. Soothing Menstrual Tea
Ingredients:

- 2 cups of cold water
- 2 tsp. of passionflower
- 2 tsp. of black haw bark or root

Directions:

1. In a pan, combine the herbs and cover with cold water; soak overnight; drain.

2. Take or serve half a cup three times a day, up to four times a day.

102. Tea for Dysmenorrhea

Ingredients:

- 1 tsp. of crampbark
- 2 tsp. of black cohosh root
- 1 tsp. of black haw bark or root
- 2 cups of water
- 1 tsp. of pulsatilla

Directions:

1. In a saucepan, combine the above herbs and cover with water.

2. Bring to a boil and cook for 10 minutes; cool and drain.

3. Take or serve half a cup, 4 times a day.

103. Cramp Relieving Tea

Ingredients:

- 1 cup of boiling water
- 1 tsp. of raspberry leaves
- 1 tsp. of St. John's wort Leaves

Directions:

1. In a glass container, combine the herbs and cover with boiling water.

2. Soak for 15 minutes; drain.

3. To ease cramps, drink or serve as required.

104. Chamomile Tea

Chamomile tea has anti-spasmodic qualities that may help reduce the unpleasant cramps that come with menstruation. It also serves to control the effects of serotonin and dopamine, which may help alleviate or at least lessen the severity of depression symptoms.

Ingredients:

- 2 to 3 tsp. of chamomile
- 2 cups of hot water
- Honey

Directions:

1. Add 2 to 3 tsp of chamomile tea to 2 cups of hot water to make this aromatic tea. Allow for 5 to 8 minutes of brewing time depending on how strong you want the tea to be. You may sweeten the tea with honey if desired.

2. Chamomile tea, made from chamomile plant blossoms, is recognized for its relaxing properties. As a result, it may be highly useful whenever it comes to premenstrual symptoms.

3. A week before menstruation, drink or serve 2 cups of tea every day. If you consume it or serve it once a month, there may be extra benefits.

105. Fennel Seeds Tea

Fennel, also known as saunf, is often ingested after a meal to promote digestion, but few people know that it may also assist with bloating and cramps. It possesses anti-inflammatory and anti-carminative effects that may aid with menstrual pain relief.

Ingredients:

- Fennel seeds
- Tea leaves
- Water

Directions:

1. Boil a cup of water with a tsp. of minced fennel seeds, including a 1/4 tsp. of tea leaves.

2. Allow for an eight to ten-minute steeping period. You may use milk instead of water. In addition, if you don't like strong tea, you might skip the tea leaves.

106. Green Tea

Green tea has been shown to help with bloating, a frequent menstrual symptom that may be quite uncomfortable. It also possesses anti-inflammatory qualities that may aid in relieving unpleasant cramps.

So, whenever Aunt Flo is bothering you or your loved one, get her or yourself a mug of soothing tea!

Ingredients:

- Green tea
- Hot water
- Honey and lemon

Directions:

1. To make a cup of this amazing herbal tea, add a spoonful or 2 of green tea to hot water and let it steep for 5 - 10 minutes.

2. If too bitter, add more honey and lemon.

Recipes Alphabetic Index

Agrimony Tincture; 159
Agrimony-Chamomile Gel; 172
Aloe Vera Gel; 149
Anti-Insomniac Elixir; 157
Antitussive Oxymel; 153
Arnica Salve; 151
Beetroot Juice; 149
Bowel-Hydrating Infusion; 145
Bowel-Motivating Tincture; 145
Bowel-Soothing Tea; 145
Calendula Toner; 171
Calming Tea; 159
Carminative Tincture; 147
Chamomile Lip Scrub; 163
Chamomile Tea; 181
Clove Application; 168
Cold Sore Balm; 165
Cold Sore Compress; 164
Cold Sore Mouthwash; 165
Cold Sore Tea; 165
Comfrey-Aloe Gel; 175
Cooling Tea for Headache; 156
Corn Infusion; 159
Cough Syrup; 154
Cramp Relieving Tea; 180
Daily Soothing Menstrual Tea; 164
Dandelion Root Tincture; 144
Echinacea and Goldenseal Tincture; 160
Elderberry Gummy Bears; 171
Elixir to Rescue; 158
Expectorating Cough And Cold Tea; 155
Fennel Seeds Tea; 181
Fever Relieving Tea #1; 166
Fever Relieving Tea #2; 166
Feverfew-Peppermint Tincture; 172
Fresh Garlic Poultice; 173
Fresh Hyssop Poultice; 150
Fresh Plantain Poultice; 174
Fresh Yarrow Poultice; 160
Garlic-Ginkgo Syrup; 173
Ginger-Peppermint Salve; 161
Ginkgo-Thyme Tea; 151
Golden Paste; 150
Goldenseal Ointment; 174
Goldenseal-Hyssop Syrup; 153
Good Dreams Tea; 157
Green Tea; 181
Hangover Infusion; 170
Hangover Tea; 170
Hawthorn Berry Tea; 160
Honey for Burn Recovery; 176
Honey-Ginger Tea; 165
Horny Goat Weed Tea; 179

Hot Infusion Tea; 164
Immunity Booster Tincture; 177
Insomnia Relieving Tea; 157
Lakota Cough And Cold Formula; 154
Lumbee Cough And Cold Formula; 154
Marshmallow Infusion; 146
Moringa Leaves Paste; 149
Mouthwash Made from Aloe Vera; 167
Mouthwash Made from Guava Leaves; 168
Mouthwash Made from Lemongrass Oil; 167
Mouthwash Made from Sage; 168
Mouthwash Made from Tea Tree Oil; 167
Nerve-Relaxing Tea; 159
Passionflower–Blue Vervain Tea; 161
Peppermint-Fennel Tea; 144
Peppermint-Rosemary Vapor Treatment; 152
Peppery Tea for Headache; 156
Poultice for Weepy Rash; 177
Pre-Emptive Bitter Tincture; 147
Preventive Bitter Tincture; 146
Purifying Digestive Tea; 146
Quick-Acting Cough And Cold Formula; 155
Quick-Acting Heartburn Tea; 147
Quick-Acting Mullein Cough Syrup; 155
Rapid-Acting Fever Tea; 166
Rapid-Acting Hangover Tea; 170
Rash Wash; 178
Rosemary–Licorice Root Vapor Treatment; 152
Salve for Dry Rash; 177
Say No to Pain Tea; 180
Sesamum Indicum (Sesame Seeds); 149
Shaking-It-Off Tea; 158
Skin-Healing Tea; 178
Soft Tissue Injury Liniment; 162
Soothing Cough And Cold Formula; 154
Soothing Heartburn Tea; 147
Soothing Menstrual Tea; 180
Soothing Tea; 158
Soothing Tea for Headache; 156
Spicy Ginger Elixir; 148
Spicy Tea; 170
Spray for Sunburns; 176
Sweet Relief Tea; 162
Swellings Tea; 178
Tea for a Steady Cycle; 179
Tea for Dysmenorrhea; 180
Topical Ointment for Burn; 176
Turmeric or Curcuma Gel Application; 169
Violet Leaf Balm; 178
Vitamin C Pills; 171
Warming Tea for Headache; 156
Witch Hazel Spray; 163

Conclusion

Various researches have shown that herbal plants are useful, helpful, valuable, and resourceful in treating various conditions and diseases. They cover different aspects of the body's health. In fact, herbalism does not focus on a single problem only, but encompasses different issues.

Traditionally, herbal medicines were the real-life saviors of numerous native people or native tribes, as they were the only existing medicines in ancient times. Moreover, with new technology and new studies, their potency became better known. More studies revealed more knowledge in regard to herbal medicine. These researches also brought a lot of visible improvements as they explore the maximum quality of each plants. There have been numerous experiments, money, budgeting, and scientific knowledge used and implemented to reach where we are today in regard to herbal medicines. However, there is still need for more studies are to get even more knowledge. There are still herbs that are not supported by facts, but they are surely supported by real life experiences.

Herbal plants are multi-functioning, whether they be on trees or on the ground and they definitely treat numerous conditions all at once. It is very reassuring to find medicines that are easily accessible in ones garden. This is cost effective and affordable. Herbs are well known as teas, pills, supplements, or creams. They are seldom used fresh due to some circumstances like poisons. Unfortunately, they are also limited based on their guidelines and there are certain factors to be considered before using a single herb plant.

Despite the benefits of herbal plants, there are still possible side effects that could last a lifetime. It is at best to follow protocols, guidelines, and even seek for professional help to make sure they are safe. They might aid almost similar conditions, but they are different in certain aspects, may it be their physical appearance, chemicals, compounds, habitat, or even their season. Some grow with poisons and others have external factors that make them harmful.

It is pleasantly surprising that herbal medicines are not fading and are in fact dominating a greater part of the world. Herbalism is the best gift given by the native people or the ancient people to their race. Herbal Plants or Herbal Medicine has been passed down from various generations, and they have never been a disappointment. Tone needs only to be quite knowledgeable about them before using any of them. Some plants must also be taken in proper timelines and proper dosages to avoid harm. Thus, it is important to stay healthy and to find the perfect medicine that would fit ones body.

BOOK 6: HERBAL DISPENSATORY VOL. 1

Introduction

Any of the plants used by Native American physicians can now be found in commercial stores around the world. This book contains steps on how to take the natural remedies that Native Americans used with regularity and incorporate them into your own life. Unlocking the secrets behind the great health practices of these ancient tribes could be the key to curing many of the diseases and illnesses that plague us today.

Native American healers worked uniquely, assisting the body and the spirit to react by themselves rather than offering an immediate cure.

Nature, being a generous mother, gave men all they need to heal within the reach of their hands filling the lands, meadows, and mountains with herbs and flowers that contain within themselves the power to stimulate the healing process.

Herbalism expands further than the historical backdrop of humanity. Everything that we realize today follows strings from the earliest times, woven together into an embroidered artwork of information that we may, in general, underestimate. However, it is normal to search out plants for medication, as creatures do.

The fact that you are putting all this effort shows a real dedication and commitment to taking matters of your health seriously. There are many prescription drugs out there. However, it doesn't mean that they are the only options available.

For simple ailments, you can always resort to herbal remedies like the ones we will discuss in this book. There is no need to create dependency on prescription drugs.

Learning herbalism and plant-based home remedies can be difficult at first, but I hope, and I'm sure, that this book has been an excellent primer for you to continue your journey, get acquainted with the plants, select which ones work best for you, and empower healing at home.

Getting Started

Personal herbal medicine would be any herbal medicine, most probably a combination, that you could rely on for getting better whenever you got a fever. With time you would feel so confident in that remedy that you would also recommend it to other people, people that you care about. This herbal medicine is not necessarily supposed to be made by you. Instead, it can be a remedy (a premade one) that you have always felt that it worked every time you used it.

Well, first of all, you will need a purpose to be making an herbal medicine; to use it as a cure. When you go through all the complicated stuff, which can be explained as the mixing process, you will have a result. This result may end up disappointing you in the end, but that will only mean that you have to try again to find a newer and better medicine.

After the successful use of a medicine that you made yourself, the feeling that you would feel right away will be priceless.

The next thing you will know is that you will be trying to make newer medicines due to the confidence in your last success, and you will find yourself constantly recommending your remedy to the people you think are in need of it.

Most of the herbs can be grown in your kitchen garden very easily. It finally comes to the point that you have to be committed to this completely. If you are, you will find yourself willing enough to plant little amounts of all of these herbs in small pots. You will also have to take responsibility for these herbs as well, so you will have to water them and take care of their fertilizers. Soon enough, this responsibility will turn into a love for those plants.

If, in any case, you don't find it easy to go through all the processes to produce herbal ingredients yourself, you can always go to the local superstore. There, you will find all the herbs you were looking for and some that you have never even heard about.

Start Your Home Apothecary

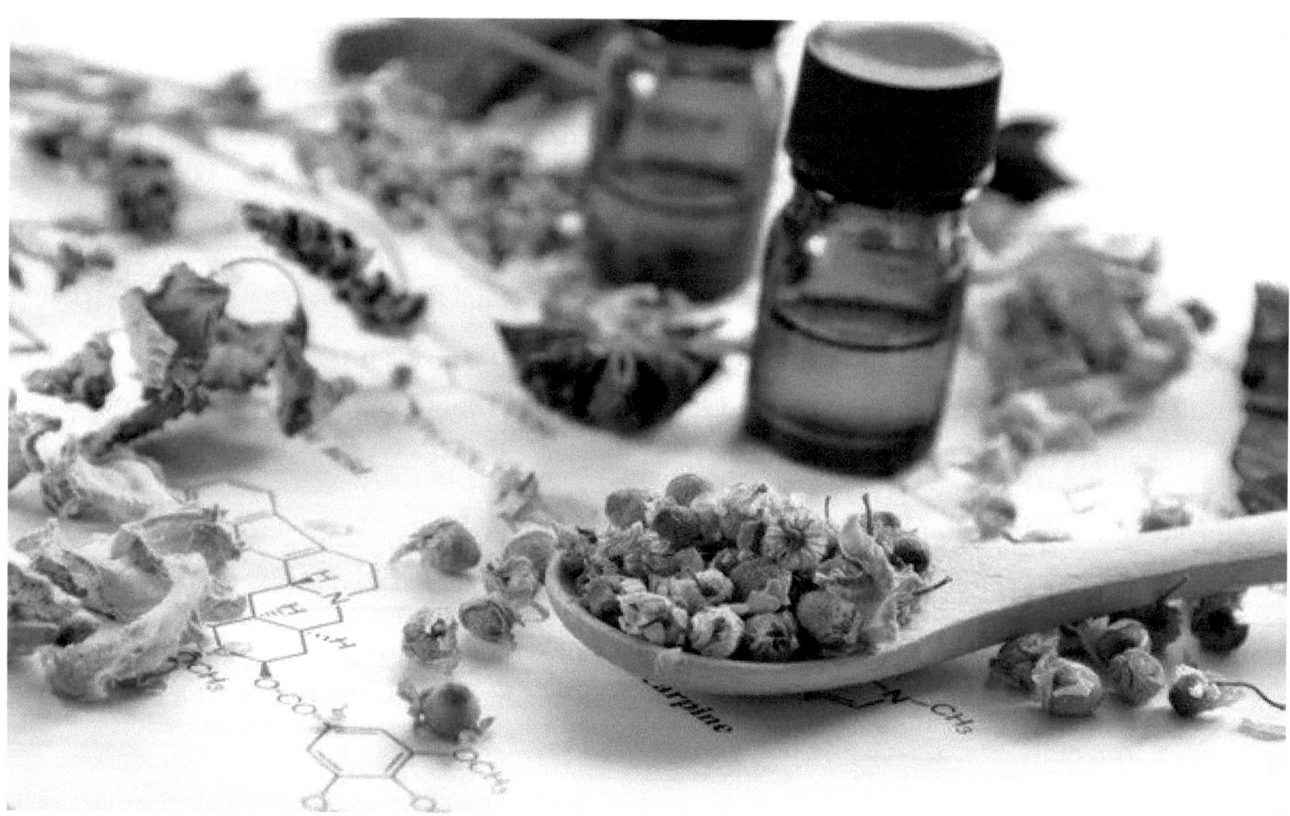

Surprisingly, only a few tools are required to begin your home apothecary. The most important things you'll need are boiling water, glass canning jars to store your products, and amber bottles to store herbal extracts. If you share a kitchen with family members or roommates, I recommend having specific tools for your home apothecary. We will cover most of the essential tools you'll need to get started, many of which are not expensive. You can start small and upgrade your tools as you gain experience.

How much herbs do you need?

Three to four ounces of an herb is usually enough to start a home apothecary. That's more than enough to create a couple of recipes and still have plenty left over for future occasions. Herbs lose potency over time, so get not too may until you understand how much you regularly use, which should be within six months to a year.

Essential Tools

To prepare high-quality herbal medicines, you don't need expensive equipment or rare, pricey components. Instead, the majority of what you'll require is likely already in your kitchen.

Mason jars

You can pour boiling water right into them to prepare tea because they're constructed of heat-resistant glass. They're also helpful for producing tinctures and keeping herbs, among other things. The most versatile jars are the quart and pint sizes, while bigger jars may be necessary for storing dried herbs. Many store-bought goods come in mason jars, washed by hand or washed in the dishwasher and dried.

Wire mesh strainers

You'll need strainers of various sizes for straining the tea or pressing out tinctures. Begin with a couple of single-mug strainers for single brewing cups of tea and a larger, bowl-size strainer to filter more significant amounts of herb-infused liquids.

Cheesecloth

This is used for straining and compressing herbs that have been infused into liquid and wrapping herbs in a poultice.

Cup, tablespoon, and teaspoon

These measures and graduated measuring cups with pour spouts that allow you to measure down to a quarter ounce are all useful.

Funnels

Getting tinctures and other liquids into bottles with narrow apertures is a breeze with a set of small funnels.

Amber or blue glass bottles

These are ideal for the long-term storage of tinctures. The "Boston round" shape is preferred for tinctures and other liquid treatments, but any form will suffice. Make it a habit to save and re-use any colored glass bottles you come across—many kombucha brands, for example, come in amber glass. Dose bottles should be one or two fluid ounces, whereas storage bottles should be four to twelve fluid ounces. Use basic bottle caps for storage, but dropper tops are required for dosing bottles.

Labels

As soon as you finish making your cures, label them. In most cases, address labels will suffice; in a pinch, masking tape will suffice.

Blender

A regular kitchen blender will blend lotions, break down bulky fresh plant stuff, and other tasks.

Other useful instruments

These tools make incorporating herbs into your life easier, especially if you have a hectic schedule, but they aren't as crucial as before.

French Press

Our preferred tool for creating herbal infusions is the French press. It is easy to clean and allows the herbs to float freely in the water, exposing a large surface area for extraction.

Thermos

A decent thermos is useful whether traveling or carrying your tea to work. There are models with a filter integrated right into the lid, allowing you to put the herbs and water in the thermos together right away.

A press pot

This is an insulated pot with a lever that you press to dispense the contents. People commonly put coffee or strained tea in them, but we've found that placing herbs right into the pot, pouring boiling water over it, and letting it infuse works just as well. It'll keep you warm all day, and you can pour it out by the cup.

Herb grinder

We use a simple, little coffee grinder for years, but if you want to prepare many herb powders, you may want to invest in a larger, dedicated machine.

Apothecary Supplies for the Home

Many treatments can be made with just herbs and water, but some preparations require extra components.

Alcohol

Tinctures are made up of a combination of botanical extracts and alcohol. Typically, we use vodka or brandy.

Apple-cider vinegar

For herb-infused vinegar, oxymels, and topical treatments, use apple cider vinegar instead of distilled white vinegar.

Honey

If you can find it, choose unprocessed/unfiltered local honey wherever feasible. Some big brands of honey are tainted or even contain high fructose corn syrup, so be cautious. Herbal honey infusions are easier to make using liquid honey, but thicker honey is better for first aid and wound care.

Oils

Olive oil can be used for almost anything, although in some cases, a lighter oil, such as grapeseed or almond oil, or a heavier oil, such as shea butter or cocoa butter, is preferable. Animal-derived fats, such as lard, tallow, or lanolin, can also be used.

Beeswax

Beeswax is used to thicken salves. Beeswax comes in rounds or pieces, which you can cut down for each usage. Beeswax pellets, which are easier to work with, are also available.

Witch Hazel extract

Look for a witch hazel extract that is alcohol-free, as this is the most versatile—especially for first aid and wound treatment.

Rose water

Rosewater is traditionally used for skin treatment, but it is also used in cooking. Rose water from the grocery store's "ethnic foods" department is just as excellent as the more expensive health and beauty area items.

Sea salt and Epsom salts

Adding a pinch of salt to baths and soaks, as well as nasal sprays and gargles, improves the treatment.

Gelatin capsules

When working with herbal powders to manufacture handmade herb capsules, it is the size is the most commonly used.

Preparations Of Native American Herbs

Mason jars are for sure the best containers to preserve your herbs and preparations: they are cheap, available in every store, and with an airtight lid.

The only problem with them is that they are transparent and allow sunlight to radiate directly to the herbs, thus compromising their medical properties. Amber or cobalt glass would be the best for the preservation of herbs and herbal remedies but unfortunately, amber glass bottles are quite expensive and not widely available.

The trick you can use, as a beginner, to avoid this problem is to use common mason jars but to store them in a cellar or any place far away from direct sunlight. With this single trick, you will increase the endurance of your herbs or preparation by 5 times.

Below the typical endurance times, you can expect using this method:

- Dried herbs: 1 to 4 years
- Tinctures: 7 years
- Oils and salves: 6-12 months

Herbal Preparations

Modern technology offers superior methods for distilling, extracting, purifying, and standardizing plant extracts, but it is beyond the scope of this book. However, for you to get the most out of this book, we'll go over some essential prerequisites for total novices.

Tea: It is made by steeping dry or fresh herbs in hot water. Typically, just the plant's soft sections are injected. Green teas, black teas, and herbal teas are some examples. One teaspoon dry herb to one cup water; four teaspoons fresh herb to 1 cup water.

Decoction: A liquid produced by simmering or boiling herbs in water is known as a decoction. Decoctions are made by extracting water-soluble chemistry from the plant's rigid portions, such as the stems, seeds, bark, and roots. Soup with garlic, for example: in a cup of water, simmer one teaspoon dry herb; four teaspoons fresh herb in a cup of water—Cook for at least five minutes before straining and using.

Percolation: It is a coffee-making technique in which water or alcohol is drizzled through a moist mass of powdered herb. Cayenne powder is dripped with hot water or alcohol, as an example. Amount: To boost concentration, drip 100 milliliters of liquid through ten grams of dry herb, then repeat the process.

Tincture: This is a mixture of chopped herbs and alcohol. Other substances, such as apple cider vinegar or glycerin, can be substituted for alcohol. A blender can be used to do the maceration. Example: To achieve about 50% alcohol, dilute a volume of 190 proof alcohol with an equal amount of water. Here, is an example: Chop fresh-cut Echinacea flowers into small pieces, place them into a bowl, cover with 50% alcohol and leave it to macerate. Refrigerate the maceration for four hours before straining and bottling. A 1:5 ratio is generally employed when producing a tincture with a dry herb, meaning one ounce of the dried herb is macerated and combined with five ounces of 50% alcohol. When working with fresh herbs, a 1:2 ration is commonly used—one gram per cubic centimeter of 50% alcohol.

Double Extraction: First, fill a container, a 32 oz. canning jar with a cup of macerated Echinacea leaves and roots. Completely cover the maceration with 7 ounces of 50 percent diluted everclear. Then cover. Set the blend in a darkened cupboard or refrigerator and shake it twice a day.

Strain off the liquid with a regular strainer. Then run it through a coffee filter (better if unbleached), squeezing out all the remains. You now have a "single extraction." Now cover the echinacea mash with water, simmer for half-hour to make a decoction (add water if necessary). Strain and blend the decoction with the tincture, creating a more vigorous "double extraction." Don't add any water to the second extraction to maintain an alcohol concentration of at least 25%. Add 10 ounces of water max for the second extraction if you poured 10 ounces of 50% alcohol over the herb in the first place.

Fomentation: Prepare an infusion of herbs or decoction, then dip a cotton cloth into the preparation. Wrap the wet cloth around an injury. Example: Wet a cloth with a mild cayenne extraction and apply it to an arthritic joint. Amount: Enough to cover the area to be healed.

Poultice: Pound and macerate fresh herbs and place the moist mass directly over the body part. Example: Put a wet and warm pounded mass of plantain over a pus-filled wound—amount: Large enough to cover the area to be treated.

Powder: Dry and finely grind the herb, then load the powder into capsules. Example: Over-the-counter dried herbs are usually powders sold in capsules. Amount: Normally 500- to 1,000-milligram capsule.

Oils and salves: These can be made with fresh or dry herbs. First, the herb is cooked in oil to extract the active principle; then, the oil is thickened or hardened with beeswax. Example: The aerial parts of the yarrow are first coated with oil, simmered, and then mixed with warm beeswax. When the blend is completely cooled, the resulting salve can be applied as a wound treatment. Amount: All you need to do is lightly pack a pan with fresh leaves and flowers and cover with olive oil or lard.

How to Get Herbs

Buying Herbs

We have a variety of choices when it comes to purchasing herbs.

Herbs can be found at the supermarket, local nursery, farmers market, online, and also in our own backyards. You can buy or get herbs at each of these locations, depending on your choice!

Let's look at each method of purchasing herbs so you'll know what to search for while you're out shopping.

Purchasing Herbs from the Grocery Store

One of the costliest ways to get new herbs is to purchase them from a drug store. Here, dried herbs can be pricey, and they add up fast! When purchasing dried herbs here, always go for organic wherever possible.

Try purchasing the least costly herbs at the drug store and looking for more expensive ones online to conserve money.

While purchasing fresh herbs from the supermarket, search for sustainable products wherever possible and inspect the herbs before purchasing. Herbs should not be wilted or brown but should be more vivid and young.

To get the best out of your grocery store order, wash all herbs before using them and store them carefully.

Purchasing Herbs from a Nursery

Local nurseries provide a wide range of quality and selection of herbs. Few nurseries use sustainable and environmentally safe growing methods, while others use chemicals and herbicides.

In order to see what you're buying, pose questions or do some testing, much as you might at a farmers' market. Ask about the type of soil used and how it is maintained.

ask also about the growing methods used, especially if chemical sprays are used.

Before buying a plant, make sure it seems to be in good health. It's a lot simpler to hold a herb plant alive than it is to save it from destruction!

Purchasing Herbs from the Farmers Market

One of the best places to find new, moderately priced herbs is the farmer's market. Herbs from here are also the freshest and most tasty choice since they are grown locally!

Always keep in mind that all herbs sold at the farmers' market are not organically cultivated. In order to see what you're buying, you can ask questions or do some testing.

Check to see how the soil has been cared for and if chemical sprays have been used on the herbs, much as you can with fruits and vegetables.

Be sure the herbs aren't slimy, dusty, or wilted to determine whether they're in decent shape. You can tell if the herbs are fresh and good with only a brief glance!

Wild/Foraged Herbs

Herbs foraged in the wild are sometimes foraged and marketed at farmer's markets. This is a great place to get tasty, unique, and eclectic local herbs, but it's a good idea to ask the farmer where the herbs forage and what they know about the property.

Chemicals or pesticides from traditional local crops, for example, may contaminate herbs collected from a ditch, pond, or field.

Buying Herbs Online

Herbs may be purchased digitally, which is an easy choice with a large range. Online shopping is available for fresh plants, plant starts, dried herbs, and seeds.

Growing Herbs In Our Garden

Herbs may be propagated in a variety of forms in your herb garden.

You may need to cultivate your herbs by planting seeds, taking cuttings, separating roots, or using runners, depending on the type of herbal plant you're attempting to develop.

Herbs Grown from Seeds

Build seedlings in pots on a sunny windowsill around six weeks before the last frost date in your region to give your garden a head start. Plant the seeds in a strong potting soil mix as directed on the box. Thin the seedlings to one per pot by removing any excess growth with tweezers or snipping the weaker seedling at the soil line.

Harden off your seedlings by bringing them outdoors for longer periods of time over the span of two weeks until all danger of frost has passed before planting them in their permanent locations in your greenhouse.

You should launch your seeds in early spring in a sunny location in your herb garden if you reside in a colder environment with a longer growing season.

Short-lived herbs used in large amounts should be sown every three to four weeks from early spring to early fall to guarantee that you have enough on hand when you need them.

If you want to save seeds from plants you've grown in your garden, bear in mind that some herbs can cross-pollinate and produce plants that aren't genetically related to their mother plant.

If you cultivate different varieties of thyme, marjoram, or lavender near together, th hybridization is most possible.

If you wish to conserve the seeds from these plants, keep the families apart as far as possible.

The following are some of the easiest and most common herbs to cultivate from seed:

- Cilantro
- Pot marigold
- Caraway
- Sweet cicely
- Borage
- Angelica

As soon as your seeds have ripened, collect them.

Clean seeds can be stored in paper envelopes for later usage. Seeds can never be stored in plastic containers since this would degrade their content.

Herbs Propagated Through Cuttings

Taking cuttings is one of the most trustworthy ways to cultivate herbs. Often cut the cuttings with a sharp pair of gardening shears and place them right away in a mixture of well-drained clay, sand, peat, or vermiculite.

When the cutting is rooting, keep it damp and warm. Another kind of cutting is layering. A stem or shoot is induced to develop roots when still attached to the mother plant. Choose a shoot that is both powerful and adaptable.

Layering is a good way to spread jasmine. Make a tiny cut on the underside of the shoot and stick it in the field with the rising tip above the dirt.

To keep it in position, use a strong object like a brick. If the stem has taken root the following fall, you can break the young plant away from its mother and replant it in a new spot.

Herb Division for Propagation

To avoid overcrowding, perennial herbs may need to be separated every few years. Although growth is small, the division should be achieved in the autumn or early spring.

To separate the herbs, dig them up carefully, cut them in half, and replant the two plants in the garden or in containers.

Water replanted separated plants thoroughly to make the soil stabilize across the root system. Herbs that ought to be propagated through division contain the following:

- Oregano
- Hyssop
- Sorrel
- Catnip

Wild Crafting

Foraging for useful plants in their normal, wild environment for edible or medicinal purposes is known as wild crafting. One of the most enjoyable activities you may engage in is wild crafting for medicinal herbs.

Not only is it useful to know where your herbal medicines come from, but it's also entertaining to learn how to recognize plants and see what they look like as they mature. Plus, you may be shocked to learn about the therapeutic properties of common plants you pass by on a daily basis!

Benefits Of Wild Crafting

Since they come from richer terrain, such as comparatively undisturbed meadows and woodland, wild plants are more potent and nutrient-dense than their monoculture equivalents. Commercial farms frequently have depleted soil or only have separate resources for the plants.

It's still a perfect place to get some fresh air. Bring a mate along for a fun adventure. When you get home, you can use your wild plant harvest to create a variety of simple herbal remedies.

Wild crafting herbs for food and medicine will help you achieve the following goals:

- eat diets that are high in nutrients
- lowering reliance on imported food and medicine
- decrease reliance on Big Agro
- Keep yourself safe with herbal tonics and cures when enjoying nature.
- You should also carry your family and friends along to help create a community.

Tips for Wild Crafting Herbs

Here are ten wild crafting medicinal herb tips to get you started on your plant foraging adventure.

Get yourself a couple of plant identification books

To help you, buy two or three decent books on plant identification. It's particularly beneficial to find books about edible and medicinal plants, and it's even better if you can find one tailored to your location. Before going out on your own, try going on a walk with a local specialist and double-check your plant identification before harvesting.

Get out of the house

The best thing about wild crafting is that it brings you outdoors and is involved in nature, even while serving a goal. Medicinal plants flourish everywhere, whether you go on a long walk through the mountains or a stroll in your own area. Everything you have to do now goes outside and start searching!

Slowly walk

When collecting wild plants, you need to take things easy so that you can really enjoy your environment. Consider bringing a kid or an older person with you while walking and exploring nature. They travel slowly by design, forcing you to run at a different speed.

Look in unusual (as well as common) locations

When you're on track, go off the beaten path for a while. If you don't want to disrupt the natural environment, be gentle while doing so. However, there are many opportunities to wild craft outside of the bush.

Sidewalks and peaceful gravel road sides, as well as empty lots and open fields, are good places to look. Often seek approval before doing something on private land, and stay away from busy roadsides to avoid chemical contamination and pollution.

Avoid places around power lines or manufacturing, and building sites, near-commercial fields where chemicals can be used, and chemical runoff can occur.

Many local locations, such as green spaces, parks, and school grounds, can be useful; just make sure that gathering wild plants is permitted before you begin.

Often verify whether foraging is permitted anywhere you pick. Make sure the plants haven't been contaminated with chemicals and aren't thriving on degraded ground.

Don't avoid the common plants

We've all grown up with a variety of medicinal plants that are readily recognized. Just a few examples are dandelion, rosehips, plantain, mullein, yarrow, and elderberry. Learn about popular plants like these first, then move to plants that are more rare or difficult to locate.

Don't take everything

Even though there are many trees, don't take them all. Leave some for future years. So always leave more than you take, and better still, grow a seed of the same type anytime you cut a plant

Prepare yourself

Prepare a backpack or bag with your plant books, water, a snack or two, spare clothes, and even a little first-aid kit before you go (make a Hiking First Aid Kit). For collecting, you'll also need a pocket knife, scissors, and tiny pruners. A tiny gardener's trowel is also useful if you assume you're going to be harvesting roots. It's also a good idea to have some kind of little baggies for your collections.

Keep your eyes open for more details

Look down while you take a long stroll. Scrutinize the trail, road, or sidewalk you're on. Look in every way, even behind you. Take a look up. Stop every now and then to drink in your surroundings. Choose a few plants and practice looking them up in your reference books. Honestly, just keep searching!

Don't go looking for a certain herb

You don't want to set yourself up for disappointment by assuming you're going to go out and harvest a whole lot of a particular plant before you know for sure that it grows in a specific location. It's half the fun to go on an adventure and not realize what you'll discover.

Plants that are uncommon or endangered can be avoided

Find out which medicinal plants are uncommon or threatened, and avoid them at all costs. Many endangered plant species may be harmed by overharvesting. Sliding elm, American ginseng, black cohosh, and goldenseal are several of the medicinal plants that are endangered.

Safety Tips and Abuse of Herbs

Native American Herbs are one of the most amazing things because they are so potent. Here, we will talk about safety tips and how people abuse herbs.

Native Americans have always had a culture that used herbal medicine to heal themselves and their family members. There are many different types of herbs that can be used for many different purposes, such as using peppermint to heal an upset stomach or cedar for a sore chest. One type of herb is tobacco, which has been used for various purposes throughout Native American history; it can be smoked, chewed or even just held in the hand for smelling. Tobacco can also be used as an offering to the Earth Mother (or any other god).

In the past, Native Americans were often poor and did not have the resources to buy quality or even effective herbs, but that doesn't mean they had no idea what herbs could be used for medicinal purposes. Many herbs grow wild on Native American reservations; these are often used for various purposes, such as cleansing or purifying.

Native American culture has been around for a long time and it is possible that they knew the healing properties of plants long before Europeans ever discovered them. As European settlers came to America in search of new lands for new crops (and more land for their own personal use), they brought with them some knowledge about medicinal plants, but most of this was simply folklore passed down from generation to generation.

Safety Tips When Using Native American Herbs

Here are a few safety tips to consider when using herbs that are Native American:

1. **Do not use herbs if you are pregnant.**

When you are pregnant, you should always check with a doctor first before taking any herbs; just because they aren't classified as a medicine doesn't mean they won't hurt or harm you during pregnancy. There are many types of herbs that can be dangerous to your baby, such as parsley and willow branches, so if you are pregnant, make sure to speak to your doctor before using any new medicinal herbs.

2. **Do not use herbal medicines unless you know what the herb is capable of doing and its purpose in Native American culture.**

There are many herbs that have different purposes in various cultures. In some cultures, they are used for healing but in others, they are for purifying or cleansing. If you know what a herb is used for in Native American culture, then you can always use this information to your advantage.

But if you don't know and just pick up a random herb and decide to use it anyway, there could be consequences; you could either do more harm than good or it could even become poisonous if used improperly.

3. **Do not start using certain herbs without the proper education.**

There are many herbs out there that can be used for the same purposes but they have different results in the body, so this means that not all of them will work the same way for everyone even if their purpose is similar. For example, a few Native American herbs such as the Stinging Nettle can be used to help with conditions such as diabetes or cancer. But if you have no education on these herbs, then how do you know if it is the right herb for your particular condition? You may find you are using the wrong herb or it might not even work for the intended purpose.

4. **Do not use too many different herbs at one time.**

When using any type of medicinal herb, you should always start out with just one and see how it affects your body before you decide to add in more types of herbs. Not only is this safe, but it will also help you to better understand how each herb effects your body and what your body needs the most at that particular time.

5. **Do not use herbs for any type of condition that is not mentioned in Native American culture.**

For example, if a certain herb was used for a specific purpose in Native American culture, then you should just stick with what works and doesn't cause any harm. But if it is used for other purposes which are something you may not be familiar with or have heard of before, then it could do more harm than good or even become poisonous. Try out the various herbs and see if they work for you.

6. **Do not use any wild herbs or plants unless you know they are edible and edible only.**

There are many different types of wild plants that can be used for medicinal purposes in Native American culture, but there are also several that can be poisonous. You need to make sure that you don't use any of these because they could have adverse effects on your body. However, if you know what the plant is used for, then everything will be okay; just make sure to do your research first before using any plant or herb from the wild.

7. Do not use too much of an herb when starting out with Native American herbal medicine.

If you start out using too much of a certain herb, then it might actually cause other problems such as nausea and vomiting. However, if you start out with the right amount, then it will help in the healing process; just be aware of how much you are taking at a time and make sure that you stick to a proper schedule.

8. **Do not use any herbs if you are out of balance.**

To use any medicinal herbs properly, you must first be in a correct state of mind, which means that you must be strict with your diet and exercise regularly. This will ensure that your body is balanced and in the proper state to heal, so it is best not to use any type of herb or plant until this has been done.

9. **Do not use too much at once; start off with a small amount.**

If you recently became interested in home remedies and Native American medicinal herbs, then you may be tempted to start off using at least a few of them right away. However, that is not the best thing to do because it will cause your body to go into shock and might actually make you sick. Instead, just try out one herb for starters and then work your way up from there when you know your body has adjusted to it.

10. Do not use any herbs that are poisonous or toxic.

There are many different types of plants which can be used as medicinal herbs in Native American culture but there are also several that can be poisonous or harmful if used improperly. If you do not know what it is used for, then it is best to completely avoid using it.

11. Do not use any herbs if they are out of season.

There are several different types of herbs which can be used for medicinal purposes in Native American culture but there are also several that need to be used during the right time of year, otherwise they will become poisonous when they aren't in their correct season. Just make sure to take this into account and only use those that are available to you at the moment.

12. Do not forget to take your medicine on time.

One of the most important things to remember when using Native American herbal medicine is to never forget about your doses. If you do, then it will not have any of the healing effects that you are hoping for. Instead, make sure that you set an alarm or use a watch so you will not miss it. Then try to repeat this process as often as possible until your condition has completely healed.

If you take these steps into account, you will find that using Native American herbal remedies can help overcome their illnesses and start healing faster than ever before. So, if you have been looking for a natural cure for your ailments, then it may be time to look into this type of herbal medicine a little bit more.

Abuse of Native American Herbs

Unfortunately, it is a common thing for people to abuse herbs for their own personal gain or to try and "self-treat" through them. Thankfully, most of these types of people are quickly caught because there are a lot of customs and laws that stem from native cultures all over the country. If you have been believing in Native American herbal remedies but have been wanting to know more about what these people were doing, then it may be time to read a book or two on the subject. You will be surprised how much information is out there, and most of it is easily available. You can easily find books on just about any topic that you are interested in.

The first thing that you should realize when reading any book on this type of topic is that these types of herbs are really dangerous when used incorrectly or improperly. Doing so can lead to serious health risks, and even death from using them incorrectly. The ways you consume these herbs are very important and they should be done in ways that were natural to the people who were using them from ancient times. If you find some of these old recipes, make sure and check the ingredients for yourself just to be sure that they are safe. Most of these herbs have been studied for hundreds of years, and a great majority of them are completely safe when used in the right way.

The first thing that you should do before starting any type of research project is to look around your house. You will want to find pages from magazines or books from medical journals. You can easily find many things related to this topic when they are kept in an old book or magazine somewhere in your home. If you happen to come across old magazines or medical journals, then it is probably best to just keep them for your own personal reference. This way, you can easily look back on them when you are trying to complete different assignments.

When looking for information relating to Native American herbal remedies, you should always be careful of what information you use because there are so many different "facts" out there; it can be hard to tell what is accurate and what is not. So, the next time you are looking for information on these types of herbs, make sure to do your homework beforehand because this will not only improve your health immensely but also help keep your body safe when working with any type of herb from this culture.

However, if you happen to be someone who has been severely injured or have been diagnosed with a disease that you cannot seem to get rid of through modern medicine, then it may be time for you to consider trying these remedies as well. After all, they have helped people in the past so why not go with it?

What You Should Know Before You Get Started With Herbal Healing

Know Before You Make a Decision

Native American medicines have been used for years even though their effects may not be as serious as they were thousands of years ago, due to poor data keeping. But people have testified to their potency.

But you can't just jump on the bandwagon; you need to get yourself educated first before taking any native medicine.

Get a diagnosis

You want to know everything as much as you can. This is why you have to work very closely with your doctor so that there will be some monitoring as you embark on this journey into healing by nature. Once you understand what you're dealing with, you can now move into the next stage.

Understand your ailment and healing options

Most people who seek native medicine think that because it is natural, it is far better than orthodox medicine. While this may be true for some medical issues, it may not be true for all. For example, there are situations or health problems that will certainly require medical surgery before it will go away. There are no alternatives.

Understanding your ailment also ensures that errors are limited or cut down to zero. No matter how determined you think you are, the nature of your ailment will always be the major determinant to know if it is something you should wholly subject to treatment through herbs.

Do research

In addition to working with your doctor, you should also try to do your own research about what is wrong with you. This is even more important for people who have been dealing with certain ailments for a very long time. Your research should be on the causes, triggers, and prevention options of your ailment. If your doctor thinks that you should try conventional medicine first, you can go on with it as long as you can afford it. If not, you still need to discuss with your doctor about herbals—and how you are going to use them the right way.

Conclusion

Herbalism is a beautiful process that allows us to heal our bodies, minds, and spirits by turning to nature. The state of nature is effective at providing us with so much of what we need to thrive when we know where to look. By learning about herbalism and learning from the Native Americans, who have continued to honor this tradition themselves, you can learn how to begin healing yourself.

We discussed how to source, harvest, prepare, dry, and store herbs. We discussed how herbs are holistic healing tools. We even went over how you can grow them at home by starting your own garden. These tools are highly effective if you know where to turn and how to use them to their fullest extent.

Remember to treat the herbs that you care for with the utmost respect. Honor the sacrifice these plants have made for us as we use them to heal our own bodies. They sacrifice their own bodies for us, and that is worthy of respect. With that in mind, you should be able to benefit greatly from your use of herbalism.

BOOK 7:
HERBAL DISPENSATORY VOL. 2

Introduction

When you have a backache, what's the first thing you do? Some people reach for ibuprofen in their medicine cabinet. Others turn to an ice pad or a hot bath to alleviate the pain. Others still turn to yoga or a massage. However, there is another option that was used centuries before.

Native American medicine is highly effective in providing relief for a wide range of ailments because rather than approaching medicine as a one-size-fits-all solution, it takes a closer look at the individuals. Instead of focusing on how to treat just the physical symptoms of how someone feels, it treats the whole person. This includes the individual's physical wellbeing, mental health, their community, and their spirituality. By emphasizing the protecting of all four corners of one's life, fostering a degree of health and wellness through a holistic approach, people remain healthier.

Much of Native American medicine draws from herbalism, the art of treating individuals with parts from plants in several different forms. These can often support the body in treating a wide range of issues, encouraging the immune system to fend off infection, or working to alleviate inflammation. They can soothe pain and help create a sensation of wellness.

Because of the community approach to wellness, often involving the family of the individual who needs health, relationships are better. Modern medicine even acknowledges that individuals with supportive and positive relationships often recover better than those without. This adds another layer to the effectiveness of Native American medical treatments.

In this book, we will delve into what Native American medicine looks like. We will discuss the common medicinal herb profiles, including the effects, common uses, and disorders they treat. We will wrap up by discussing how to administer herbs in several different forms. Herbal remedies often come in many forms, including capsules, dried herbs, extracts, and more. Being able to identify the most common forms and knowing how to prepare them is a crucial part of learning how to use Native American medicine.

Learning these methods comes with more than just discovering which herbs are used for what. It also involves discovering how to begin getting in touch with the ancient art of herbalism. It involves learning how to treat many of the most common minor ailments yourself, alleviating pain, inflammation, and often infection. So many ailments that do not require massive treatment can be handled at home if you know which herbs to turn to and what to do about it.

Remember, this book specifically delves into Native American traditions. While these are not the only herbalistic approaches to treating the mind and body, they are the emphasis here. Other forms of herbalism exist in just about every culture around the world. You just have to look in the right places.

Preparations of Remedies Using Fresh Herbs

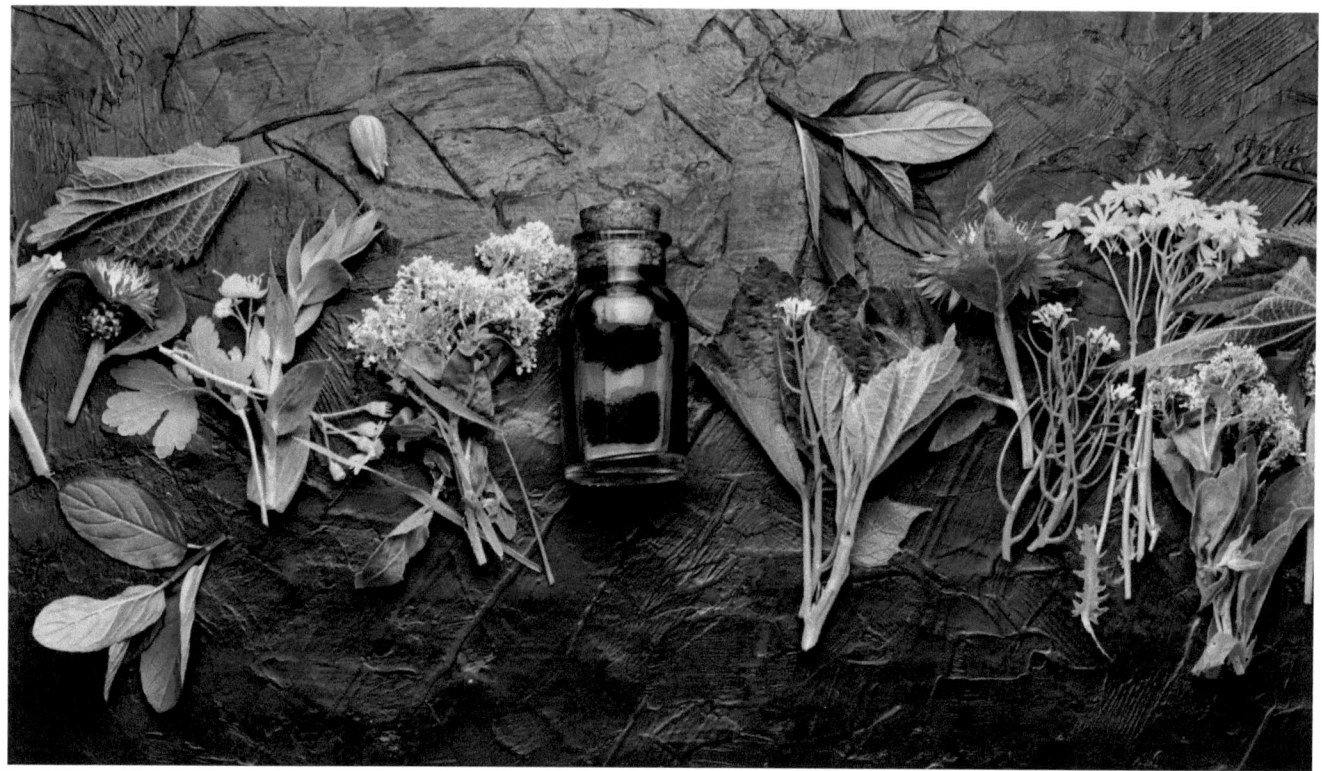

When you are planning to use fresh herbs or plants medicinally, you need to be aware of the nature of these substances. The herbs and plants that you will utilize need to be harvested in a way that is consistent with their energetics, which is different for each plant or herb.

A few herbs are not harvested at all because they are too difficult to process. These include burdock roots, red clover tops, and horsetail (not the hemlocks!).

One thing to consider when harvesting fresh herbs is how much yield you want in relation to your container size. If you plan on using fresh ingredients in liquid form and don't want them sitting on the counter, then a small amount is better. If you want to make a larger container with herbs or plants, then you should plan on having a greater amount of ingredients.

The next thing to consider is the energetics or flavor of the fresh plant or herb. For example, if you are using fresh mugwort leaves in an infusion, it will taste very different if you harvest it before the flowers bloom. The energetics for this plant are largely based on its lightness and clarity, and that comes from its flowers. Harvesting mugwort before its flowers have blossomed will result in a somewhat astringent taste.

Equipment Needed

The following is a list of equipment that you need:

- Container of some kind to hold the plant or herb.
- A knife or scissors for harvesting.

- A strainer for the container. This allows you to pour off the liquid while leaving the solid parts in your container while filtering out any debris that might be inside of it, such as dirt, small twigs, and leaves.
- A bowl or cup to hold your herbs and a spoon if necessary to scoop them out with while transferring them into your strainer container or storage container.
- A drying rack that can be used to dry.
- A cutting board for harvesting.
- A clean cloth to place over your container and dry the herbs while they are still moist, such as a dish towel or handkerchief.
- A jar that can be easily cleaned with dish soap and water. If you plan on using fresh herbs in liquid form, then you will need to transfer them into a glass container that will fit into your refrigerator after they are harvested and dried.

Harvesting: Step by Step Guide

Harvesting at the right time

Most herbs and plants need to be harvested at the right time in order to have the best overall outcome. Some will tolerate more than others depending on their light needs, but for most, their maximum growth and potency are when they are receiving the right amount of light.

Although it is recommended that you harvest your plant or herb before its flowers blossom, this does not mean that you cannot harvest from it after it has bloomed. Once it has bloomed, you can rest assured that it will continue to send its energy into the air around itself as a form of sexual pollen or seeds for each flower. If you harvest early enough in the season, the energy from the plant will continue. If it is only just beginning to bloom, you might have trouble with its energy leaving you through its leaves and flowers.

Therefore, consider harvesting your fresh herbs and plants at different times in order to harvest from them at their peak of potency before they begin to pass their energy on to the next generation, or if that is not a concern, then be sure that your container has no stagnant air or water or grime (dirt) in it.

Harvesting the right part of an herb

When harvesting an herb, you need to consider where the main part of the herb is, and this is what will determine how you process it. To do this, make sure that all of the leaves are removed from a plant or herb before harvesting any parts of it. The stems, woody underside, and flowers can be left on the plant or gathered after your plant or herb has bloomed. Try not to tear off too many leaves because this can cause damage to the growth, and the leaves will eventually dry out and die off anyway.

The main part of a plant or herb is often the middle or any lower part, such as a root, tuber, stem, leafy underside (no flowers), and sometimes bark. Harvest from the middle downward to get the most for your effort.

It is also important that you know if your plant or herb is harvested in certain ways, then you will change its energetic potential. Harvesting an herb at certain times will affect its energetics, and this can cause them to be more potent at certain times than others.

Best way to bundle and label plants after harvesting

You can bundle the stems together with string, thread, yarn, or rubber bands to keep them together and label your bundles with a pen, so you know what each bundle is for.

Harvesting the fresh herbs and plants is a good time to take a moment and thank the plant or herb for sharing its energetic potential with you. You can also give them a blessing or ask their permission before harvesting them, which will go a long way in making your herbs more potent when it comes time to use them.

To make sure that you have the most for your effort, harvest in accordance with the energetics of each plant or herb. Plan on drying half of everything that you harvest, as many herbs need to be dried out quickly before their energetic potential drops significantly.

Drying: Step by Step Guide

Best Time And Practice To Dry Herbs

Herbs and plants need to be dried out to get the maximum energetic potential from them during the time they are being harvested. This is because their freshness and energy are being held in their outermost layers of leaf, stem, or root (the outside part of live things). If you wait until they have dried more than halfway before removing them from the ground, then it might take a very long time for their energetic potential to dry out completely.

Hanging herbs upside down is the simplest way to dry them. The gravity will pull all of the moisture out of them. This process is called drying. The best time for this is early morning at first light, just as the sun comes up brightening the day with its productive energy.

Methods to Dry Herbs

- Air Drying: This is done by spreading your herbs on a screen, bed sheet, or on paper towels and letting them sit in a breezy spot for about two weeks. You can also dry them with the aid of an electric fan.
- Microwave Drying: Prepping herbs for microwave drying is much like prepping vegetables for the oven: you want to remove any dirt and cut off leaves that are too large, so they don't burn during microwaving. Then, place your herb sprigs in a paper towel-lined bowl and cover it with another paper towel, so the steam from the microwave doesn't escape from all sides of the bowl. Cook on high heat for 4 minutes or until most of their water has been dried up.
- Oven Drying: Doing this can take anywhere from 5–20 hours, so you'll have to keep checking to see if the process is done. You also want to make sure that your oven is not too hot as you don't want your herbs to burn. Once done, you can store the dried herbs in air-tight containers.

- The Sun and Air: This method is ideal for those living in regions with warm climates and who do not own a microwave or electric fan. This method will take about two weeks and requires your herbs to be spread across a screen and placed outside in an area that receives direct sunlight throughout the day. You can also dry fresh herbs by placing them in large sponges or between clean rags placed on a sturdy surface.

To dry fresh herbs without losing any of the leafy green colors, you can place them between two clean sheets of paper towels or a piece of cloth, and you can also use glass containers with air space for your drying method. If you choose to use glass containers, then be sure that they have no cracks or chips in the glass itself to prevent your dried herbs from absorbing harmful radiation.

Remedies Preparation Using Dried Herbs

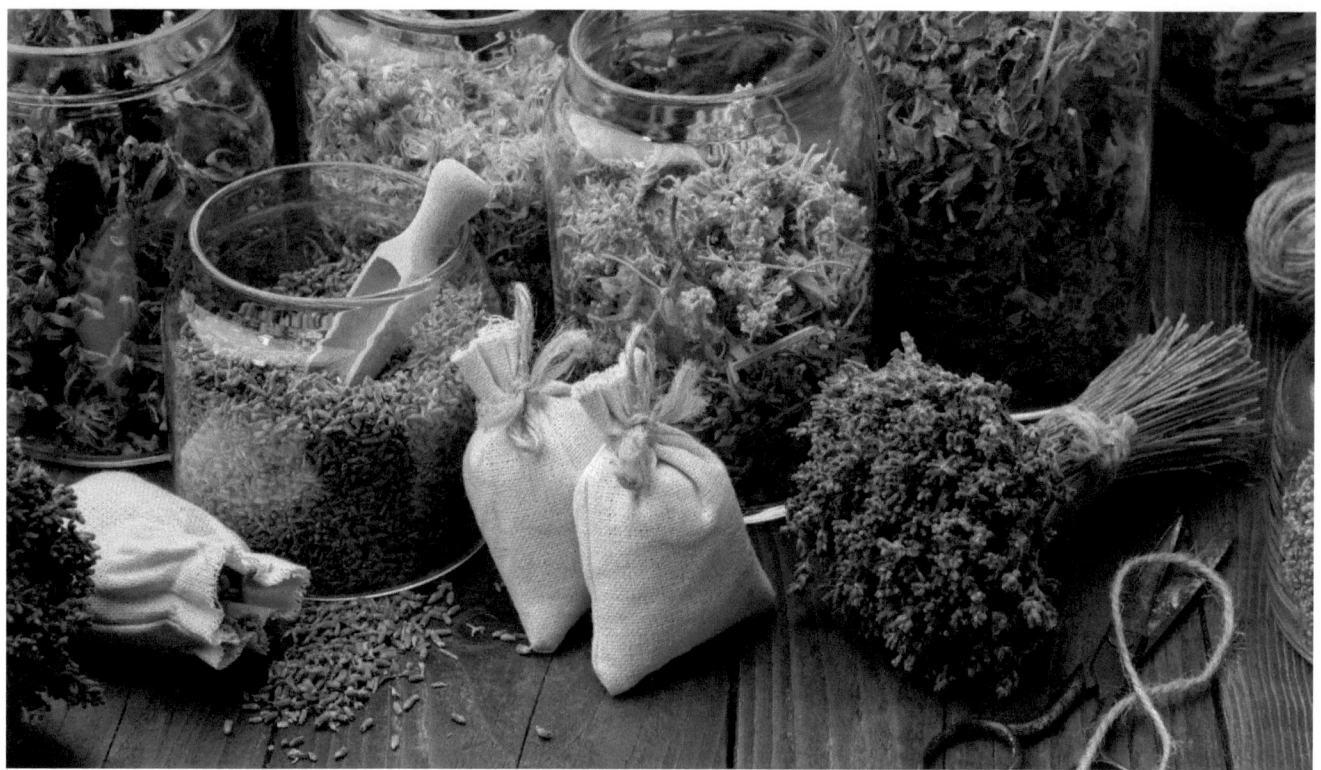

All herbs should be dried in direct sunlight, in a dehydrator, or in the oven at 180°F for 4–10 hours until dry. The oven must be turned off when herbs are fully dried.

The best way to store dried herbs is sealed in airtight jars. If you prefer to put them away in sealed packets, you can use aluminum foil or plastic wrap over the top of the packet.

Make sure that your jar lids are airtight before sealing them shut so that nothing can react with the herbs and cause chemical changes during storage which will alter their natural properties.

Remove any stems from freshly picked herbs. Any stems that remain on the plant will become bitter and will not store well.

A great deal of the healing power of herbs is lost when they are used as cooking ingredients. When using herbs as spices, it is best to use them fresh, as most of their medicinal properties are lost within a few days after drying. However, there are some exceptions, such as spearmint and thyme.

Equipment Needed

Here is the equipment needed when you use dried herbs:

- A mortar and pestle (or electric grinder)
- A large bowl or casserole dish to hold the herbs
- A spoon to help mix the herbs with the liquid
- Funnel to help pour your tincture into a bottle or container.

Bulk Herbs

Using bulk herbs is an excellent way to save money because you can buy them in bulk and make your own herbal medicine for the entire year. Herbs, however, are a living things, and each batch of herbs has a life span. If you purchase your herbs from the same dealer each time, then you'll get herbs with similar properties and potency. You can also purchase bulk herbs at a discount if you buy them in larger quantities, say by the pound or half-pound.

Quality Control Issues when Buying Dried Herbs

When buying dried herbs, a common complaint is that the quality can vary greatly from one batch to another because different herb suppliers may use different methods. Although this may be the case, you can still purchase herbs and mix them with alcohol and make a tincture that will work for any diseases that your family may be developing or dealing with.

To buy bulk herbs, you might have to visit herb shops in your area on occasion because each herbalist will use their own method of drying the plant material so that it doesn't lose its properties when you dry it out. In order to prepare the herb for use, you'll need to grind it with a mortar and pestle.

Unfortunately, herbalists don't label their herbs with what diseases they are good for. Because of this, you'll have to do some research into each plant l so that you will know how they can be used.

Capsules

The first step is to grind the herbs and then fill empty capsules with them. You can buy empty gelatin capsules at most health food stores;they usually carry a variety of sizes that you'll need when you create your herbal medicine.

Many herbs are too bitter or strongly tasting to take raw. For these herbs, it can be more pleasant to take them in capsule form.

Step-by-step instructions:

- In a mortar and pestle or in a blender, crush the chosen herb into approximately the consistency of a coarse meal. Store in a glass jar.
- Add a small amount of powdered vegetable glycerin. This adds to the body of the capsule so that it will dissolve more easily when swallowed, or it can be used along with an enema for cleansing.
- Fill the capsules 2/3 full with this paste. After this is done, add the remaining mixture to fill them completely (an extra 1/3).
- Store in a cool place until ready to use.

Tablets

You can also create tablets for acute problems such as an upset stomach. To do this, you'll mix an herb with gelatin and then shape the mixture into a tablet. You can crush the tablet into a powder before swallowing it, or you can mix it with water and drink it like tea.

Tablets are simpler to use than capsules, but they are less stable over time. You can get a longer duration from the more stable capsules.

Step-by-step instructions:

• Make an infusion. Using the method described in Making Infusions, combine dried or fresh herbs with filtered water to produce your mixture.

• For each tablet, combine the correct quantity of herb powder with powdered vegetable glycerin.

• Fold in a kitchen towel for several minutes until all the grains are completely embedded in the substance.

• Add approximately 1/2 teaspoon of any flavoring oil or butter to help facilitate swallowing. This may be necessary if you are having problems with tablets sticking to your tongue or throat after taking them.

• Using a spoon, scoop one-fourth of the mixture into rounded flat cherry-sized balls. These consist of about 1/8–1/4 teaspoon each.

• When done, wash your hands and dry them. To minimize the possibility of transmission, use your bare hands instead of a spoon to scoop up the mixture.

If you are unsure how these will affect you, first begin with 1/8th teaspoon doses for 24 hours, diluting if necessary with water on the second day. If it affects you adversely, increase to 1/4 teaspoon or less for 24 hours, then dilute again, if necessary, on the third morning.

Nut Butter Balls

You can make nut butter balls, which can be used to help heal coughs such as whooping coughs or to ease sore throats. You'll need to grind the nuts first, and then you'll mix them with organic honey or date syrup. The next step is to mix with dried herbs and then form the mixture into small balls before putting them into their containers.

Some people prefer the taste of nut butter. With the addition of a little powdered vegetable glycerin, it is possible to make nut butter-like balls yourself.

Step-by-step instructions:

• Combine the herb powder with powdered vegetable glycerin, just as you would for tablets-infused oil or butter. These are much tastier than plain nuts and have many times the potency of tablets eaten alone.

• Use 4–8 servings per batch for more potent medicine.

• Roll these into balls about 1/2" across and place them on a cookie sheet covered with waxed paper or tin foil to protect them from exposure to air or moisture.

• Refrigerate until you are ready to eat them or store them in a cool place for a longer time.

If you have trouble swallowing the nut butter balls, grate a little over-ripe banana on top of each one, and they will dissolve in your mouth without too much effort.

In conclusion, it is important to have a good herbal medicine cabinet because it contains natural medicines that will help your family when they are dealing with certain issues.

Remedies Preparations Making Extraction

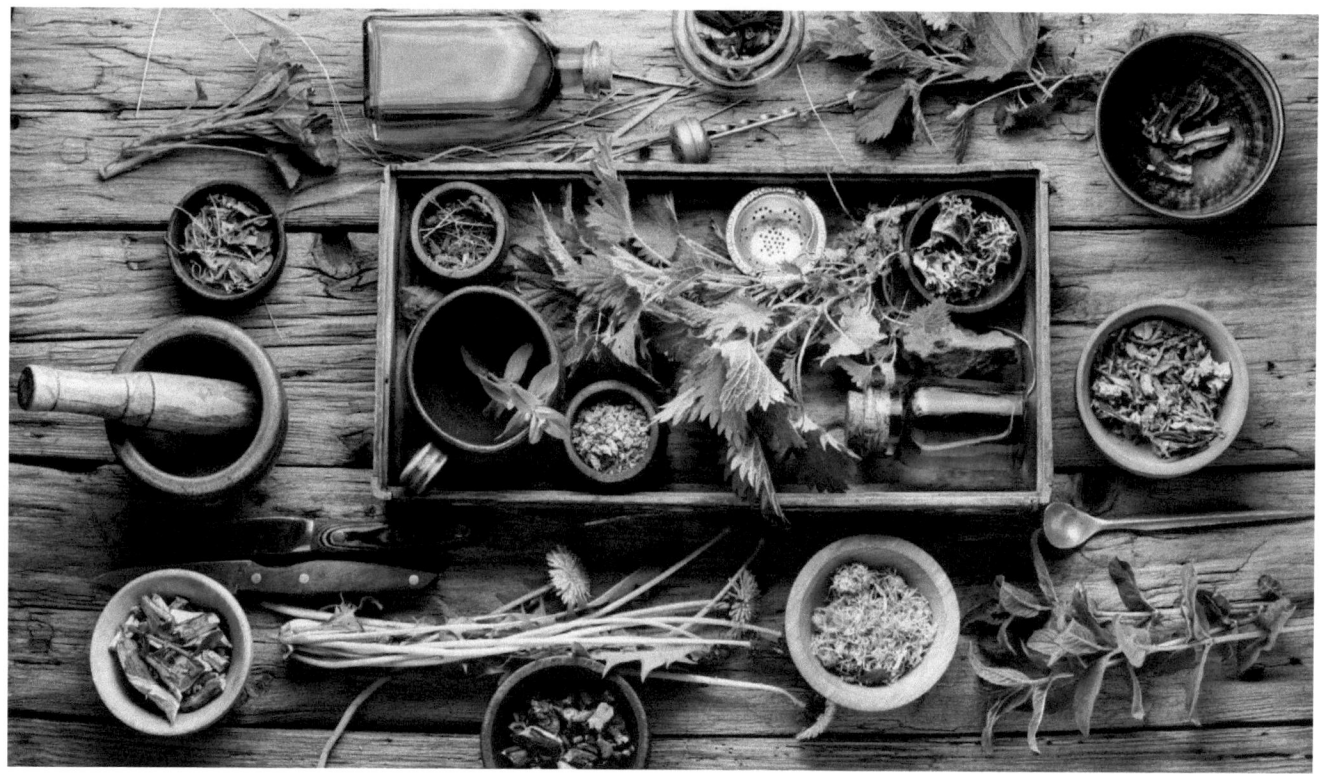

Water-Based Extractions

This is the most common method and is probably the easiest to use. For this type of extraction, it is best to prepare your herbs in the whole form or loosely ground so they will be easier to work with. Following these simple steps will help reduce the chances of killing off some of the plant's beneficial substances. Additionally, it may be helpful to choose high-proof alcohol that is suited for your intended use, such as Everclear (190 proof) or Everard (210 proof).

Infusions

Unless your herb is a leafy type, you will want to chop it up. If it is a leafy type, then you may simply tear or break off a piece to use in the infusion.

3. Fill a small saucepan with water and turn on medium heat.

4. Add your herbs to the water and let boil.

5. Simmer for 10–15 minutes according to your recipe or until water has absorbed all of the essential oils from the plant material.

6. Turn off the heat and set aside to cool before straining out herbs with a cheesecloth or fine mesh strainer.

Decoctions

7. Chop your herbs into small pieces to help release the active components within.

8. Place herbs in a pot and cover with water, then bring to a boil while reducing the heat as needed (you may need to add more water during this process).

9. Let it simmer until very little liquid remains, about 15–20 minutes; At this point, do not allow it to evaporate off completely to avoid the risk of burning off some of the plant's beneficial substances.

10. Strain through cheesecloth or muslin cloth into another container, squeezing any remaining liquids out of your herbs.

11. Decanting: Pour the mixture from your cloth or cheesecloth back into the pot, then fill a container with alcohol and pour it over the herbs.

12. Cap and label, letting it sit for 2–3 weeks in a dark place at a warm temperature such as 65°-85°. Shake it daily, if possible, to extract all of the beneficial substances out of the herbs.

Syrups

13. Place your herbs in a pot with water, then bring to a boil while reducing the heat as needed (you may need to add more water during this process).

14. Let it simmer until very little liquid remains, about 15–20 minutes; At this point, do not allow it to evaporate off completely else to avoid burning off some of the plant's beneficial substances.

15. Strain through cheesecloth or muslin cloth into another container, squeezing any remaining liquids out of your herbs.

16. To make a syrup, combine 1 part water to 1 part alcohol in a saucepan; boil until it reaches the desired consistency and strength of your desired herbal remedy.

17. Decanting: Pour the mixture from your cloth or cheesecloth back into the pot, then fill a container with alcohol and pour it over the herbs.

18. Cap and label, letting it sit for 2–3 weeks in a dark place at a warm temperature such as 65°-85°. Shak it daily, if possible, to extract all of the beneficial substances out of the herbs.

Alcohol Extractions

There are two distinct ways of making alcohol extracts. The first is by using a double boiler in which the herb sits directly on top of the boiling alcohol. This method works best when the herb is finely ground to release as many of its beneficial components as possible. Alcohol burns off at a higher rate than water, so it'll need to be reduced somewhat after you have added your ground herbs into the pot.

The alcohol types that you can use for this purpose are wine, vodka, beer, and brandy. Some strains of the plant will work with less alcohol than others. The key with these extracts is to make sure they are not too hot, and that you do not let the herb sit too long at a high temperature as this can actually damage your extract.

Tinctures

For this process, it is best to use Everclear (190 proof), Everard (210 proof), or any higher-proof alcohol you can find.

19. Place your herbs in a pot with alcohol and place the pot on the stove on medium-high heat. Add enough alcohol to just cover the herbs; occasionally stir until all of the material has been dissolved. Adding hot water can help build pressure and release more of the active components from your herbs, while cold water will slow down this process.

20. If necessary, reduce the heat to low and let it simmer for about 40–60 minutes; ensure that the alcohol does not burn off during this process.

21. Strain through cheesecloth or muslin cloth into another container, squeezing any remaining liquids out of your herbs.

22. To make a tincture, add 1 part alcohol to 1 part water in a jar and shake for 30 seconds before placing the lid on tight and keeping it in a dark, room-temperature area for at least 2 months before using; shake well before each use to extract all of the beneficial substances out of the herbs.

Dried Herbs Tinctures (Macerations)

This process is similar to making tinctures, but instead of using alcohol-primarily, the herb is soaked in an herbal liquid for 1–2 months. The goal in this process is to release as many of the active components as possible while preserving their original beneficial properties.

23. Place your herbs in a jar and fill with a concentrated herbal liquid such as alcohol or vinegar; cover with the lid and shake well before each use to extract all of the beneficial substances out of the herbs.

24. Allow it to sit for 30 days, shaking daily if possible. After 30 days, strain through cheesecloth or muslin cloth into another container, squeezing any remaining liquids out of your herbs.

25. To make a tincture, add 1 part alcohol to 1 part liquid in a jar and shake well before each use to extract all of the beneficial substances out of the herbs.

Fresh Plant Tinctures (Macerations)

26. Grind your fresh herb

27. Fill a jar a little less than halfway with your ground herb.

28. Fill the empty space in the bottle with a high-proof alcohol (Everclear should be used if you are just starting out.) but keep an eye out for this as it evaporates faster than water.

29. Shake the bottle to blend the components well for around 10 minutes, then close with a lid and let it sit in a warm place for at least 4 weeks. Shake regularly every few days to help release active ingredients from plant material, etc.

30. After 4 weeks, strain through cheesecloth or muslin into another clean bottle, then add 1/4 cup of glycerin (optional) and re-cap tightly.

31. Label and date your new herbal extract and store it in a dark place (kitchen cabinet) for future use.

Glycerin Extracts (Glycerites)

Glycerin is an emollient; it acts to soften skin, making it more supple by helping the skin retain moisture. Glycerin also increases smoothness in formulations for the treatment of rough, dry, or cracked skin.

How Glycerites Are Made

32. In a jar, cover your herbs with vegetable glycerin; close with the lid and shake well before each use to extract all of the beneficial substances out of the herbs.

33. Allow it to sit for 2–4 weeks, shaking daily if possible; after this time has passed, strain the mixture through cheesecloth or muslin cloth into another container, squeezing any remaining liquid out of your herbs.

34. Cap and label, letting it sit for 2–3 weeks in a dark place at room temperature before using; shake well before each use to extract all of the beneficial substances out of the herbs.

Seales Simmer

This method of extracting a medical tincture follows the same principles and methods as above but with great modifications. For instance, in this method, the herbs are placed into a simmering pot on low heat instead of the oven, filtered through a muslin cloth or cheesecloth before placing into an amber jar.

35. Place your herbs in a container with water and calcium water (1 teaspoon of calcium carbonate for every quart); place the pot on the stove on low heat to begin the heating process.

36. Continue to heat the water throughout the duration of your mixture while stirring every few minutes; then turn off the heat and allow to cool before placing the herbs in a freezer.

37. Place the herbs in the freezer for 3–5 days, stirring daily to ensure that all of the beneficial substances are extracted from your herbs.

38. After 3–5 days, remove your herbs from the freezer and place them through a muslin cloth or cheesecloth into another container, squeezing any remaining liquids out of your herbs.

39. Cap and label, letting it sit for 2–3 weeks in a dark place at room temperature before using; shake well before each use to extract all of the beneficial substances out of the herbs.

Extracting in Vinegar

40. Place your herbs in a pot with vinegar; place on stove on medium-low heat to begin heating process.

41. Continue to heat the vinegar throughout the duration of your mixture while stirring every few minutes; then turn off the heat and allow to cool before placing the herbs in a freezer.

42. Place herbs in the freezer for 3–5 days, stirring daily to ensure that all of the beneficial substances are extracted from your herbs.

43. After 3–5 days, remove your herbs from the freezer and place them through a muslin cloth or cheesecloth into another container, squeezing any remaining liquids out of your herbs.

44. Cap and label, letting it sit for 2–3 weeks in a dark place at room temperature before using; shake well before each use to extract all of the beneficial substances out of the herbs.

Topical Preparations

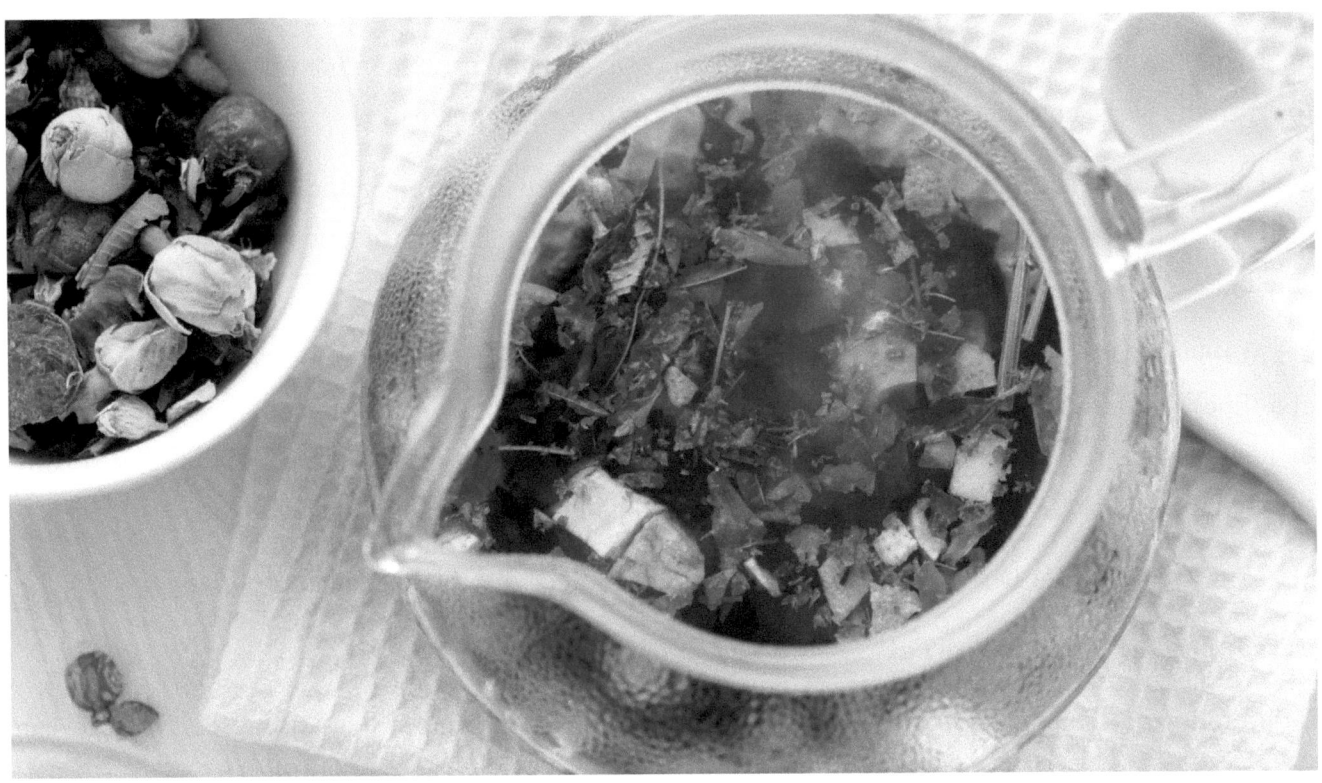

What Is a Topical Preparation?

Topical preparations are made from plant material that is prepared in a way so that it can work topically on the body. For example, a topically applied preparation could be made by macerating herbs in a carrier oil and then applying the oil to the skin (a topical ointment) or by grinding herbs into powder and then applying that powder to the skin (a topical scrub) or by boiling plants whole, seeds, bark, leaves, etc. of their appropriate genus in water and then applying the solution to dry areas of skin for local application (for example foot soak). This preparation would typically be applied before bedtime or during hot weather for foot care.

Oil-Based Herbal Preparation

Making an herb oil preparation is fairly easy and only takes a few minutes to a few hours of your time and small equipment.

Equipment

- Mason jar with lid, grinder (mortar and pestle, coffee grinder, hammer, or stone)
- Stainless steel or glass pot/pan (if using stovetop)
- Spoon, cheesecloth, or other strainer bags (like a coffee filter)
- Funnel
- Glass bottle to store finished product in

Ingredients:

- Fresh herbs that can be ground finely or have leaves that can be chopped easily. A good ratio is 2–6 tablespoons of herb to 1 cup of carrier oil.

Process:

45. Grind the herbs in a mortar or coffee grinder if possible. If not, use a hammer or stone in a glass bowl to crush the herbs until fine and then transfer the herbs to a small pot/pan.

46. One of my favorite methods is to put everything but the oil in a mason jar and then put that jar on top of a stove burner on low heat and leave it simmering for about an hour until it starts to change color and smell.

47. At this point, you can remove the lid and pour off about half of the liquid into a strainer bag (1/2 cup at a time) to remove debris and let it drain. When you have strained out all the liquid, pour it into your blender with the rest of your oil. Blend everything at low speed until it is fully mixed and then strain again through a cheesecloth or other strainer bag to remove all of the ground herb bits and pieces.

48. Now you have your herbal-infused oil! Pour it into storage bottles and label appropriately.

Extracting Herbs in Oil or Fat

A different way to prepare a topical herbal preparation is to soak the herbs in oil or fat. This method can be very simple or very complex, depending on what you want out of your preparation. If you are making a salve, then the process should be fairly quick and simple. If you are making an infused oil for internal use, then it should take considerably longer. For a salve, simply combine equal parts herb and oil (or fat) and heat until the herbs become saturated.

Local Applications

The most commonly used topical applications are salves and ointments. Salves are greasier and typically made with beeswax, lanolin, or other plant waxes as a base. Ointments are typically oilier and can be made in a variety of ways but typically include some sort of vegetable oils or animal fat (like lard). Another easy way to make an herbal ointment is to mix melted shea butter or cocoa butter with an infused oil.

Herbal salves and ointments have been used historically for both internal and external applications such as scrapes, cuts, burns, dry/cracked skin, bleeding wounds, bug bites/stings, etc.

Other Applications

- **Concentrates:** with the term concentrate, herbalists refer to a type of medicinal preparation which possesses a high concentration of the beneficial ingredient, or active principle that can be found in a certain strain of herb. Concentrates can be used in different ways: they can be ingested when dealing with problems such as an upset stomach or some kind of infection, they can be used when making teas or they can be used to make baths. Concentrates can often be found in the form of infusions or decoctions, the difference between these two preparations is that infusions are prepared mixing dried herbs with hot water, while decoctions are made using the same principle but instead of using dried herbs, herbalists use fresh plants. Concentrates are very versatile and can be used to make tinctures, tease and baths.

- **Lozenges:** these types of medicinal preparations are usually found in the shape of small tablets that can be placed inside the mouth and sucked on in order to slowly release their active principles. Mostly, they consist of finely powdered medicinal herbs combined with an emulsifier, water, volatile oils and a sweetener, like for example honey. Lozenges' medical use is to treat conditions that affect the mouth or the respiratory tract, like a cough or a sore throat.

- **Chinese Preparations:** Chinese school of traditional medicine is characterized by a large amount of different types of preparations. Some of the most common techniques to consume medicinal herbs is to use raw or heated herbs for tea balls or tea bags. These balls or bags can either be placed and steeped in hot water as infusions, or they can be placed in boiling water to make extracts. An interesting technique coming from this school of medicine is the use of bamboo baskets that are filled with hot water and herbs in order to make healing teas.

How to Store Herbs and Keep Them Safe

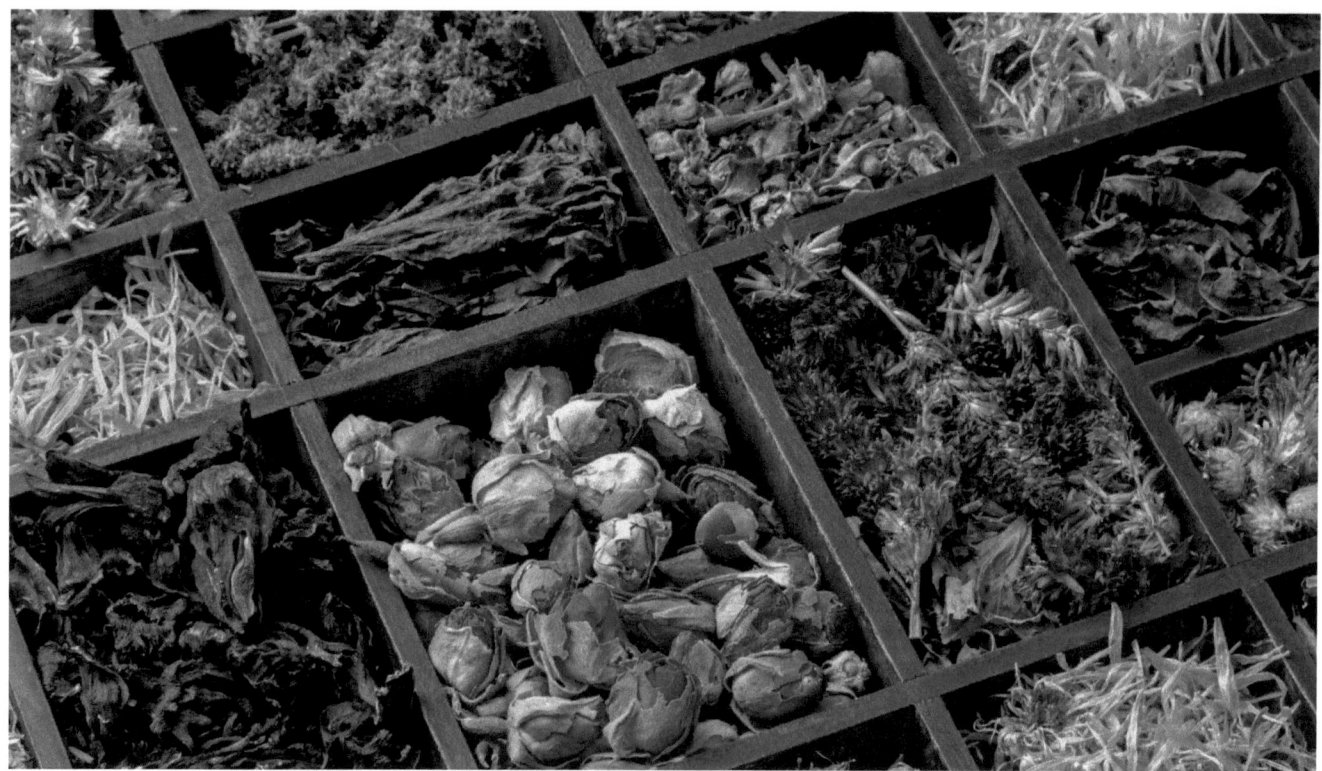

Herbs, even when dry, are highly perishable and will easily lose their benefits if not properly prepared and stored.

Since fresh herbs lose their potency in just a few days, most herbalists dry them for storage. To dry herbs, remove the leaves from the stems and spread them out on a clean, flat surface in loose, single layers.

Plants that are bulkier may be hang from a line in a dry area like a warm basement or attic. Since flies and other insects may be drawn to herbs, you should cover them with cheesecloth.

The shorter the drying time, the better because herbs lose their potency very easily. It takes around a week on average.

When an herb has lost its fragrance but is still dry enough to crack, it is considered sufficiently dry. You dried it too long if it crumbles absolutely when you treat it.

Roots, which should be thoroughly washed before drying, take a little longer to dry than leaves and flowers—about three weeks on average.

Store them in glazed ceramic, dark glass, or metal containers with tight-fitting lids until they've dried. The essential oils can be absorbed by plastic bags or food storage containers.

Keep Your Herbs Potent

Your stored herbs are vulnerable to sunlight, air, heat, moisture, and reactive metals like aluminum, tin, and copper.

They deplete the herbs' strength and potency over time. Herbs should be kept in a cool, quiet, and well-ventilated place, such as a kitchen cabinet, pantry, or cellar.

We all know the difference between vine-ripened and gassed tomatoes because we've eaten and compared them. Always use the best-quality herb you can find when making medicinal for long-term storage, such as tinctures, oils, and salves, and make small quantities before you get a feel for the medication.

Nothing is more frustrating than finding a five-year supply of ineffective tinctures on hand. It isa waste of your time, the plant's resources, and your money, and it may even be dangerous if you are using the tincture for medicinal purposes.

Storing Herbs

Prepare your herbs for storage as soon as possible after harvesting them. Herbs left out for even a few hours can deteriorate in quality.

Shake the Dirt Off

Remove any dead leaves or debris. Remove the stems from the leaves and the seeds from the chaff. Roots should be washed and blotted dry before being spread out to dry. Roots should be cut into 1-inch-thick sections, while leaves and flowers should be left whole as much as possible.

The Benefit of Clear Glass Jars

Consider storing your herbs in clear glass jars to keep a close eye on them. Then you will be able to spot some color changes, which are a sure sign of corruption. Just make sure the jars are kept hidden behind a curtain or door in the dark.

Different Methods of Storage

There are many ways to preserve your herbs.

Drying

The simplest and most effective way to store your harvest is to dry it. It does not necessitate any special materials or equipment.

You just need a well-ventilated area away from direct sunlight and wind. To allow air to flow through the drying plants, gather the herbs into 1-inch-diameter bundles and secure them with rubber bands or strings.

Then hang them in a shady, dry location with good ventilation.

The essential oils are drawn into the leaves by hanging them upside down. Keep several bunches of herbs well-spaced when drying them on a line.

Tiny quantities of herbs may also be placed inside paper bags.

The bags absorb a lot of moisture while still protecting the herbs from the light. Every day, shake or stir the herbs until they are dry. When drying seeds, this is particularly useful. Cut a drainage hole in the top of the bag if the plant has a lot of moisture.

Stapling sheer curtains to a frame can also be used to create simple screens. Lay the herbs out to dry on a thin sheet.

For loose blossoms and leaves, this screen is ideal. Simply pass the herbs to airtight containers such as glass jars once they are crispy-dry.

You might make a birch-bark box if you're a purist. Mold-inhibiting agents are found in the bark of the paper birch, making storage easier.

Freezing

Another method of storing and preserving the harvest is to freeze it. For a minute, blanch the herb in boiling water. Then drain the herb and quickly immerse it in ice water to cool it down. Drain once more.

Spread the herb in a thin layer on a tray and put it in the freezer to quick-freeze to avoid a quart-size lump of frozen herb. Place it in freezer containers and just take out as much herb as you need at a time.

Extracting or Tincturing

Tincturing is one of the most basic and time-honored methods of preserving herbs for medicinal use. A tincture is a liquid herbal extract that can preserve your herbs for months or even years if done correctly. Apple cider vinegar and alcohol are the two most popular substances for making tinctures.

If you're going to use alcohol, make sure it's at least 40%. If you don't want to use alcohol or have liver issues, raw, organic apple cider vinegar can be used instead.

Vinegar-based tinctures have a shorter shelf life, whereas alcohol-based tinctures will last for years. If you're looking for a particular action or part of the herb you're using, you should select your solvent carefully.

Infusions of Herbs

One of my favorite apothecary techniques is herb-infused oils. Most of them can be used in the kitchen to enhance the flavor of dishes, while others are ideal for use in herbal skincare items.

Canning

Some herbs can be made into syrups, jams, or preserves, which can then be canned to prolong their shelf life. Consider Elderberry preserves, Hawthorn berry jam, and violet flower syrup, both of which are medicinally useful and can be easily stored.

Herbal Butter

Another traditional way of preserving herbs for use in the kitchen is to make herbal kinds of butter. Chop down your herbs and fold them into the butter before freezing them for later use.

You can either spread the herbal butter out on a sheet of the freezer or parchment paper, form the butter into a cylinder, and freeze that for later use.

Conclusion

From foregoing discussions, it clear how important it is to acquire enough knowledge, not only about the herbal plants that could treat numerous medical conditions, but also about the diseases that they could possibly treat. It might be surprising that the common beliefs are wrong, correcting these beliefs is a start. Learning and studying these health conditions would make a person realize how different they are when they were first presented or taught. Nothing is simple, they could all lead to severe complications, and this also sheds some light on the importance of the right diagnosis. A normal person might see a headache as just a headache without thinking that there are numerous types that could result to different effects. Proper diagnosis is important and getting the right knowledge about It must be ongoing.

Herbal medicine never fails. It could cover much more than what a hospital could, in terms of treating inoperable conditions. It is also a beautiful sight to see a single herb treating various conditions, considering the fact that they could be harvested anytime and anywhere. They are reliable and they were also proven through time. It is one of the greatest inheritances given to the twenty first century world. The magic that herbal plants have will make a person believe. They might start by just a mere belief to believing that traditional medicine conquered its superiority through time by garnering its position back. Moreover, it is best to use these herbal plants because they are cheaper, and a person can have overall control from planting, to harvesting, to preparation, to storing, and to applying, it can all be done by a simple person.

Medical conditions are always there, they will go away, same with how quick the population of herbal plants spread. It is important to focus on organic and fresh treatment, because too much processing and too many chemicals could harm the body. It is also great to learn about the treatments of common diseases that could occur any day or any time. And with the limitations raised to humans these days, it is great to know that they have a remedy near their homes, protecting them.

Herbal plants will always work on these diseases. They will not fail. Nonetheless, they must be taken carefully and thoroughly. Learn them, how they work, how they are prepared, and how they are made. They must also be taken in the right manner and with proper guidelines. With these knowledge, a person could also automatically know which diseases they could possibly treat and they can live with pure nature and less chemicals. And in this age, that is one of the healthiest lifestyles that is offered freely.

BOOK 8: HERBAL REMEDIES FOR CHILDREN

Introduction

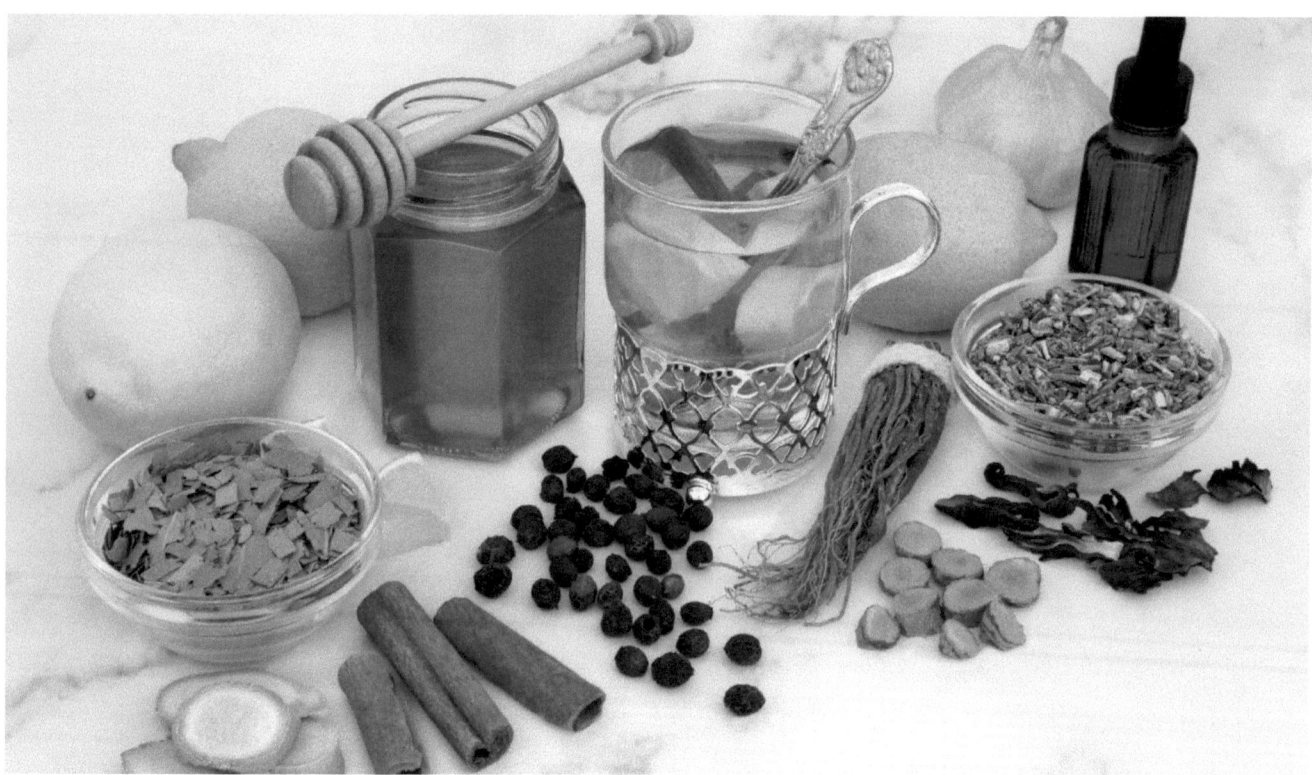

Native American herbalists were powerful healers and herbal remedies for the Native Americans are still used today. Many easy-to-find herbs can effectively combat a variety of childhood ailments, such as colds, headaches, fever, bruises, and sprains.

There are many cost-saving ways in which parents can help their children stay healthy without going out of pocket to purchase expensive medicines or vitamins. One such way is by using Native American Herbalism Remedies for Children.

When children come down with an ailment, they often want immediate results. Native American herbal remedies are easy and convenient to administer, also most of the time, they do not require exact measurements. Parents should note that although these types of remedies are natural and free from harmful chemicals and preservatives, herbs can cause mild side effects. Parents should closely monitor adjustments to the normal dosages of herbs, as some may have adverse reactions to medications. It is also important for parents to keep an updated list of their children's allergies in a prominent location in their homes so that they do not inadvertently give their children any harmful substances or medications.

Native American herbal remedies are made of easy-to-find plants and usually have a single active ingredient that can cure the ailments of many children. To administer these types of medications, all needed is boiling water, 1 glass or plastic cup, and some key ingredients. The way the remedy is prepared varies depending on the type of ailment being treated and the form it takes, such as balm or tea. For example, when treating fever and colds, it is best to use herbal tea to help soothe the throat.

There are no specific ingredients in herbs that are harmful or dangerous for children in almost any dosage. The main concern with herbal remedies is that they are not regulated by the Food and Drug Administration (FDA), so there may be harmful or poisonous substances or misapplication of an herb for a certain ailment. Native American herbal practitioners use herbs that have been used for generations, but parents should note that herbs are not a substitute for medicine. Herbal remedies have different effects from person to person depending on the individual's body chemistry.

The most common household plants used as Native American herbal remedies are St. John's Wort, plantain, and chamomile.

To prepare the herbal remedy; boil water, steep the herbs, and strain. Do not add any sugar or milk because Native Americans did not use those additives. Alcohol is never used in these remedies.

Native American herbal remedies for children when used properly can help treat many childhood maladies. Parents need to choose an herb for their ailment and take it at the proper dosage. There are also many ways to apply herbal remedies that make them more convenient for parents and children, such as applying them topically.

It is also important to remember that some herbs may have side effects, so it is best to check with a pediatrician to rule out any other causes of the ailment before administering herbal remedies.

Although Native American Herbalism Remedies for Children can have some beneficial effects and may be used to help an adult, they should not be used to treat an infant. Native American herbalists recommend that precautions should always be taken when using any remedies or natural plant-based products for children. For example, one must attempt to rule out other causes of a child's illness before giving them herbs. Also, it is important to note that even though these types of medications can help a child sleep better, they should still expose him or her to natural sunlight daily.

Native American herbalists and doctors do not prescribe Native American Herbalism Remedies for Children without first researching the possibilities and side effects of each herb. Many of these herbalists will test each herb individually on themselves to rule out any allergies or reactions before using it. Some individual herbs can have some side effects, such as stomach upsets or diarrhea, but may be taken from a small dosage or used in a certain way to prevent these symptoms from occurring.

The word of a Native American herbalist or doctor is considered sacred and should be relied upon for any diagnosis or treatment of any ailment. Although Native American herbalists have been using these remedies for centuries, scientists still have not completely studied every herb in detail and so, some unknown dangers could exist. One must consult a doctor at least before embarking on any course of action, although indigenous people do not place much faith in Western medicine and do not recommend it.

When used properly, these remedies can treat many ailments in children. They help the child feel well and encourage him or her to stay healthy, which can allow them to fight certain illnesses with their immune system a little more effectively. As long as these remedies are used by people who have extensive experience in using them, they can be very beneficial to both the child and his or her community.

15 Herbs Perfect For Your Children's Health

Almost every herb safe for an adult is also safe for a child if the dosage is modified to account for the child's smaller size and weight. On the other hand, herbs with a gentler action are better suited to children's sensitive constitutions. The herbs in this chapter are the ones most frequently suggested for children. They're typically thought to be safe and harmless, with no lingering effects or side effects in the body. These "gentle" plants can be extremely powerful and effective, but they are less abrasive than other therapeutic herbs or medications. These herbs generally promote the body's intrinsic ability to repair itself through strengthening the immune system, fortifying the neurological system, and in a variety of other ways. They should be the cornerstone of children's natural health care.

1. Anise (*Pimpinella anisum*)

Parts used: The seeds are the most important part, but the leaves are also useful.

Benefits: Anise has been cultivated for over 4,000 years and has a long medicinal plant and culinary spice history. It is generally used as a warming digestive aid and carminative (gas-expelling) herb. It can also treat minor urinary infections and as an expectorant (a substance that helps discharge mucus) for respiratory problems. It has a sweet licorice flavour that most kids appreciate.

Suggested uses: Tea can be used to treat colic and other digestive issues. Anise is frequently combined with less tasty herbs to make them more appealing due to its sweet flavour. It makes a delicious syrup.

2. Astragalus (*Astragalus membranaceus*)

Part used: roots

Benefits: Astragalus is the young person's ginseng because of its adaptogenic (resistance-building) and toning properties. Astragalus stimulates the deep immune system by helping to repair the bone marrow reserve that regenerates the body's protective shield, while echinacea helps the immune system's initial line of protection. Numerous studies have demonstrated its efficacy in assisting young children who are undergoing chemotherapy or radiation therapy.

Suggested uses: Astragalus is best used as a tea to assist patients in overcoming long-term illness and poor energy and to maintain and strengthen immunity. The root resembles the tongue depressants prescribed by doctors, and children may enjoy chewing on it like a licorice stick. It can be added to soups and broths by simply placing a root or two (whole or chopped) in a pot and simmering for several hours.

3. Catnip (*Nepeta cataria*)

Parts used: leaves and flowers

Benefits: While catnip causes pleasure spasms in cats, it is a wonderfully soothing herb for humans and is used to alleviate a variety of stress. It is particularly good for decreasing fevers and alleviating teething pain. It is also a digestive medicine that helps with indigestion, diarrhoea, and colic. Because catnip is peaceful, relaxing, pain alleviating, and mild, it is widely suggested for youngsters.

Suggested uses: Teething pain might be relieved by drinking this tea throughout the day. To make catnip more appetizing, combine it with plants with a pleasant flavour, such as oats and lemon balm, or mix it with fruit juice. Before meals, take a few drops of catnip tincture as a digestive help. Before sleep, a few drops of the tincture can help settle a cranky kid. This is one of the greatest herbs for reducing childhood fevers; it can be used as a tincture or an enema.

4. Chamomile (*Matricaria recutita, Anthemis nobilis*, and related species)

Parts used: The blooms are the most important part, although the leaves are also useful.

Benefits: This tiny plant is a miracle worker when it comes to healing. It possesses a high concentration of essential oil that functions as a potent anti-inflammatory agent in its flowering tops. The flowers produce a beautifully relaxing tea that is also helpful for the digestive system. It is especially beneficial for digestive issues brought on by stress, such as colic.

Suggested uses: To soothe a tense or nervous youngster, provide chamomile tea sweetened with honey throughout the day. A massage oil prepared with chamomile essential oil can be used for similar relaxing benefits and it also relieves painful, achy muscles. A few drops of chamomile tincture before feeding time will assist digestion.

Caution: Even though chamomile is generally believed to be safe, it is a part of a composite family, and some people are allergic to plants in this family. Do a test before introducing chamomile to your child if he or she is really sensitive and allergic.

5. Dill (*Anethum graveolens*)

Parts used: primarily the seeds, but the leaves are tasty.

Benefits: Dill gets its name from the Old Norse word Dilla, which means "to lull," It has a reputation for relaxing and reassuring babies and toddlers. Dill is a terrific digestive aid, and it is even better in getting rid of gas. It is one of the most well-known herbs for helping youngsters with gastrointestinal discomfort, colic, and anxious digestion. Dill is high in manganese, magnesium, and iron, and it also includes calcium.

Suggested uses: Dill is a widely used culinary herb. It is also good in tea, either alone or in combination with other herbs.

6. Echinacea (*Echinacea angustifolia, E. purpurea*, and related species)

Parts used: roots, leaves, flowers, and seeds.

Benefits: Echinacea boosts the body's first line of defense against infection by enhancing macrophage T-cell activation. It is one of our most vital immunity boosters and infection fighters. Despite its potency and effectiveness, it is safe for youngsters to use, with no documented negative effects or residue buildup.

Suggested uses: Echinacea is most effective when administered at the outset of infection or when precautions are necessary (for example, if everyone at daycare is sick, keep your child home and give her echinacea!). Give echinacea in tea or in tincture form at the first sign of a cold or flu to increase immunity and help ward off the infection. It works best when given in tiny, frequent doses; for example, adults should take a teaspoon of tincture or a cup of tea every 30 to 40 minutes, with a child's dosage adjusted appropriately. It can also be used as a tea or tincture to treat respiratory and bronchial infections in children, as well as in a spray to relieve sore throats. Use the tea or diluted tincture as a mouthwash flavoured with peppermint or spearmint essential oil for sore gums and oral inflammation. While echinacea is most effective when taken orally, it can also be used externally to treat skin diseases as a wash or poultice.

Caution: Echinacea, like chamomile, belongs to the composite family and can produce allergic reactions in some people. Do a test before introducing echinacea to your child if he or she is really sensitive and allergic. Note: Due to the high demand for this herb, it has been ruthlessly plundered from its natural environment and is becoming increasingly scarce in the wilds; therefore, avoid wild-harvested echinacea. Instead, go with a reputable company that sells cultivated echinacea, preferably organically grown. Even better, cultivate your own.

7. Elder (*Sambucus nigra*)

Parts used: berries and flowers.

Benefits: During the flu season in Europe, you will see a wide range of elderberry remedies on drugstore shelves. Though every part of the plant has a purpose, my favourite is the rich blueberries. The berries are high in both vitamin A and vitamin C, and they play an important role in immune system health. They also have a lot of flavonoids and anthocyanins, which protect the heart and boost the immune system. In addition, the berries (as well as the blossoms) have antiviral qualities. Elder is typically used to treat colds and flu, but it can also treat upper respiratory infections. It is frequently mixed with echinacea in immune-boosting treatments.

Suggested uses: Elderberries provide some of the greatest syrup you will ever taste, and it is also useful as a medicine. Elderberries also create a pleasant and colourful immune-boosting tea (it will need to be sweetened or mixed with fruit juice to appeal to most children). The blossoms are frequently used in fever-relieving drinks.

Caution: There are numerous types of an elder; choose the one with blue blossoms rather than red. The red elder is a somewhat poisonous plant. Blue elderberries should be cooked rather than taken raw, as the seeds contain a minor toxin that can cause gastrointestinal discomfort and even poisoning if consumed uncooked in large quantities.

8. Elecampane (*Inula helenium*)

Part used: roots.

Benefits: Elecampane is an expectorant (a substance that clears mucus from the lungs and relieves congestion in the respiratory system) that can be used to treat coughs, bronchitis, and persistent lung infections. When used with echinacea, licorice, and marshmallow root, it is extremely beneficial for coughs. Add a little valerian, a muscle relaxant, to the combination if the cough is extremely spastic or repetitive. Try treating a respiratory or bronchial infection with a mixture of elecampane and pleurisy root if it does not respond well; this combination is often successful for even the most stubborn lung infections.

Suggested uses: Elecampane is not extremely tasty, so use your imagination when cooking it for kids. To make tea, it can be combined with other more flavorful herbs, such as licorice and marshmallow root. Sweeten with honey or maple syrup and a pinch of cinnamon. If you are going to use the elecampane-pleurisy combo, combine the tinctures in equal parts and let the child drink it with water, tea, or fruit juice.

9. Fennel (*Foeniculum vulgare*)

Parts used: primarily the seeds, but the leaves and flowers are also used.

Benefits: This licorice-flavored herb is well-known as a carminative and digestive aid and for its capacity to enhance and enrich milk flow in nursing mothers. Fennel is also an effective antacid, neutralizing excess acid in the stomach and intestines and clearing uric acid from the joints, reducing inflammation and arthritic pain. It is a wonderful digestive aid that helps with digestion, appetite regulation, and gas relief.

Suggested uses: Fennel tea is a delicious way to cure colic, improve digestion, and eliminate gas from the system. Nursing moms can boost and enrich their milk flow by drinking two to four cups of tea every day. Use a wash of warm fennel tea that has been strained well through a fine-mesh strainer to treat eye irritation and conjunctivitis. Fennel is frequently mixed with other less aromatic herbs to make them more appealing because of its sweet licorice-like flavor.

10. Hawthorn (*Crataegus oxyacantha, C. monogyna,* and related species)

Parts used: fruits, flowers, leaves, and young twigs.

Benefits: Hawthorn, which is high in antioxidants, aids in developing a strong immune system. It is thought to be a superb heart tonic since it strengthens and nourishes the heart. Hawthorn is effective as a preventative for heart disease and treatment for heart disease, oedema, angina, and arrhythmia. It can also be helpful in times of loss and can help us get through difficult situations in life. Hawthorn is a wonderful herb for youngsters, despite its reputation for adults with heart problems and the elderly. It nourishes the blood, boosts the immune system, promotes clear vision, and can help a youngster cope with grief and loss.

Suggested uses: When turned into a sweetened syrup or jam, hawthorn is delicious. When combined with other herbs like hibiscus, oats, and lemon balm, it produces a delicious tea. Because it has an astringent flavour, it may need to be sweetened. Alternatively, you might use it as a tincture.

11. Hibiscus (*Hibiscus sabdariffa* and related species)

Part used: flowers.

Benefits: Vitamin C, bioflavonoids, and antioxidants are abundant in hibiscus flowers. It aids in restoring and maintaining overall health and immune support function and prevents colds and cases of flu. It can also treat mild anaemia and impaired circulation because of its high bioflavonoid and vitamin C content. The brilliant red colouration of the hibiscus flower makes it a great source of anthocyanins, which are beneficial to vascular health. The flower has long been used in North Africa to preserve respiratory health and treat respiratory infections and sore throats. Aside from that, hibiscus tea is one of the most beautiful natural beverages, and most youngsters appreciate it.

Suggested uses: The ruby-red tea is made from the huge hibiscus blossoms. The flavour is tart with a sweet aftertaste, and children may prefer it sweetened. Make a thick syrup out of hibiscus flowers and mix it with sparkling water for a brilliant red drink. It is tasty and refreshing, plus it is also good for you!

12. Lemon balm (*Melissa officinalis*)

Part used: leaves.

Benefits: This delightfully scented member of the mint family is one of nature's best nervine herbs, calming, antiviral, and antibacterial. It is one of the most important natural antiviral plants, and it is used as a light sedative in times of depression and mourning. It is very good for recurrent herpes, shingles, and thrush outbreaks, and it can also be used as a preventative if taken regularly.

Suggested uses: Though lemon balm can be dried, the flavour is finest when it is fresh. Lemon balm can be tinctured or encapsulated, but it is most commonly used as tea due to its refreshing, agreeable flavour. The tea can be used with lemon and honey throughout the day to relieve stress and anxiety and prevent herpes, shingles, and thrush (all related viral infections). Any viral infection, including measles and mumps, requires this treatment. Combine equal parts lemon balm, oats, and chamomile to make a delightful nervine tonic tea. Hawthorn can be added to this blend to help someone who is grieving. To treat mild to moderate depression, add St. John's wort to the mix. Fresh lemon balm makes a wonderful syrup (see), which may be used to make a delightful spritzer or all-natural soda by mixing it with sparkling water.

13. Licorice (*Glycyrrhiza glabra*)

Part used: roots.

Benefits: Licorice has high antiviral qualities, making it a great treatment for herpes, shingles, thrush, measles, and mumps, among other viral infections. For this purpose, it is frequently mixed with lemon balm. It is a calming and therapeutic cure for sore throats, respiratory, viral, and gastrointestinal inflammations such as ulcers due to its high gummy content and anti-viral and anti-inflammatory qualities. It also has modest laxative qualities, making it useful for mild constipation.

Suggested uses: Licorice is a sweet herb frequently mixed with other herbs to make them more appealing. On the other hand, licorice root is often overly sweet when consumed alone; therefore, it is combined with other herbs to reduce the sweetness. Licorice makes a delicious syrup (see) that can be used with sparkling water to make a refreshing soda. Children adore chewing on licorice sticks, and you can even give a teething baby a "stick" of licorice root to gnaw on — though you may need to give the root a few "chews" yourself to soften it enough for the child to bite on. It can usually keep a teething baby occupied for a short period.

Caution: Those with hypertension or Syrups renal/bladder problems, as well as anyone undergoing steroid therapy or using the medicine for a heart or kidney ailment, should avoid licorice.

14. Marshmallow (*Althaea Officinalis*)

Parts used: The roots are the most valuable part, but the leaves and blooms are also useful.

Benefits: Marshmallow, like slippery elm, can be used in herbal medicines as a relaxing, cooling demulcent, but it is much more readily available and easy to grow. Marshmallow root is anti-microbial as well as anti-inflammatory. It soothes swollen, irritated membranes and is frequently used in tea blends and tinctures to treat sore throats, respiratory infections, and digestive irritation.

Suggested uses: For sore throat, digestive irritation, bronchial inflammation, diarrhoea, or constipation, make a tea with it. Marshmallow is a urinary tract tonic that is frequently prescribed for urinary tract and bladder infections. It can also be used externally: make a thick paste with water to heal burns and irritated skin, or mix it with oatmeal to make a soothing wash or bath for irritated, itchy, dry skin.

15. Nettle (*Urtica dioica*)

Parts used: Fresh leaves and young tops are the most common ingredients, but roots and seeds are often used.

Benefits: Nettle has a wealth of vitamins and minerals. It is a particularly good source of iron and calcium, and it is used to help pregnant and nursing women regain these vital nutrients (for this purpose, mix it with raspberry leaf, another good nutritious and a female reproductive tonic). The calcium in the nettle is in a biochelated state that is easy to absorb, making it particularly beneficial for stress relief and nerve healing. When combined with creamy green oats, it is extremely good for nerves. Nettle is also beneficial for tissue and bone healing and is frequently used with oats and horsetail for this purpose. It helps maintain dense bone growth and can help ease growing pains in young children due to its high calcium and mineral content. It is also a great treatment for allergies and hay fever, and some people have reported that it works wonderfully for them. The herb nettle root is well-known among men for its ability to enhance prostate and sexual health.

Suggested uses: Nettle is commonly boiled, tossed with olive oil, lemon juice, and a pinch of feta cheese, and served as a mineral-rich side dish during meals. It can be used in any recipe that calls for spinach or other cooked greens. It must, however, be steamed entirely and thoroughly; otherwise, it will "sting" if undercooked. The little hairs on the underside of the nettle leaf and the stems are packed with formic acid, which causes the skin to swell and results in a painful, itchy rash, similar to that caused by bee stings. Wear gloves when picking nettles, avoid brushing up against them, and teach your children to appreciate this plant. If someone is stung, use a poultice made from plantain leaves to pull the poisons out. Although nettle can be used as a tincture or tea to treat allergies, freeze-dried nettle appears to be the most beneficial. Combine freeze-dried nettle capsules with nettle tea and tincture when possible for a more potent impact.

Herbal Remedies for Children of 0-2 Months

Gripe Water

Ingredients:

- 2 1/3 cups water
- 1 ½ slice ginger
- 2 tsp. chamomile, dried
- 1/2 tsp. cardamom, dried
- 2 tsp. crushed fennel
- ½ tsp. coconut sugar
- ¼ tsp. cinnamon
- ¼ tsp. clove

Instructions:

1. Pour water into a deep pot at a high flame and let it boil.

2. Add all the ingredients except for cinnamon, sugar, and clove in a cloth and tie a knot.

3. Place the tied cloth in boiling water and remove the pot from the flame.

4. Cover the pot and let it steep for 1 hour.

5. Take out the cloth from the water and stir in the remaining ingredients and mix well.

6. Transfer the solution into the glass jar and seal it.

7. Place the jar in the freezer and freeze it.

8. Shake well before using and give ½ teaspoon to your child.

Homemade Powder for the Soft Skin of Newborn

Ingredients:

- 2 tbsp. kaolin clay (natural absorbent, uses as the base for baby powder)
- 2 tbsp. powder arrowroot (natural adsorbent)
- 3 drops essential oil, chamomile (safe to use with soothing and anti-inflammatory properties)
- 3 drops lavender oil

Instructions:

1. Add the kaolin clay and arrowroot to a bowl and mix well.

2. Now, mix in the oils and combine the mixture well.

3. Shift the powder into a bottle.

Yarrow Recipe for Babies

Ingredients:

- 1 tbsp. elderflower
- 1 tbsp. yarrow
- 1 tbsp. peppermint

Instructions:

1. Mix the flour, peppermint, and yarrow in a bowl and toss well.

2. Shift the mixture to a storage container.

3. The yarrow balm is ready!

Note: The balm can be used as an anti-inflammatory and anti-microbial agent in case of fever or injury.

Herbal Remedies for Children Of 2-12 Months

Creamsicle Bath

Ingredients:

- 3 tsp. sweet orange essential oil
- ¼ cup lukewarm water
- 2 tsp. vanilla oleoresin essential oil

Instructions:

1. Add sweet orange essential oil, about 3 drops, with 2 drops of vanilla oleoresin essential oil in lukewarm water and stir well.

2. Bathe your child with this water and let him enjoy the freshness and soothiness that he will get after taking a bath.

Herbal Bath

Ingredients:

- 1 tbsp. peppermint
- 1 tbsp. lavender
- 1 tbsp. chamomile
- 1 tbsp. lemon balm
- Warm water, as required

Instructions:

1. Add a mixture of peppermint, lavender, chamomile, and lemon balm into a cloth and tie a knot to keep the content inside.

2. Place the knotted cloth in warm water that you will use to give a bath to your baby. Stir well.

3. First, clean the burnt area with cold water using a cotton cloth.

4. Then, add a few drops of lavender in water and wash the burnt area with this lavender water.

Note: Lavender gives a soothing effect on the burnt area, acts as an anti-microbial, and enhances the skin repair system. This herbal bath is a good source of antiseptic and skincare for your baby.

Remedy for Teething

Ingredients:

- 5 tsp. chamomile
- 3 tsp. vegetable oil

Instructions:

1. Combine a few drops of chamomile and vegetable oil in a small bowl.

2. Now, take 2 teaspoons of the blend in a mini bowl and add cool water. Mix well.

3. Apply the mixture over the baby's gum using a cotton cloth.

4. Massage the area well. This will help to soothe the area and make the gum soft and reduce teething pain.

Baby Powder

Ingredients:

- 4 cups cornstarch
- 1 tbsp. kaolin clay
- 1 tbsp. rose geranium essential oil
- 4 cups arrowroot powder
- 1 tbsp. sweet orange essential oil
- ½ tbsp. ylang-ylang essential oil

Instructions:

1. Combine cornstarch, kaolin clay, and essential oil of rose geranium, arrowroot powder, essential oil of sweet orange, and essential oil of ylang-ylang in a bottle.

2. Close the lid of the powder bottle and shake well to blend all the ingredients.

3. Apply on the skin of the baby but remember, don't apply directly. First, transfer the powder into your hands and then use them to apply the powder to the desired area.

Note: This powder absorbs unnecessary moisture from the skin, and rose geranium will give a floral essence to the skin. The powder will keep the skin of the baby smooth and silky.

Herbal Remedies For Children Of 12 Months-5 Years

Rosy Roll-on

Ingredients:

- 3 tsp. rosewood
- 2 tsp. rosehip oil
- 2 tsp. rose absolute

Instructions:

1. Combine rosewood, rosehip oil, and rose absolute in a bowl and mix well.

2. Transfer the mixture into the roll-on bottle and apply when required by the kid in the summer.

Leg Roller

Ingredients:

- 3 tsp. cedar wood
- 2 tsp. jojoba oil
- 2 tsp. rosewood
- 3 tsp. sweet marjoram

Instructions:

1. To give relief to your kid in bed from itching or any restlessness, mix cedar wood, jojoba oil, rosewood, and sweet marjoram. Shake them well and transfer them into the roll-on bottle.

2. Apply before bedtime and enjoy your sleep.

Yoga Ground Inhaler

Ingredients:

- 5 tsp. frankincense
- 3 tsp. cypress
- 3 tsp. rosewood

Instructions:

1. Combine frankincense, cypress, and rosewood in an inhaler. Use it to enhance the immune system of your kid.

Palmarosa Calming Aroma

Ingredients:

- 6 tsp. coconut oil
- 2 tsp. jojoba oil
- 4 tsp. sandalwood
- 4 tsp. Palmarosa oil
- 1 tsp. patchouli
- 1 tsp. rose geranium
- 1 tsp. absolute oil

Instructions:

1. Combine any body lotion (unscented) with coconut oil and jojoba oil along with sandalwood and Palmarosa oil each. Also, add patchouli, rose geranium, and absolute oil.

2. Shake everything well to get a smoothly blended mixture.

3. Apply when needed to soothe the body of your kid.

Herbal Remedies for Children of 5 Years to 12 Years

Carrot Puree

Ingredients:

- 2 cups chopped carrots
- ¾ cup water
- ¼ tsp. nutmeg

Instructions:

1. Boil water in a pot over a medium flame.

2. Add the carrots and cover to cook it for 10 minutes. Let it cool.

3. Place the boiled carrots, 1/2 cup of liquid, and nutmeg into a food processor.

4. Add liquid to adjust the consistency of the mixture to the desired level.

5. Serve your child and let him enjoy it.

Note: It is a source of beta-carotene, which protects the health of the eyes, and an antioxidant source to keep immunity strong and provides calcium to keep bones strong.

Apple Nutmeg

Ingredients:

- 2 cups chopped apple
- ¼ tsp. nutmeg

Instructions:

1. Combine nutmeg and chopped apple in a bowl and steam it for 20 minutes to get a puree.

2. The apple-nutmeg puree is ready to use for your baby.

Note: Apples are a rich source of vitamin C, antioxidants, and fibers and strengthen the immune system. While nutmeg has inflammatory and antioxidant properties.

Pear-Nutmeg Puree

Ingredients:

- 1/3 cup water
- 1 tsp. nutmeg
- 2 cups pear, chopped

Instructions:

1. Add 1/3 cup of water, a pinch of nutmeg, and 2 cups of chopped pear in a pan and mix well.

2. Cover the pan and let it cook for 20 minutes over medium flame with occasional stirring.

3. Remove the pan from the flame and let it cool down.

4. Blend the mixture in the food processor to obtain a smooth puree.

Note: The combination of nutmeg and pear will help your baby in digestion and give relief to his tummy.

Colic

Ingredients:

- 2 tsp. chamomile
- 2 tbsp. lavender
- 2 tbsp. almond oil

Instructions:

5. Add 2 drops of chamomile and lavender in a bowl with 2 tablespoons of almond oil. Mix them well.

6. Rub this oil as messaging oil over the tummy and the back of the baby to give a soothing effect to make him relax.

Ear Aches

Ingredients:

- 1 tsp. almond oil
- 1 tsp. lavender oil

Instructions:

1. Combine 1 teaspoon of almond oil and 1 drop of lavender oil.

2. Use cotton buds to clean the ears of the baby using the solution you just made.

3. Secondly, you can also use the mixture to massage the baby's ear from the backside of the ear to soothe him.

Fevers

Ingredients:

- 6 tsp. chamomile
- 5 tsp. lavender
- Lukewarm water, as required

Instructions:

1. Combine lukewarm water with 6 drops of chamomile and lavender in a bowl.

2. Dip the baby wipe in the water mixture and wipe your baby to reduce the temperature.

3. Be patient and continue using the mixture to lower the temperature.

Lemon Bath

Ingredients:

- 3 tsp. grapefruit essential oil
- 3 tsp. lemon juice

Instructions:

1. Add 3 drops of grapefruit essential oil and lemon in warm water and stir well.

2. Bathe your baby with this water to keep his skin healthy.

Baby Lotion

Ingredients:

- 2 tbsp. coconut oil
- 2 tbsp. coconut butter
- 3 tsp. lavender essential oil
- 2 tsp. chamomile essential oil

Instructions:

1. Melt coconut oil and coconut butter in steam water and stir in 3 teaspoons of essential oil of lavender and 2 teaspoons of chamomile oil. Mix to combine well.

2. Keep the mixture aside for a while to cool down.

3. When cooled down, beat the mixture using a beater till the mixture is fully whipped.

4. Shift the mixture into the container. The baby lotion is ready.

Conclusion

As stated repeatedly throughout this book, it would be foolish to consider natural remedies as a substitute for conventional medications, especially when it comes to children and their illnesses. Children can't always communicate effectively, so it is critical that parents understand the seriousness of what is happening and, as a first option, decide to seek medical attention to figure out how best to help their child.

However, children often suffer from minor ailments or discomforts that can easily be treated with all-natural, homemade remedies. These remedies can give them relief, whether it is a skin rush or an intestinal disorder. And we can give them relief without using medicines that are sometimes unnecessary.

Nature offers us so many remedies that we just need to know and use them. And we can do it even when it comes to our children, instilling in them the healthy habit of daily care of the body in a natural way.

This is in no way in conflict with traditional medicine, but rather is a complementary way to give wellness to our body, even and especially when it is not sick.

I hope the remedies listed in this book will help alleviate yours and your children's discomfort.

BOOK 9: EVERYDAY HERBAL REMEDIES

Introduction

Herbal treatments help the body mend itself naturally and ease discomfort. If you have a medical problem, there are a number of herbal medicines that can safely ease your discomfort without causing any negative side effects.

The wonderful thing about herbal medicines is that they solely include organic components. There are no chemicals or medications in them. To address your medical concerns, herbal remedies employ natural therapies rather than chemicals or prescription pharmaceuticals.

Similar to how people now utilize herbal treatments to treat a variety of problems, ancient people employed herbal medicines to treat illnesses and afflictions. In reality, in ancient cultures, it was usual to locate natural plants and plant extract-based cures for ailments.

We are constantly assaulted with advertisements that claim to make our bodies younger, slimmer, and fitter. Modern medicine, we're taught, can treat almost every condition. Because herbs are so easy and natural, many of us turn to them for health and longevity.

Herbal medicines aren't just beneficial for your health; they're also good for your mind. Herbal medicines have been utilized for a range of conditions throughout history, including pain reduction and healing. Herbal treatments are being used to treat tiredness, sleeplessness, nausea, and other ailments.

Because they're so popular these days, it's a good idea to use them at least twice a week to enjoy the advantages. Herbal medicines and recipes have the advantage of being adaptable to your specific needs. Depending on your needs, you can reduce or enhance the dosage of herbs. You should always see a doctor before beginning to use herbs, but herbal formulas may be trusted to give the desired outcomes.

Herbal medicines are available in a variety of formats, such as tablets, teas, and powders. For added advantages, many individuals opt to take herbal treatments as teas or mix them with water.

The following are some of the benefits of taking herbal remedies:

- they often have no side effects or adverse consequences
- they are inexpensive
- They are sealed to keep them fresher for longer.
- There are several herbal cures for a variety of ailments, including sore throats, colds, toothaches, stomach aches, and more.
- Many do not require a prescription or doctor's clearance since they are natural solutions to many common diseases.

Best Common DIY Herbal Tea Recipes

Herbal teas make up a wide range of medicinal treatments used by Native Americans. These are sometimes pleasant to enjoy, and other times a bit bitter. Whenever you enjoy one of these teas or drinks, if necessary, you can adjust the taste through the use of some honey. A bit of honey or stevia allows you to sweeten up the drink without adding artificial or processed sugars.

As you read over these herbal teas, remember that you can always adjust the time that you steep the drink. You can also change the amount of herbs if desired to make a tea stronger or weaker. Before you consume any herbal teas, however, make sure they are safe for you and your usage. Pregnant and nursing women should always check whether the herbs they are consuming are safe.

Juniper Tea

The juniper tree has been known as the medicine tree for a good reason. Native Americans relied on it to provide them with food, medicine, and shelter. However, keep in mind that juniper tea and berries can be dangerous during pregnancy.

Treats:

High blood sugar, digestion problems, bloating, intestinal worms, UTIs, and kidney and bladder stones.

Ingredients

- Juniper (20 tender sprigs; they should be young)
- Water (2 quarts)

Instructions

1. Prepare the sprigs, washing them gently to ensure there is no debris or insects left on the leaves.

2. Place the clean sprigs and water into a big enough pot to fit it all. Allow the water to come to a boil.

3. Once boiling, cover the pot, then reduce the temperature and leave it to simmer for 15 minutes.

4. Take the pot off of the heat and leave steeping for 15 minutes.

5. Strain the liquid, then serve. It can be sweetened with honey or sugar.

Mint Tea

Mint was used regularly by Ojibwe women. It was regarded as medicinal and enjoyable.

Treats:

Burns, boils, worms, or parasites

Ingredients

- Fresh mint sprigs (10 large stalks)
- Water (2 quarts)

Instructions

1. Begin by preparing the herbs. Give them a gentle clean to remove any dirt or debris.

2. Fill a saucepan with water. Then, place the mint in the pan.

3. Bring the water to a boil. Then remove from the heat and leave steeping for 5 minutes, covered.

4. Strain the liquid and serve. Sweeten if necessary.

Honey Drink

This drink was enjoyed in the summer months and was a favorite for children.

Treats:

Sore throats

Ingredients

- Water (1 quart)
- Honey (⅔ cup)

Instructions

1. Combine honey and water in a large container that will fit both with an airtight lid.

2. Shake well to combine the ingredients.

3. Chill and serve iced.

Apricot Tea

Apricots were introduced by English settlers in the 17th century. They were quickly adopted for the healing properties of the apricot oil, known to be good for treating swelling and ulcers.

Treats:

Constipation, inflammation, heart issues

Ingredients

- Apricots (20 fresh)
- Water (2 quarts)

Instructions

1. Boil water. While the water is boiling, wash the fresh apricots well. Then, place the apricots into a large pot.

2. Pour the hot water over the apricots.

3. Let cool just enough so you can touch the mixture without burning yourself. It should still be hot. Place a straining cloth over another pot, then strain the mixture through it, smashing the pulp out of the apricots as you go.

4. Enjoy it while it's still warm.

Sassafras Tea

Sassafras tea tastes like a light root beer. It has been used widely to treat many different ailments noy just because it tastes good, but it has great benefits for the people as well.

Treats:

Colds and fevers

Ingredients

- Water (4 cups)
- Sassafras (6 roots)

Instructions

1. Ensure the sassafras roots are well-washed and clean from any remaining soil.

2. While washing the roots, bring water to a boil in a big enough saucepan to fit everything.

3. Once the water comes to a boil, place the roots in the pot. Allow the roots to boil until the water is red and aromatic.

4. Enjoy sweetened with honey if desired.

Medicinal Pine Needle Tea

White pine has been used medicinally by many Native American tribes. Turning it into tea allows for the treatment of many colds and the flu.

Treats:

Colds and cases of the flu. Serves as an expectorant and decongestant.

Ingredients

- Water (1 cup)

- Chopped fresh pine needles (1 Tbsp.)

Instructions

1. Gather your pine needles. They should be young. Then, remove the papery brown bits that sit at the base of the needles, where they attach to the twigs. They should come right off.

2. Chop up the needles into little pieces, roughly ¼ inch long.

3. Begin boiling your water in a small saucepan. When the water comes to a boil, place the needles into the water and cover with a lid.

4. Leave the needles to boil for 3 minutes.

5. Take the saucepan off of the heat and leave the water steeping while covered up until the liquid is cool enough to begin drinking. Enjoy fresh and warm.

Burdock Root Tea

This tea was used by the Lakota tribe to help treat a wide range of ailments.

Treats:

Liver disease, inflammation, respiratory infections, and stomach disorders.

Ingredients

- Burdock roots (8 to 10)
- Water (2 cups, distilled)
- Honey (1 tsp, or to taste)

Instructions

1. Put burdock root into a teapot. In a saucepan, bring water to a boil.

2. Let the boiling water cool for a moment or two before pouring it into the teapot.

3. Steep tea for 10 minutes. Then, enjoy the tea with sweeteners added to taste.

Lung Tea

This tea combines several herbs known and commonly known to be effective in clearing out lungs in many cases.

Treats:

Congestion and lung issues

Ingredients

- Bee balm (1 tsp, dried)
- Anise hyssop (1 tsp, dried)
- Peppermint leaf (1 tsp, dried)
- Mullein leaf (1 tsp, dried)
- Marshmallow leaf (1 tsp, dried)
- Water (2 cups)

Instructions

1. Bring two cups of water to a boil. Then, pour in the dried herbs.

2. Leave the mixture steeping for 15 minutes, while inhaling the steam.

3. Strain the tea, then sweeten it with honey as needed.

Hawthorn Tea

Hawthorn tea is commonly used by Native Americans for many medicinal uses. The flowers and leaves are easily brewed into a tea that has been used to treat ailments of the heart.

Treats:

Heart conditions

Ingredients

- Hawthorn leaves (½ tsp)
- Hawthorn flowers (½ tsp)
- Boiling water

Instructions

1. Place the herbs into the bottom of a cup.

2. Boil water. When boiling, pour it into the cup, over the herbs.

3. Let the tea steep for at least 15 minutes (up to 30 minutes).

4. Strain the tea leaves. Then enjoy, sweetening with honey if necessary.

Buck Brush Tea

Cherokee healers recognized buck brush as an effective kidney stimulant that gives a diuretic effect. They used this to help flush out the kidneys and lower blood pressure.

Treats:

High blood pressure

Ingredients

- Buckbrush root (dried and ground, 2 tsp)
- Water (1 cup)

Instructions

1. Place two tsp. of dried buck brush root that has been ground into each cup being used. Then, for every cup, add in 1 cup of boiled water. Let the water steep for 5-15 minutes, then strain.

2. Enjoy sweetened with honey if desired.

DIY Personal Care Herbal Recipes

This chapter will offer you an overview of the various herbal recipes and strategies for personal care.

Yucca Shampoo

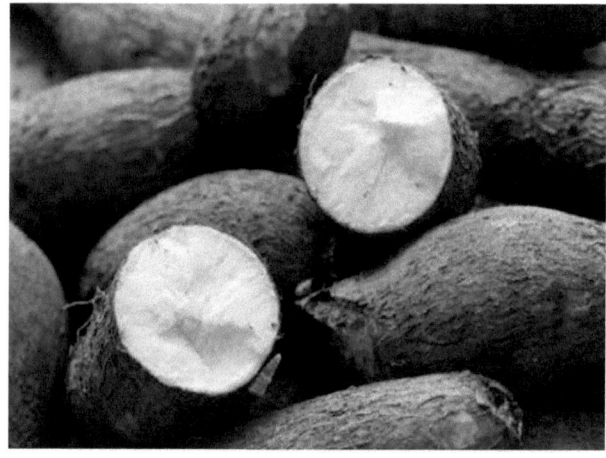

Yucca is indeed the common title for the genus Yucca, which contains over 40 plant species. Medicine is created from the non-flowering plant's root.

Osteoarthritis, migraine headaches, high blood pressure, high cholesterol, intestinal inflammation (colitis), diabetes, stomach issues, gallbladder diseases, and liver are all treated with yucca.

Some individuals apply yucca straight to the skin for wounds, sprains, skin problems, joint discomfort, bleeding, dandruff, and balding.

In producing carbonated beverages, yucca extract is utilized as a foaming plus flavoring ingredient. Many yucca chemicals have been employed in the development of novel medications.

Chemicals found in yucca may aid in the reduction of high blood pressure as well as cholesterol. It may also help alleviate arthritic symptoms, including pain, edema, and stiffness.

Yucca was a vital plant for the Ancestor Pueblo people due to its numerous users. The plant's roots were peeled and mashed to make a frothy pulp. The pulp was combined with water and employed in the production of soap or shampoo.

Ingredients

- Tap water/ distilled water 4 cups
- Yucca root 1/2 cup/ medium size roots 2

Directions

1. Wash your hands.

2. Chop the roots into large chunks.

3. Cut up the dice into little pieces. Because the pulp is rather stringy, blending it in little pieces is the best option.

4. Fill the blender halfway with water.

5. Toss in the yucca root.

6. To get as much soap as possible, blend everything together completely.

7. Drain the liquid and filter the particles using a strainer.

8. Save the pulp for your garden or use it to produce paper.

9. Fill the bottle with liquid soap using a funnel.

Wild Rose

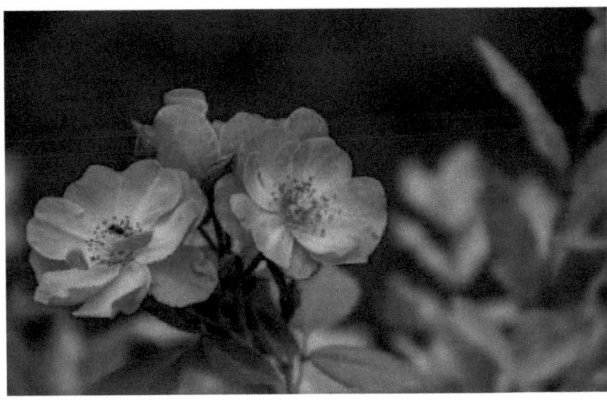

Rose exudes a legendary aura. She symbolizes love, beauty, protection, and elegance and is linked with saints and gods. Rose legends are deeply linked in human history wherever she blooms — from China towards the Middle East through Europe to the native Americas. After all, she seems to be an old soul who has lived for 35 million years and witnessed the fall and rise of numerous civilizations. Since ancient times, her tremendous presence has reigned in poetry, art, song, and religious ceremonial, and her influence continues to reign now.

Ingredients

- Honey 1 jar
- Wild rose ½ cup

Directions

1. Gather fragrant petals and let them wilt for a day or two till they become half-dry. Fill a glass jar using petals and a tight-fitting cover.

2. Warm honey gradually upon the stovetop till it is extremely liquid but not hot.

3. Fill the container with enough honey to fully surround the flowers. Cap.

4. Put in a warm location in the garden or on the vent.

5. Give it a good stir and wipe the moisture from underneath the lid. This will be beneficial.

6. Get rid of any extra water in your honey.

7. After about 2-3 weeks, strain using a muslin cloth. Tea may be produced from the crushed petals and sipped or soaked in for a delightful "rose honey" bath.

8. Honey should be kept inside a glass jar together in a cold, dark location. Some people prefer to keep their honey in the refrigerator, although this isn't required if your honey doesn't contain too much water.

Wild Rose Toner

Rose is said to be the most skin-balancing of all plants. This old-fashioned formula can compete with today's high-priced face care products. The bark of a witch hazel tree is both astringent and therapeutic. Water is used to extract it, with around 15% alcohol added as a preservative. Several herb shops, natural food stores, and pharmacies carry it.

Ingredients

- Wild rose ½ cup
- Witch hazel extract 1 jar

Directions

1. Put wilted/wild rose dried petals in a glass jar.

2. Using witch hazel extract, fully cover the surface.

3. Put a cover on the rose mixed with witch hazel jar and set it aside for at minimum two weeks.

Shake every couple of days to ensure that the drug is evenly distributed throughout the fluid.

4. Strain and store inside one glass jar/spray bottle with a muslin cloth. Label. To tighten pores and for balanced skin, spray or apply this liquid upon the face as a pleasant astringent. If you wish to add more rose aroma and medication to this extract, you may put 25% rose water.

Honey Face Mask

This face mask works wonders upon the scars and dark areas. It's also quite simple to make. The usage of honey as a face mask by Native Americans is depicted in this recipe.

Its anti-inflammatory properties help eliminate excess oil from the surface; when used daily, it will balance your skin's micro-organisms. It may be used as a spot remedy to help with obstinate outbreaks and even autoimmune skin disorders like eczema and psoriasis.

Ingredients

- Lemon Juice ½ tsp.
- Raw Honey 2 tsp.

Directions

5. Mix the lemon juice plus honey in one mixing bowl.

6. Allow this mix to settle on your face for several minutes.

7. Allow for almost 20-30 minutes of resting time.

8. Rinse.

9. Because lemon juice is such a powerful substance, you should only use it 1-2 times each week.

Aloe Vera and Almond Oil Face Mask

Almond oil is used to manage dry skin problems such as eczema and psoriasis for ages. Acne is reduced. Fatty acids in the oil might help break down excess oil upon the skin, while retinoids in the oil help decrease acne and enhance cell turnover. Aids in the reversal of sun damage.

Enzymes, antioxidants, and vitamins A plus C are abounding in Aloe Vera, which could also help with burns, dry skin, acne, and various other skin problems. It's also quite inflammatory. Aloe Vera is unquestionably beneficial to the skin with all of such advantages.

Ingredients

- Aloe Vera Gel 1 tsp.
- Banana 1 tsp.
- Almond Oil ½ tsp.

Directions

1. This mask is excellent for moisturizing and hydrating as well as addressing dry, flaky skin.

2. Mash a banana using a fork inside one mixing dish.

3. Put 2 tbsp. of aloe vera gel into the mix.

4. Stir till all the items are well blended.

5. Mix 3 tablespoons containing almond oil to the mix.

6. Make a thorough mix.

7. Apply to a clean surface.

8. Allow approximately 15 minutes of resting time.

9. Rinse

Coffee and Turmeric Face Mask

Caffeine and antioxidants are the two key advantages of this mask. Caffeine aids in alleviating inflammation, such as puffy eyes, whereas antioxidants make the skin brighten. Turmeric's most active ingredient, curcumin, has a long list of scientifically documented health benefits, involving the ability to boost heart health and protection against Alzheimer's and cancer diseases. It has anti-inflammatory/antioxidant properties. It may also assist in dealing with depression and arthritic problems.

Ingredients

- Instant/ Ground Coffee 1 tbsp.
- Greek Yogurt 1 tbsp.
- Powdered Turmeric 1tbsp

Directions

1. Mix all the items.

2. Apply to the entire face, including the area around the eyes.

3. Allow for a 20-minute rest period.

4. Using a warm, wet cloth, remove it

DIY Herbal Remedies for Pets

Pet care is essential since pets are an integral part of our lives. Our dogs have a variety of issues, which can be treated naturally by following herbal recipes.

Treatment for Fleas

Ticks and fleas are most commonly seen in cats and dogs, and they can be treated by bathing them in the following solution:

Flea Treatment with a Body Bath

Ingredients:

- 40 drops rosemary extracts, essential oil
- 40 drops sage extracts, essential oil
- 1 cup unaromatic herbal conditioner

Directions:

1. In a large mixing basin, combine the solution and the basic oil, stirring thoroughly with a whisk or a beater.

2. Transfer it to a plastic jug with a pressing top using a pipe.

3. While washing your pet, add a small amount of the body bath to your pet's body, changing the amount used to cover it completely.

4. Wait for 2 to 5 minutes before washing away the body bath with cold water. Increase your use of it for better results.

Diarrhea

Diarrhea is common in pets, and it can be readily treated by following the recipe below:

Catnip and Sienna Tea for Diarrhea in Pets

Ingredients:

- 1 oz. dried senna leaves
- 1 cup water
- 1 tsp. dried catnip
- 1 tbsp. honey

Directions:

1. Bring the water to a boil and pour it into a cup.

2. Place all the herbs in the cup and cover it with a lid for a few minutes.

3. After a while, strain the tea and add the honey when the herbs have beautifully mingled in the water.

4. Drink this tea 3 to 4 times a day, and your pet's ailment will be solved.

Animal Injuries

Our pets are prone to getting bruises and injuries from time to time. The following solution is simple to use in treating this condition.

Hyssop Poultice for Pet Injuries

Ingredients:

- 2 tsp. fresh hyssop leaves

Directions:

1. Apply the fresh hyssop leaves to the injury and massage for 15 minutes.

In just a few days, you'll get extraordinary results.

Coughing in Animals

Cough is also fairly prevalent in many pets, and the following recipes can readily cure it.

Elecampane Root Tea for Cough in Dogs and Cats

Ingredients:

- 1 cup water
- 1 tsp. dried elecampane root
- 1 tbsp. honey

Directions:

1. Bring the water to a boil and pour it into a cup.

2. Place all the herbs in the cup and cover it with a lid for a few minutes.

3. After a while, strain the tea and add honey when the herbs have beautifully mingled in the water.

4. If you give this tea to your pet 3 to 4 times a day, it will cure their cough.

Home Herbal Recipes

The purification of a home is a priority for every single person. However, as noted below, numerous concerns frequently develop in our homes and must be addressed.

Mold Production on The Ceiling

Mold growth can be a problem, especially when the rainy season begins because mold growth begins quickly, and our ceilings and walls can be a hotspot for this unpleasant growth.

Garlic and Thyme Compress to Prevent Mold Growth on Walls and Ceilings

Ingredients:

- 1 cup water
- 2 tsp. dried thyme
- 2 tsp. fresh garlic

Directions:

1. Fill a pan halfway with water and bring it to a boil.

2. Add the garlic and thyme and cook for a few minutes, covered.

3. Strain the infused water into a mug using a cheesecloth.

4. Clean the moldy spots with a cotton swab dipped in the compress for fifteen minutes. Within a few days, you will notice extraordinary results.

Keeping Lizards Away

Lizards and other wall-crawling insects can be unsanitary and even frightening to some people. But, following this excellent natural recipe, you may not need to use synthetic products to keep them away any longer.

Keeping Lizards Away from Your Home with Black Pepper and Coffee Balls

Ingredients:

- 1 tsp. coffee
- 1 tbsp. black pepper
- Water, as needed

Directions:

1. You can combine all the ingredients to form round ball structures.

2. Store these balls in a netted pouch in various parts of the house. Lizards will no longer be a resident of your home.

Mosquitoes in the House

Mosquitoes are common in homes and can be quite dangerous since they spread malaria. To get rid of them, use the herbal remedies listed below:

Lavender and Lemongrass Candles for Mosquito Repellent in the Home

Ingredients:

- 1 tsp. lemongrass essential oil
- 1 tsp. lavender essential oil
- 1 cup candle wax

Directions:

3. In a double boiler, combine all the ingredients.

4. Remove the mixture from the bowl and place it in a dark-colored jar with a thread for lighting the candle.

5. Now, every day, light this candle to keep your home mosquito-free.

Killing Bugs

Bugs can become a big part of your home, and different bugs can irritate you a lot. To get rid of these bugs, use the recipes below:

Bug Spray with Witch Hazel, Peppermint, Spearmint, Lavender, and Lemongrass

Ingredients:

- 20 drops lavender essential oil
- 1 tbsp. natural vodka
- ½ cup vinegar
- 1 tbsp. lemongrass
- 1 cup water
- ½ cup rubbing alcohol or witch hazel
- 20 drops peppermint essential oil
- 20 drops spearmint essential oil

Directions:

1. Combine all the ingredients in a mixing bowl.

2. Pour the mixture into a dark spray bottle with a spray head.

3. Spray the mixture around your home to keep it fresh, fragrant, and bug-free.

Conclusion

Native American medicine is an opportunity for people to discover new ways to tackle their ailments and find a natural solution to their health challenges. Many herbs can be used to tackle this. Before you make a move, it is important that you consider getting some knowledge first. Know what it is exactly that you're suffering from. Discuss with your doctor about options and choose what will best work for you. Always ensure that whatever you consume is in the right proportion.

If you have gone through conventional means without any positive result, you should try Native American medicines. Many ailments that we have today were treated long ago. It is just that the application process may have been lost due to many factors that include disrupting the natural lifestyle of the Native American tribes.

For simple ailments, you can always resort to herbal remedies like the ones we have discussed in this book. There is no need to create dependency on prescription drugs. Going herbal is much safer and healthier most of the time. If you are in doubt, always consult your physician first.

Starting out learning herbalism and plant-based home remedies can be difficult, but I hope—and I'm sure—that this book has been an excellent primer for you to continue your journey, get acquainted with the plants, select which ones work best for you—and to empower healing at home.

Native American medicine addresses the healing of the whole person and uses the holistic approach to healing and cure. We know that health requires some kind of balance. These days we come across medical problems like some types of cancer, which defy all types of treatments.

Many medical problems can be resolved by changing our lifestyle and the social connections we have with those around us. With this book on your shelf, you will always have the ancient wisdom of Native Americans at your fingertips. Remember to investigate every substance you take and don't delegate responsibility for your healing to anyone but experts.

Good luck!!!

BOOK 10: ESSENTIAL OILS

Introduction

Native Americans are well-known for their understanding of medicinal plants. People claim to have first learned about the healing properties of plants and herbs after seeing animals consume certain plants when they were unwell. It was customary for medicine men to pluck every third plant they came across to prevent the overharvesting of these plants. People who lived in the Native American tradition had a spiritual vision of life, and to be healthy, they had to be motivated and pursued a virtuous, harmonious, and balanced route through life. According to them, certain ailments were just life lessons that the individual needed to learn without intervening.

Many current cures and medications are founded on Native Americans' understanding of the many plants and herbs they have utilized for thousands of years to treat various ailments. Herbs have a wide range of applications, including culinary, healing, and in some instances, spiritual applications. Green, leafy parts of plants are often utilized in culinary preparations, but for herbal medicine, the plant's root bark and inner bark, the berries and occasionally the pericarp or other parts of the plant, may be used instead. When you think about herbs, you probably think of popular herbs like Basil and Rosemary, among others.

However, there is a plethora of less widespread plants, herbs that have a wide range of applications. In this book, we have endeavored to present several well-known and some lesser-known herbs and describe their qualities, applications, growing tactics, and other aspects of their usage. Before the invention of pharmaceutical factories, people depended on herbal cures created from plants. Among the most effective therapeutic agents available in nature are essential oils, extracted from plants and flowers.

These oils are fragrant compounds extracted from the plants' leaves, flowers, bark and roots. They are formed deep within plant cells and they protect against disease and hungry pests and make plants more attractive to pollinating insects. Such oils are obtained from plants' leaves, roots, flower petals, and bark.

Essential oils are also the most natural approach for you to prevent and cure problems of your own and improve your health and promote overall well-being via aromatherapy. These oils were considered holy by the ancient Egyptians and essential to Ayurvedic procedures in India. They were also widely employed by Roman and Greek doctors, who passed on their expertise to academics from other areas of the world, including the United States.

Essential oils may be good for your health, mind and soul, and even your budget. Anxiety, frustration, and insomnia are all unpleasant states of being that may be managed using aromatherapy to benefit your entire health. Aromatherapy is a very effective type of treatment because of its ability to impact both the body and the brain. Many of these applications are covered in further detail in this book, including treating illnesses, generalized anxiety to blisters, and enhancing general well-being via various means.

Essential Oils. The History

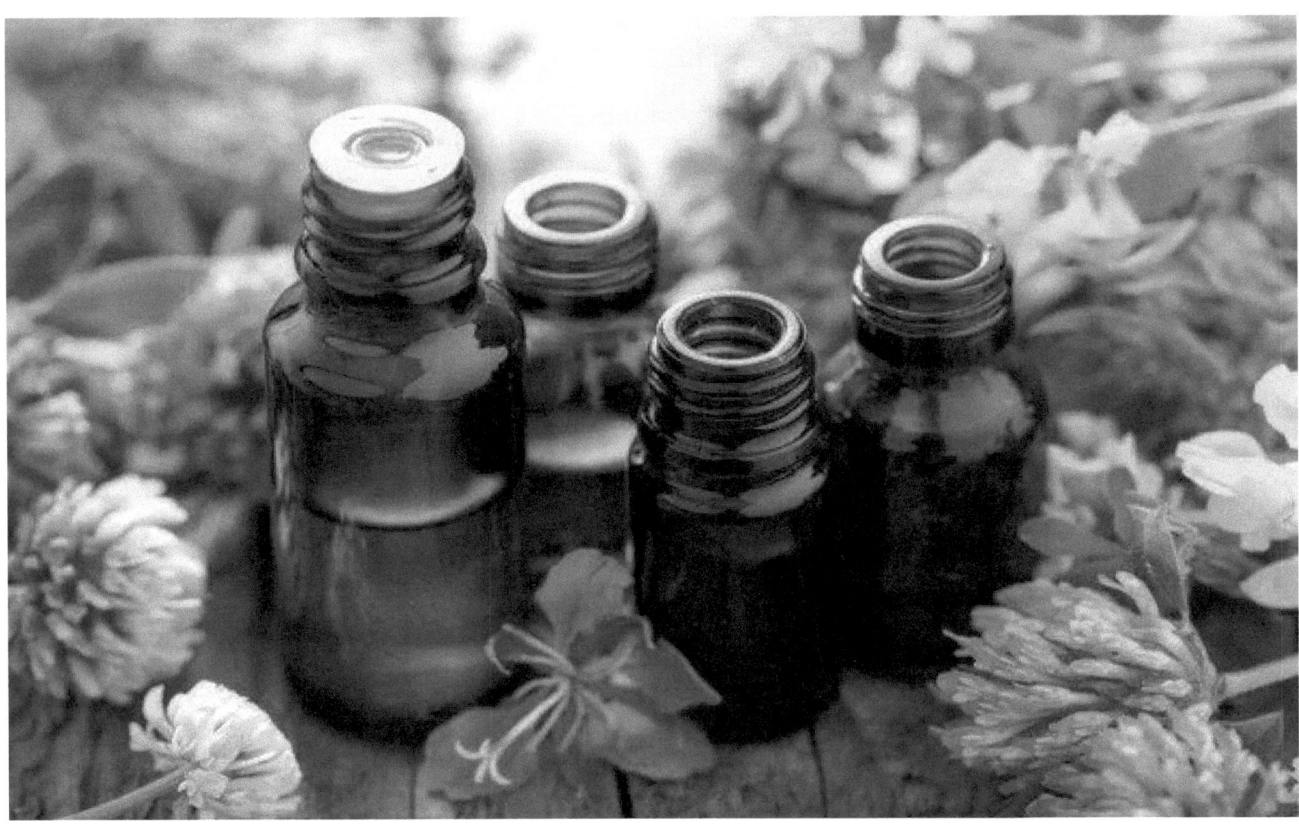

Essential oils have long been used by Native Americans and ancient civilizations in their everyday routines and spiritual/domestic rituals. They have a deep respect for Mother Nature and utilize only natural products in their daily lives. They think that essential oils, with their potent scents, may ward off evil spirits while also improving their overall health. Aromatic herbs and oils are used in Native American cleaning rituals. Aromatic herbs such as Sage, Juniper, Pine/Pinion needles, Cedarwood, Sweetgrass, and others aid in the purification and removal of negative energy from the air, as well as the attraction of positivity into one's life.

Plants are used to obtain essential oils. The oils capture the "essence" of the plant, which includes its aroma and flavor. Every essential oil has a distinct aroma due to the aromatic chemicals. Distillation (steam and/or water) or mechanical processes, like cold pressing, extract essential oils.

Throughout history, essential oils have been employed in folk medicine. Essential oils, also known as ethereal or volatile oils, are fragrant oily liquids derived from different parts of plants and used mostly as culinary flavorings. Essential oils are "essential" in the sense that they carry the essence of various fragrances as well as the qualities of the plants from which they are extracted. These volatile oils demonstrated antibiotic, antioxidant, antiviral, insecticidal, and other biological properties.

Some of these oils are used in food preservation, aromatherapy, and fragrance sectors, while others are employed for cancer treatment. Essential oil's anti-bacterial and anti-oxidant properties are used in various applications, including processed and fresh food preservation, natural remedies, pharmaceuticals, and complementary and alternative medicine. Because of the aromatic chemicals inherent in essential oils, they are employed in aromatherapy as an alternative source of wound healing. They are also used for relaxation.

Numerous attempts are being undertaken to investigate the use of essential oils in the treatment of multiple infectious disorders that are unresponsive to pharmacological therapies. Medicinal or fragrant plants are widely employed as natural organic chemicals and medications. Essential oils have previously been used to treat various infectious disorders worldwide. Essential oils are becoming increasingly important in our century. They are widely employed in the beverage and food sectors, the cosmetics and fragrance industries for creating excellent scents, and various biological activities.

Various essential oils have been employed for insecticidal activities against pests; however, detailed research has revealed that they lack repellence, avicidal, phytochemistry, antifungal, and oviposition properties. The essential oils do not have the characteristics listed above. However, there is still a pressing need to work on this side of the research and study in vivo and in vitro to control pests, and most of the oils have demonstrated high antioxidant activity. Essential oils have a defensive role for unsaturated lipids in animal tissue, and hepatoprotective negotiators in mammals have been discovered. Because oxygen is a toxic element that can change metabolic activities into the most reactive form of oxygen, such as hydrogen peroxide, superoxide, hydroxyl free radicals, and singlet oxygen, collectively known as active oxygen, antioxidant substances are essential for humans.

Essential oils are most known for their anti-spasmodic, anti-viral negotiators, anti-bacterial, and carminative properties. Essential oil composition varies, as do their effects, mainly dependent on chemotypes.

Since ancient times, essential oils have been employed in folk medicine. Ibn Sina, known in Europe as Avicenna, was the first to distill floral attar, whereas Ibn al-Baitar (1188–1248), an Arab Al-Andalusian (Muslim Spain) pharmacist, physician, and chemist, is thought to be the first to discuss the processes and methods used to manufacture essential oils.

Rather than referring to essential oils as a whole, current publications usually refer to the chemical components that make up the essential oils, such as methyl salicylate rather than "wintergreen oil."

Aromatherapy, a type of alternative medicine that employs essential oils and other aromatic substances, has sparked renewed interest in essential oils in recent decades. Volatilized oils are massaged, disseminated in the air with a nebulizer or diffuser, heated over a candle flame, or burned as incense.

Medical applications from those who sell medicinal oils range from skin treatments to cancer treatments. They are frequently based purely on historical records of Native American essential oils used for these purposes. Most countries currently regulate claims about the efficacy of medical therapies, especially cancer therapy.

A concentrated liquid that is hydrophobic and contains volatile (evaporated quickly at temperatures even when it is normal) chemical components from plants is referred to as an essential oil. These oils are volatile, ethereal oils, petroleum, or simply the oil derived from the plant, such as clove oil. Such oil is "essential" in the sense that it contains the "essence of" the plant's fragrance—the distinctive scent of the plant from which it was extracted. The word "essential" in this context does not signify "indispensable" or "useful" by the human body like it does in the case of essential amino acids and essential fatty acids, which are named because these are necessary nutritionally by a live creature.

Distillation is one of the most practiced methods for essential oils, commonly done with steam. Solvent extraction, expression, wax embedding, sfumatura, resin tapping, absolute extraction of oil, and cold pressing are other techniques. They are found in fragrances, soaps, air fresheners, cosmetics, other items, drink flavoring, food, and incense and cleaning products. The Essential Oils shouldn't be mistaken with perfumes, fragrances, or other similar products since the latter typically include chemical components, but essential oils will be made from plants.

Aromatherapy is a form of alternative medicine in which aromatic chemicals have healing properties. Essential oils are often used in aromatherapy. Aromatherapy can help you relax, but there isn't enough data to suggest that Essential Oils effectively treat many conditions. Improper usage of Essential Oils can result in allergic responses, skin irritation, and inflammation, with youngsters being particularly vulnerable to the hazardous effects.

Aromatherapy was employed in ancient ceremonies to combat negativity and evil. According to our forefathers, good scents fend off evil spirits and keep wicked creatures at a distance. Essential oils were employed to get rid of bad items for people's health and well-being. Aromatherapy, it was strongly argued, had a significant impact on one's life and so should be included in all types of cleansing - physical, emotional, spiritual, or psychological.

Essential oils were first recorded in ancient Persia, Egypt, and India, and both Rome and Greece engaged in considerable trade in the ointments and odoriferous oils with the Orient. These were most likely extracts made by soaking flowers, leaves, and roots in fatty oils. Odorous plants or their derivatives (resinous) were used directly in most ancient cultures. With the arrival of Arab culture's only golden period, a technique for distilling essential oils emerged. Arabs were the first to distillate ethyl alcohol through fermented sugar, creating a new and simple solvent for essential oil extraction that replaced the fatty oils used for millennia.

During the Middle Ages, distillation became more well known in Europe, and the isolation of essential oils through distillation was reported between the 11th and 13th centuries. These distilled goods became the specialty of medieval European pharmacies. Around 1500, oils of calamus, cedarwood, rose, costus, rosemary, incense, turpentine, spike, sage, benzoin, cinnamon, and myrrh had been introduced. Pharmacists and Physicians were inspired to explore essential oils through woods, fragrant leaves, and roots thanks to the alchemical beliefs of Swiss physician and alchemist Paracelsus.

Since Marco Polo's day, the highly sought spices of China, India, and the Indies have been the driving force behind European trading with the Orient. Spices like sage, cardamom, nutmeg, and cinnamon were naturally submitted to the pharmacists' stills. Around 100 essential oils had been imported in Europe by the mid 18th century, despite a scant understanding of the items' nature. Many famous chemists participated in chemical characterization for essential oils as chemical knowledge grew in the late 1800s and early 1900s. Essential oil expertise improved, resulting in a dramatic increase in production. The use of volatile oil in medicine was pushed aside in favor of beverages, foods, and perfumes.

Before 1800, peppermint and turpentine oils were produced in the United States; over the next decades, oils from four American plants that are indigenous, namely sassafras, sweet birch, wormwood, and wintergreen, became commercially important. Many essential oils have been created since 1800, but only some have become commercially significant.

The diversity of essential oils is currently receiving worldwide attention, yet their use is not new. Botanicals have been used as healers for thousands of years. Essential oils and other botanicals have been employed in wellness practices for at least 5,000 years.

Introducing Essential Oils Therapy

How Do Essential Oils Work?

There are many distinct components in every essential oil, each of which has a particular effect on the body. Anthracene and its derivatives, such as phenylpropane, serve as the precursors of amino acids, which link together to build practically all of the body's structures.

When it comes to the chemistry of things, our bodies and essential oils are both composed of many of the same substances. These include complex chemicals known as terpineols, which are naturally occurring alcohols that play an important role in producing vitamins, energy, and hormones in the body. Their production takes place as a byproduct of the continuous cellular respiration process. They contribute to the body's cellular energy source by assisting with functions such as metabolism and healing. Because plants manufacture these crucial compounds throughout their development, they may be found in various essential oils. They are very simple for the human body to absorb and use for nutrition and therapeutic purposes.

Despite their intricacy, these oils are, for the most part, non-invasive and harmless, except a couple that are derived from deadly nightshades and which should only be used under the strictest of conditions. Aside from that, essential oils have a beneficial influence on blood circulation. They have the potential to play a significant role in the delivery of oxygen and key nutrients to the body's tissues and the effective elimination of waste products generated by regular metabolic processes. As a result of improving blood flow, essential oils increase immune system effectiveness while simultaneously decreasing blood viscosity, which has a beneficial effect on the whole body, including the brain.

While essential oils are sweet-smelling and sometimes employed just for their pleasant smells, they contain the most potent molecules that plants can generate from the sun, water, and soil that provide them with nourishment and protection. However, even though their chemical structures are highly complicated and potent, essential oils are simple and enjoyable to use.

What Are Essential Oils Used For?

Many essential oils have adaptogenic properties, which work as natural balancers. When taken orally, they cause the body to undergo a balancing response, which may impact various systems, including blood pressure, the autonomic nerve system, the endocrine system, and the digestive system.

Many essential oils are natural painkillers, which relieve pain by working on the peripheral and central neural systems and the central nervous system. Wintergreen and birch were thought to be the finest pain relievers until synthetic pain medications were developed in the 1900s; in fact, Native Americans employed both plants long before written records were ever utilized.

While contemporary medicines play a significant role in pain management, most of these medications fall short of the potency of analgesic essential oils in that they are generally used to treat just physical pain.

As well as being able to foster emotions of self-acceptance, wintergreen essential oil is also recognized for its capacity to block pain. Peppermint essential oil, which has been proven beneficial in pain relief, is also known for its ability to produce an overall sense of peace and well-being.

Although most antiseptics on the market today include a range of chemicals, antiseptic essential oils are entirely natural. Lavender oil and clove oil are just a few of the anti-bacterial essential oils that have been shown to work. There are many ways to combine antiseptic essential oils to increase their effectiveness. There are many other ways to use them, like infusing them in a hot bath, applying them to small wounds, and adding them to herbal remedies or compresses.

Inflammation is a normal aspect of the body's natural defensive mechanism against pathogens, and many essential oils have anti-inflammatory qualities. For example, thyme essential oil is a valuable addition in mixes meant to relieve muscular tiredness, while pure, unadulterated rose otto oil is excellent in healing dry or irritated skin and reducing the appearance of brokenness capillaries if applied topically.

Aromatherapy and Flower Essences

Flower essences are the most popular home remedies for anxiety. These remedies were founded by Edward Bach, a homeopath in England during the early 1900s, who was fascinated with the idea that flowers had healing properties. He did not believe in chemical medicine and even said that "in letting nature take its course, we are letting God take his." He aimed to find a way to heal people without using medicine, which he believed led to a dependency on more and more drugs.

He found that when he placed a flower in a bowl of water and allowed it to sit overnight, the flower's energy would infuse the water. When taken internally, this water could treat what he called a "specific condition", such as fear or guilt.

A few drops of these flower essences are usually taken under the tongue four times daily (or as directed by an herbalist). They are supposed to change our vibration from fear to love through their unique vibrational frequencies.

Some people who experience synesthesia and the sense of a different color when they hear sounds also see colored shapes and forms or get numbers as sounds. Others might have what is referred to as "visual sound," where they see words blend while reading them.

Synesthetes often develop synesthesia later in life and are highly intelligent and creative individuals who can even use their unique abilities to help them solve puzzles. Synesthetes also tend to have an excellent imagination and an affinity for art.

Aromatherapy is the use of certain plant essences as medicine through their scent. These are also known as essential oils and are extracted using either distillation or expression. The word "aromatherapy" is a combination of the Greek word for aroma, "aroma," and the French word for therapy, "therapies."

Distillation involves steeping a plant in water and collecting its components that evaporate, which can then be used to make the essential oils. The distillation process is extremely time-consuming and expensive but is the most effective way of extracting essential oils.

The expression uses steam to extract the resin from the plant, which is then pressed and dried for storage. The concept behind the expression is very similar to that of distillation – where the plant's essence (essence meaning life force) is released into the steam so it can be collected and used.

Not: Kindly see your doctor if you suspect you might have some form of synesthesia.

Essential Oil Safety

Essential oils are highly concentrated, particularly from the leaves, flowers, roots, and fruit of aromatic plants that come from the world of plants. While the number of plants required to produce oil varies, for example, 3.6 million- or 1,000-pounds jasmine flowers are needed to produce a pound of jasmine oil. Rose oil is more concentrated, and more than 10,000 pounds of rose petals are required to produce 1 pound of rose oil! These two examples demonstrate both why these oils are costly and why it's so important to use them with expertise and care due to their concentrated nature.

Dilute Before Usage

Always dilute essential oils before adding them to the skin, as they can cause skin irritation, rashes, and allergic reactions if they are "neat" in their pure form. Lavender and tea tree oils are commonly listed as exceptions to this law, but diluting these oils remains the preferred approach in most circumstances. A common rule is to add a drop of essential oil, like sweet almond or grapeseed oil, in high-quality, cold-pressed vegetable oil per teaspoon. When creating a bath with aromatherapy, add 2 to 4 drops in a warm (not hot) bath. In other words, use either four drops in a bath or one drop in the mix to a teaspoon of vegetable oil.

Check Patch

It is a reasonable idea to first test a patch for new flavoring oil, particularly if you have allergies or sensitive skin. Mix one drop of oil tested in a tea cubicle of base oil and dab a small amount on the inside of the arm or wrist. Wait 24 hours to ensure there is no redness or discomfort.

Matters of Consistency

It is necessary to purchase high-quality oils and not to confuse essential oils with synthetic, not natural, fragrance oils. Some products marketed as pure oils are diluted or adulterated in cheaper oils. Read product labels carefully but know that brands may not disclose complete information. Get to know the botanical names of the oils you want to use and never buy an oil not marked by its botanical name or by the common name.

Aromatherapy Essential Oil Safety Tips

Aromatherapy is one of the best treatments used under the supervision of a trained doctor. Essential oils are natural plant extracts produced by steam, expression, or chemical extraction of particular plant species.

Particular attention should be paid to the application of essential oil. Sometimes, certain essential oils should be avoided, and other oils should be treated with caution. Some safety tips on the use of aromatherapy oils are provided here.

• Be very mindful of the pure essential oil. Never put it in a pure state on your skin. Still dilute crucial oils with compact oils like almond and baby oil. If you manufacture your oils plan plant carrier oil, the resulting oil is weak enough to use on your skin. If you have epilepsy or allergic skin, are pregnant, are homeopathic or take another prescription drug, or have a heart condition, please contact your general health care provider before you use some essential oil. If you go out in the sun, you should not add any product with citrus oils to your skin. The essential citrus oils may cause the skin to burn and redden.

• Don't take essential oils by mouth. If you intend to work with oil, do a small skin test on your arm. Stop it if irritation occurs. Avoid eucalyptus, fennel, hyssop, sage, pennyroyal, juniper, tansy, thuja, tempestuous, and rosemary because of the possibility of seizures in such oils. Rosemary, wise, and thyme should be avoided by people with high blood pressure.

As an assault this may cause, asthmatics should avoid the direct inhalation of essential oils.

• Stop contact with the eyes with essential oils. Essential oils are highly irritating to the eyes and should not be used close to them. Don't even rub your eyes with hands that still have oil traces. You should never blaze pure oil in the oil heater and place the water in the tank and put a little drop of Aotearoa. It is worth noting. Keep your oils in a cool, dark place or refrigerator. Some essential organic oils are hazardous and should not be used at all, but are still sold. Before you purchase, always check the safety of any oil product. Most of the time, you can confidently use widely available essential oils like lavender.

• Keep essential oils out of children's reach. It is safer to place it in a closed case than in a locked case. If a child ingests unintentional essential oils, don't induce vomit, let them drink a glass of cold water, and seek medical advice promptly and urgently.

The great advantage of aromatherapy is that most real Utica herbs are those that smell healthy, so it is not too difficult to avoid those that smell bad and are potentially dangerous!

Many oils are available for children and babies under the age of 12. It is advisable to dilute these oils with other tools, which can be used for babies and young children.

Any essential oil can lead to dermatitis and sensitivity, especially when used repeatedly.. Stop this at any time by using only minimal quantities of the oil.You should also practice substituting the oils from time to time instead of using the same oils every day.

When choosing essential oils, always make sure you use the correct oil by testing the Latin or botanical names. Many essential oils can have the same common name but may have numerous functions. There are also several essential oils with familiar names.

Some Safety Tips to Note before Buying Essential Oils

Essential oils are not meant to be used by any Tom, Dick, and Harry. This is because they are very potent chemical substances with great health benefits and medicinal value, but could become harmful to the body if used indiscriminately, and excessively, and could easily become a health hazard if used by certain persons on whom essential oils are not meant to be used without the direction and guidance of a qualified physician.

Essential oils can be used by almost everyone, except pregnant women, breastfeeding mothers, children and persons that are suffering from, or have a history of diabetes, epilepsy, and seizures.

Essential Oils on Diabetics

Essential oils that have a high ketone content generally should not be used in large quantities, or for an extended period of time. This is because ketones are not easily metabolized by the liver, and tend to accumulate in it with dire consequences on the liver and kidneys.

Persons suffering from diabetes, or who have a history of diabetes should not use essential oils with a high ketone content. This is because the accumulation of ketones in the liver leads to a disruption of the hormonal balance of the body, which is quite a bit of a dangerous situation for a diabetic.

Some of such essential oils that contain ketones in high concentration include lavender, peppermint, rosemary, spikenard, spearmint, clary sage, turmeric, etc.

Essential Oils on Pregnant Women

There are differing opinions amongst aromatherapists on the use of essential oils on pregnant women. Some say that essential oils can be safely used on pregnant women if used minimally and under the guidance of a physician. On the other hand, some say that essential oils should be totally avoided by both pregnant women and breastfeeding mothers.

The second group of aroma therapists sounds more reasonable. Essential oils are just too strong to be used by pregnant women, especially during the period of the first trimester of pregnancy. During this period, the baby passes through a vital and delicate developmental process, using a strong substance such as essential oils during this period is not safe. This is because the essential oil could interfere with or disrupt this developmental process, which could be dangerous to the health and growth of the baby.

After the first trimester of pregnancy, some essential oils can be used minimally and for only a short period of time. Tobe on the safe side though, essential oils should be completely avoided from the beginning to the end of the pregnancy. Some of the essential oils that should be avoided include wintergreen, lemongrass, clary sage, thyme, eucalyptus, peppermint, ginger, rosemary, marjoram, basil, clove, nutmeg, cinnamon, cassia, etc.

Essential Oils on Epileptics

Persons suffering from epilepsy or who have a history of epilepsy can use essential oils, though minimally and under the watchful eyes of a qualified physician, and get some relief from some of the symptoms of epilepsy. However, essential oils that have neurotoxic qualities, such as lavender, eucalyptus, rosemary, hyssop, clary sage, camphor, etc., should be avoided.

Topical Use of Essential Oils

There are various ways by which essential oils can be safely used which include topical application, aerial diffusion, and direct inhalation. It is important to note that essential oils should not be ingested as this can cause a myriad of problems. The essential oil molecules are tiny enough and strong enough to pass through the skin and nostrils and carry out their function at the target location in the body.

When applying essential oils topically for the very first time, it is important to conduct a skin patch test to ensure that you do not react negatively with that particular essential oil. To conduct a skin patch test, first, apply about 2–3 drops of a particular essential oil to the back of your wrist or the sole of your feet, and then cover it with a bandage for a whole day and then watch out for any reaction. If that area of your skin becomes irritated or itchy or turns red, apply vegetable oil to wash off the offending essential oil. The reaction shows that your skin does not agree with that particular essential oil, or that you need to dilute the essential oil before use. You can also repeat the skin patch test using the diluted oil to confirm if your skin agrees with the oil at all.

Also note that some citrus essential oils such as orange, lime, lemon, etc., can be phototoxic. That is, when such essential oils are applied topically, they make the skin become more susceptible to sunburns, and irritations when you are out in the sun. So, it is necessary to limit how much you go out in the sun whenever you use such essential oils.

Using Essential Oils on Pets

Pets react very differently to essential oils than humans; they are more sensitive to essential oils, especially cats. So, when using essential oils on pets, we need to be cognizance of how it reacts to that particular essential oil. Whichever essential oil you are using on your pets, make sure to use only a very little amount at a time.

You need to gently introduce new essential oils to your dog before using them. Add a drop on a handkerchief, then bring it close to the dog and watch how it responds. If it shows a lack of interest in that particular essential oil, or backs away from the handkerchief, that is an indication that it has had enough of that oil, or does not like it at all. If on the other hand, the dog licks its lips or blinks rapidly, that is an indication that it enjoys that particular essential oil. Most importantly, do not force any oil on your pet, but it should be used on them on their terms.

If you have pets around, be sure not to use essential oils on your hand or skin. This is to prevent the dog from licking and ingesting essential oil from your hand or skin. Also, do not rub essential oils on the fur or skin of your dog, and avoid using them close to its eyes and nose, especially when spraying or using a hydrosol. Speaking of hydrosols, hydrosols are safer to be used on dogs compared to essential oils, they can be sprayed directly on the skin or fur of the dog.

How to Prepare Essential Oils DIY

If you are willing to extract the essential oils in the comfort of your home to be sure of the quality and purity, then you must grow the Native American herbs in your garden.

As you grow them, you need to be sure that your plants are not exposed to herbicides, pesticides, or any chemical fertilizers. This is because if any of such chemicals exist in your plants, the steam distillation process of extraction will allow some of the chemicals to seep into the essential oils that you eventually collect. If your house garden is near power lines or roads, then be aware of the spraying that is done occasionally by the city management vehicles. The herb plants should not be sprayed with any kind of chemical fertilizer at any cost if you intend to extract essential oils out of them.

You need to first be aware of the perfect time for harvesting the plants. If you are willing to extract essential oils out of the herbs, then you should harvest the plants just before they flower completely. You should actually harvest them when the flowers are half-open. There are a few herbs that go by the exception of this rule. Lavender is a prime herb that is highly preferable for essential oils. If you have lavender in your garden, then you can harvest it when the flowers are half-bloomed. But on the other hand, the rosemary plant should have the best oils if it is harvested in full bloom.

This happens because different plants have varying times when their essences are at their peak. And these essences are what you are about to extract from those plants while adapting the process of extracting essential oils. The first step that you need to acquire before getting into the actual methods of extracting essential oils is to let the herbs or flowers dry. You don't need to put them into the extraction process while they are fragile and might get crumbled in your hands. Wait until you feel the flowers or herbs dry on your fingers. Do not let the herbs dry out in hot spaces, but hang them in warm areas of the house. Environments that are too hot can damage the volatile essence of those herbs or flowers, and the final outcome might lack efficiency.

You will need many herbs or plant materials to process the essential oils. To give you a basic idea, you might have to process hundreds of pounds of herbs or plant parts to produce around one or two ounces of oil. Most of the stills (processing containers) that are widely available for use at home cannot process such a big amount of plant materials. Therefore, you will have to prepare your essential oils in batches. Proper drying of the herbs before processing the extraction will let you obtain essential oil in each processing batch. But this reference is just based upon the method of still distillation. The detailed steps of execution for it and an alternative method are highlighted below:

Still or Steam Distillation Method of Extracting Essential Oils

- A large container called still is used for the process. If you are extracting oil from plants at your residence, there are smaller non-commercial containers available for the process.

- The plant material is added to that container, and steam will be added to it. Remember not to chop the plant material while adding the same to the still because you might just lose some of the oils from plant material.
- In a different container or still, add water and heat it up to form steam. It will then be injected into the still with herbal extracts through an inlet. It will then release the aromatic molecules of the plant and turn them into vapor.
- The vaporized plant compounds will travel to that of the condensation flask and the condenser. There are two different pipes that are accountable for exiting the hot water and allowing the cold water to enter the condenser chamber. You will get the condenser chamber with the steam distillation kit. Hence, this will allow the vapor to cool back into liquid form.
- The aromatic liquid will then drop from the condenser chamber and be collected in a container underneath that is termed as a separator. The water and oil don't mix as the essential oil will be floating on top of the water. Most of the essential oils will be found on the top of the water, while some of them are heavier than that, for which they are found at the bottom of the separator container.

Hence, this is how you collect essential oils through the steam distillation method at home! You can get the equipment online or from any herbal store. There are many other industrial methods of extracting the essential oils, such as solvent extraction, CO_2 extraction, Maceration, Enfleurage, cold-press extraction, and others, that cannot be used by commoners who are just herbal enthusiasts and are not running a business out of the medicinal plants. Moreover, these types of equipment are expensive and are not affordable for most people. Therefore, people who are willing to extract essential oils for their personal medicinal use can either use the miniature steam distillation units or the alternative methods below!

Alternative Methods of Extracting Essential Oils

There are two homely alternative methods to extract essential oils from Native American herbs. Still, distillation is an industrial or commercial method of extracting the oil, which most individuals want to ignore for its complexity. Even though a miniature version is prepared for people with herbal gardens to extract their own oil, it is still complex and expensive. Therefore, here are alternative methods that are easy to adapt and are quick as well. The only drawback is that the quality of essential oil derived from these methods won't be as rich as that of the other industrial methods.

The methods are:

- Crockpot Extraction Method- You need to first place a handful of dried herbal plant material in a crockpot. I prefer a larger one! Now fill the pot with distilled water and leave just an inch over the top. Cook on low heat for around 24 to 36 hours, and then shut it off and leave the top open. Now, cover the same with cheesecloth and let it settle somewhere out from the direct heat of the sun. The solution should sit idle for a week, after which you can remove the oils that have collected over the water top. It can then be transferred into another blue glass jar or an amber. Allow the jar to stay open for the next week while covered with the cloth to allow the rest of the water to evaporate. You can now seal the jar/bottle properly to store and use the oil when needed. Remember that the shelf life of the extracted oil is only 12 months!

- Preparing Essential Oils on Stovetop- Use a regular pot over the stovetop to repeat the same process as specified in the above method. The only difference is that you should place the plant material in some porous mesh bag before adding it to the boiling water. You should then simmer your plant material for the next 24 hours and add sufficient water every time when needed. Now, strain and remove oil that gets collected over the water surface. Follow the same instructions as in the previous method for evaporating the excessive water.

The Process of Blending Different Essential Oils

Essential oils should be used or mixed separately for different purposes such as scent skin scrubs, perfumes, body butter, and others. Mixing these oils can really be a fun activity if you intend to do everything with the herb plants all by yourself. The essential oils should be diluted with that of the carrier oil, alcohol, and dispersing agent before they can be used over the skin. After you mix these oils, you should count on safely storing the oil if you are planning upon aging the blend. The process of blending different essential oils involves certain steps, which are as follows:

Formulating the Blend

Step 1: Determining the type of Aroma or Scent you want

There are various types of scents that you often use for alleviating different health issues. You need to think about what specific type of scent you basically want. There are many categories of herbs from which unique essential oils are extracted. You may prefer to mix the scents from varying categories. The categories of scents listed from that of the essential oils are flora, earthy, herbal, minty, spicy, and citrus. For instance, lavender, jasmine, and rose are accountable for product floral scents; Peppermint, sage, and spearmint are accountable for offering minty scents, and so on. Pick two herbal essential oils of the same or different categories based upon your herbalist's recommendation or your medicinal knowledge.

Step 2: Pick the Top, Middle and Base Notes

The note of the oil refers to the length of time that it needs for evaporation. The top notes are accountable for evaporating the quickest, while the base notes take the most time for evaporation. If you intend to let your oils hold onto the aroma for a specific amount of time, go with a good base note that will pair well with that of the middle and top notes. Consider the following:

- The top notes will evaporate within a couple of hours. Some herbs that fall under this category are basil, citronella, eucalyptus, spearmint, lavender, lemongrass, and orange.
- The middle notes will evaporate within 4 hours. Some herbs that fall under this category are nutmeg, tea tree, fennel, chamomile, and jasmine.
- The base notes will last for up to a few days before evaporating. Some herbs that fall under this category are oakmoss, ginger, cedarwood, patchouli, and balsam.

Step 3: Test the Blend before Final Mixing

- Take a cotton swab and dip it into each oil bottle. Do not use a single swap for all the oil bottles! Use one swap per bottle!
- Hold the swab at least a foot away from your nose and swirl it in circles around the air.
- It will give you an idea of what scent you would get upon combining the scent of all of these oils.
- If you do not like the aroma, then you can count on removing one of the swabs and then try again. Try another separate oil by dipping another swab into it and repeating the same process.
- With this, you will be able to find the perfect blend of oils in terms of scent.

Step 4: Mix the Oils

After you have determined what blend would be best for your need in terms of scent and their medicinal properties, you can now add them together. Here are the steps for you to do the same:

- You must use a dropper or a pipette for the mixing process.
- Drop the picked measurable amount of your base, middle and top notes of oil in a clean bowl or in some glass vial.
- Drop the correct amount of drops as per the recipe. If you want a specific understanding of how much oil you should use in a specific blend to attend to your health adversities, then you can talk to an aroma therapist or an herbalist.
- If you are willing to do this measurement manually, then you can use either the 30-5-20 rule or the 1-2-3 rule.
- The 30-50-20 rule states that your blend should be 30% of the top note essential oil, 50% of the middle note essential oil, and 20% of the base note essential oil.
- The 1-2-3 rule states that for every one drop of the base essential oil, you will have two drops of the middle oil and three drops of the top oil.
- I prefer to mix all of the essential oils together before adding any diluting agents or carriers to it.

<u>Diluting the Essential Oil Blends</u>

Step 1: Look for a Carrier Oil

You need to look for a carrier oil to make the blend good for application on the skin. Diluting the oil blends or essential oils is pretty much important because they are in high concentration form when raw. If you intend to apply those oil blends to your skin directly without diluting agents, you might impose permanent damage on your skin. The carrier oils can typically be the usual vegetable oils! Some of the common carrier oils preferred for this purpose include almond oil, sunflower oil, coconut oil, grape seed oil, and others.

Step 2: Add any Dispersing Agent

If you are planning on using the essential oil blend in your bath, then you should dilute the same with a dispersing agent. These agents help the oil spread throughout the bath safely. Some of the vegetable oils are ideal for being used as dispersing agents while others are not. For instance, coconut oil cannot be used as a dispersing agent because of its thickness, which does not make it ideal for use in the bath. You can go with lighter vegetable oils that consist of higher liquid viscosity. Some of the options that you can use are jojoba oil, milk, honey, or sweet almond oil.

Step 3: Mix the Blend with Alcohol

You can dilute the essential oil blend with alcohol as well if you prefer to use the same as perfume. The mixture ratio should be around 10 to 15 drops of essential oil blend to every 15ml of alcohol. You can also use jojoba oil for making a perfume, but alcohol is the preferred agent.

Finish the Essential Oil Blend

Step 1: Decide on the Proportion Based upon Needs

- If you are blending for massages, then use around 15 to 20 drops of essential oil for every ounce of carrier oil.
- If you are blending lotions or different skin oils, use around 3 and 15 drops for every ounce of carrier oil.
- If you are using the essential oil on children, then you should blend 3 to 6 drops of the blend to every ounce of the carrier oil.
- If you are using the essential oil blend for the bath, then the mixture should be 2 to 15 drops of oil blend to every ounce of the dispersing agent.

If you are using the oil blend for inhaling or smelling only, you do not need to blend it with any of the carrier oils.

Step 2: Store it in a Bottle

You can store the oil blend in vials, sprayers, or bottles, which will be a good way of storing the essential oil blends. The amber bottles with a specific volume of 2 to 4 mm are often recommended for storage of the essential oils. You need to carefully pour the blended oil into your container. If it seems difficult for your trembling hands, use a funnel for the same. Make sure you are storing the bottle in a cool or dark area.

When diluting the essential oils with vegetable oils, keep in mind that the vegetable oils might expire more quickly than the essential oils, and that might make the bottle useless. Therefore, if you are diluting the essential oil blend with sesame, sweet almond oil, or rosehip, then it can only be stored for around 6 to 12 months. Coconut and jojoba oil are quite stable and have the possibility of lasting indefinitely.

You can also store your blended oil in the refrigerator, unless you have mixed the blend with avocado oil in which case you should not store the bottle in the fridge. Avoid oils that smell either bitter or rancid and avoid storing the bottles under direct sunlight or anywhere near the stove. Heat can spoil the medicinal effects of your essential oil blend and might also hamper its aroma.

Step 3: Let the Oils Settle

The scent of an essential oil blend is more likely to change and improve when the oils settle down. Therefore, you can wait for around 3 to 4 days before you try smelling your blend again. Keeping the changes in mind, decide how the oils will blend. By imposing the aging aspects on your oil blends, you will eventually obtain more satisfying aromas out of your bottles.

So, this is how you can extract the oils from your herbs and plant materials and blend different oils to enhance their medicinal or aromatic outcomes. Both of these processes go hand in hand! Most peoplegrowing herbs in their gardens are often eager to learn the process of extracting oils and blending them to get the perfect scent for aesthetic purposes. Apart from the aesthetic and scent benefits, the oil blends also multiply their medicinal capabilities which is yet another important reason why you should know how to blend these oils. If your prime motive is to attain health relaxation upon some condition, you can talk to your aroma therapist or herbalist to get a prescription on which oils you should blend and the mode of consumption.

Even if you are not growing herbs in your garden, you can still buy pure essential oils from many online and offline stores. You just have to dig deeper to find trustworthy brands for the same! The herbal enthusiasts will stay strong on growing their own herbs and extracting their own oils to use their benefits.

Essential Oils Benefits

Essential oils are good for your health, mind and soul, and even your budget. They have many applications, including treating illnesses, generalized anxiety to shingles, and enhancing general well-being. Native Americans use essential oils for the following purposes.

Healing

Adaptogens are present in all essential oils. An adaptogen is a natural drug that stimulates a balanced response in the body, enhancing the body's capacity to cope with stress and exhaustion, both known to be risk factors for chronic illness. Some adaptogens promote healing, while others inhibit infections and yet others aid in recovery from disease or accident. It has been proved in several studies that such herbs may restore balance to the body's activities without producing disruptions or negative effects to the body's functioning.

Pain Relief

A large number of essential oils are painkillers. When it comes to pain, analgesics operate directly on the nerve system to relieve it.

Aromatherapy essential oils such as clove, peppermint, birch, and thyme are examples of natural painkillers that are safe and effective.

Reducing Inflammation

A large number of essential oils have anti-inflammatory properties. Following exposure to chemicals or accidents, inflammation is a critical component of the body's natural defense mechanism, assisting in healing. Swelling, redness, and discomfort at the location of the inflammation are all common symptoms of this condition. Essential oils such as thyme, bergamot and clove are well-known for their anti-inflammatory effects, as are other citrus fruits. In many circumstances, you will discover that it is not essential to use over-the-counter medications since these oils can deliver efficient inflammation treatment without using hazardous chemicals.

Antiseptic

Antiseptic properties are found in several essential oils. An antiseptic is an anti-microbial chemical which minimizes the likelihood of infection when administered to live tissue. All natural antiseptics such as clove, lavender, and tea tree essential oils are among the most potent on the market. Besides being effective for healing minor injuries, these ingredients may also be used to make natural cleaning products.

Stress Relief

Some of these oils are known to provide relaxation and stress relief. For many people, stress is an unavoidable aspect of everyday existence. Anyone who has experienced excessive stress understands how negativity can take over, causing turmoil and anxiety while also causing physical problems such as migraines, indigestion, and even itching, red rashes on the face and body. Stress-relieving essential oils such as peppermint, rosemary, and ylang-ylang are the best available. Others are good for encouraging relaxation, boosting meditation, and expediting sleep, among other things.

Using Essential Oils

There are a variety of ways to use essential oils. You might even be able to come up with a few on your own.

Just remember to be alert for signs of sensitivity whenever introducing a new oil to your regimen. And, of course, avoid consuming the oils!

Use a method of administration that works for your situation:

- Inhale the scent directly. This is the easiest way to get started. Place a couple of drops of essential oil on a tissue or paper towel. Hold the tissue close to your face and inhale through your nose.
- Bath. Just 5 drops in one ounce of carrier oil, such as almond oil, can be added to your bathwater. Ensure that you're choosing an appropriate essential oil.
- Inhale via steam. Boil two cups of water and then transfer the water to a bowl. Add approximately five drops of essential oil to the water. Keep the bowl close to you and enjoy the scent. Stop if you experience any discomfort.
- The room method. Follow the previous method, but use 10 drops of essential oil. Place the bowl near the center of the room.
- Massage. Add 10–20 drops of essential oil to 1/8 cup of carrier oil. Almond or jojoba oil are acceptable carrier oils. Ideally, have a partner massage the oil into your skin keeping away from the eyes and mucous membranes.

Try all the different methods and see which works best for you.

There's no method that is universally superior to another. Keep an open mind and experiment. You will likely find one method that you prefer over the others.

Diluting Oils

Essential oils are very powerful. They can make breathing easier, relieve pain, and even combat cancer. You willl want to dilute them in some kind of carrier oil before applying them to your skin in order to provide a barrier between the delicate membranes of your body and the potent oils.

We are often asked, "How much oil should I put in my blend?" as a general guideline, we recommend using 1 to 2 teaspoons of essential oil per 10 ml of the carrier. Keep in mind that this is only a guideline, and some oils can be used at higher concentrations.

Topical Use

Oils can be rubbed or massaged into the skin or into clothing. They can also be dispensed through a dropper, but that is more difficult.

For external use only—not for ingestion! Do not use essential oils directly to your eyes. If you are allergic to any of the oils, do not use them topically. Essential oils are very concentrated, and if you apply too much, they could burn your skin or cause an adverse reaction.

When using essential oils on the skin, always dilute the oil before applying it. The easiest way to do this is to place your carrier oil in a bowl and slowly add the essential oil, making sure it is well mixed before adding more—this will prevent clumping of the carrier oil at the bottom of the bowl. The preferred method by most people is to add about 10 drops of essential oil to 1/4 cup (60 ml) of a good quality carrier oil.

Diffusion

The aroma of an oil blend will be affected by the amount of air that comes into contact with the oils. Some oils diffuse very easily, and some can take hours or even days to fully release their fragrance. It's best to keep your blends in a glass bottle or a stainless steel atomizer to prevent evaporation.

We recommend that you perform your blends in a well-ventilated space if possible. You'll want to work with a fan or an oscillating fan going at high speed. If you don't have a fan, set your burner on low, but never leave your home without ventilation.

Bottles of spice oils are very effective for diffusion, and they come in small bottles that can easily be tucked into a handbag. The oils will dissolve and disperse into the air, and people around you will breathe in the therapeutic benefits of the essential oils that you've blended.

Inhalation

The aromatic benefits of the oils are most effectively absorbed through the mucous membranes of the sinuses. Simply inhale the aroma of your blend for a minute or two, and you should feel some immediate benefits. If you feel light-headed, stop immediately and take deep, even breaths until feeling better.

For children, place a few drops on a tissue and breathe in slowly to smell the fragrance.

Inhaling oils can be very relaxing, and many people like to add 1 or 2 drops to a hot bath before getting in for 20 minutes. This is an excellent way to benefit from essential oils while soaking in a tub of hot, soothing water.

Internal Use

Before ingesting essential oils for internal usage, they must be diluted in a carrier oil. Follow this ratio for internal use:

- 3 drops of essential oil per teaspoon (5 ml) of carrier oil.

Essential oils should never be swallowed undiluted. Keep out of reach of children and pets.

Shake well before each use to disperse the natural essential oils that might have settled on the bottom of the container. Avoid heat, light, and air as much as possible to preserve your essence.

Makes 24 capsules with 100 mg each:

- Put the gelatin capsules in a bowl of hot water for 5 minutes to soften them. Once they are soft, drain the water out of the bowl. You can use a small funnel to pour in the contents of your bottle if you would prefer not to shake all the oil out.
- Gently shake out as much of the carrier oil as possible without shortening the life of your capsules by breaking them open and spilling their contents into the gelatin capsules.
- Add the drops of essential oils, be sure to shake the bottle first, and fill each capsule with your blend.
- Once the capsules have been filled with an even amount of oil on each one, you can use a wet toothpick to scrape away any excess oil from the opening on the top of each capsule. This will help them from sticking together in storage. Cap tightly and place in a cool dark place until ready for use or into a bottle for daily use or into another container of your choice for storage—I like to use old film containers with lids.

You may also create your own roller bottle by using an empty 10 ml glass bottle and a roll-on cover.

7 Must-Know Essential Oils Remedies

Now that you have a basic grasp of how to use essential oils, you should be able to put this newfound knowledge to use, so get to work! Throughout this chapter, you will learn which oils are useful against various conditions, ranging from gastric reflux to whooping cough, as well as how to make treatments.

Essential oils should not be used as a replacement for professional medical treatment. This kind of treatment should always be used in conjunction with a medical approach, particularly for chronic disorders such as asthma, headaches, depression, diabetes and heart disease, and should never be used instead of medical treatment. Before using any essential oil, please consult with your doctor to ensure that it will not interact with any medications you are taking or plan to take. If your illness worsens, you should seek medical attention as soon as possible.

Here are some easy and effective essential oil recipes for you.

Anti-Allergen Essential Oil

Allergies are a kind of reaction to something. The symptoms may be effectively treated with drugs, but they come with several unpleasant side effects, such as dry mouth, sleepiness, and other discomforts. Alternatives to pharmaceuticals include natural therapies such as using essential oils.

Ingredients

- 8 to 10 drops of lavender essential oil

Directions

- Add the lavender oil to the water in your diffuser and turn on the machine.
- Set it to run for about 15 minutes every two hours for the next day.
- To get an ongoing therapy, position the diffuser next to your bed and leave it running throughout the night.

Essential Oil for Arthritis

Using essential oils to massage into tight, painful joints may provide relief from the discomfort of arthritis whenever and wherever it manifests itself.

Ingredients

- 1 tsp. of primrose carrier oil
- 10 drops of wintergreen or clove oil

Directions

- Place the primrose oil in a small glass dish and set it aside.
- Stir the wintergreen oil into the carrier oil until it is well incorporated.
- Apply the mixture to the afflicted region with your hands, massaging it into the skin with your fingertips.

Body Pain Relief Oil

Lavender, cedarwood, and peppermint oils all have elements to reduce swelling and eliminate inflammation-related pain.

Ingredients

- 2 drops of lavender oil
- 1 tbsp of carrier oil
- 4 drops of peppermint oil
- 2 drops of cedarwood oil

Directions

- Mix all the ingredients in a glass dish.
- Apply to the concerned area as needed.

Minty Oil for Swelling

This is one of the basic oil recipes on our list that only has a few elements, making it quicker to make at home.

Ingredients

- 6 drops of carrier oil
- 8 drops of wintergreen oil
- 12 drops of peppermint oil

Directions

- Mix all the oils.
- Store in an airtight bottle.
- Apply on the inflamed area three times a day.

Essential Oil for Menstrual Pain

The ingredients of this oil help improve blood circulation, which then helps reduce pain, muscle spasms, and menstrual cramps.

Ingredients

- 5 drops of carrier oil
- 10 drops of cypress
- 5 drops of lavender oil
- 10 drops of peppermint oil

Directions

- Blend all the ingredients in a small dish.
- Store in a bottle.

- Apply on your pelvic area in a circular motion.

Essential Oil for Headache

What do you normally do when you get a headache? Instead of taking medicines, use this essential oil recipe.

Ingredients

- 8 drops of peppermint oil
- A 10ml roller bottle
- 6 drops of lavender oil
- 5 drops of jojoba or avocado oil

Directions

- Fill the roller bottle halfway with a carrier oil.
- Add the essential oils on top of that.
- If necessary, apply to the back of your neck and temples, as well as the wrists and hands.

Essential Oil for Coughs

Coughs may be dry and annoying at times. However, they are often accompanied by mucus production. You should see your doctor if you have a persistent cough since it might indicate a more severe underlying ailment. Lavender and peppermint oils help relieve the pain that comes with coughing, clear congestion and help to decrease mucus production.

Ingredients

- 2 drops of peppermint oil
- 1 ounce of lukewarm water
- 2 drops of lavender oil

Directions

- Combine the water with the lavender oil in a small drinking glass.
- Add peppermint and lavender oil with water into a mixing bowl and whisk until well combined.
- Gargle and swish with little quantities of the therapy until it is completely gone.
- Repeat this therapy as many times as necessary during your sickness, up to three times every day.

Conclusion

This book has introduced you to the world of essential oils, right from the beginnings when people were merely experimenting with a range of products. It has established a scientific basis for using these products, as well as the inherent challenges of finding the right balance. Ultimately, this book has laid the foundation for any future efforts to professionalize the art and science of aromatherapy. This is the age when we are reconsidering virtually everything that relates to traditional medicine. It is, therefore, not surprising that remedies, which were once dismissed as being nothing more than amateurish science, have come to dominate the market. In fact, essential oils have led to the development of new professions that were previously considered to be unworkable. Moreover, these oils allow people to treat their conditions in a way that is safe, cost-effective and efficient. The book readily acknowledges it is not always easy to get the best out of the products marketed as essential oils. For example, there are many potential side effects, depending on the health of the person and the way they use the product. Moreover, the fact there is very limited information about the potential benefits and downsides of these oils means many people are, effectively, operating in the dark. To bring balance to the book, there is no claim that essential oils are the solution to all the ailments of humanity. Rather, the argument is that this is an alternative solution for people, who want to think outside the box.

The next stage is to start thinking about how you can apply these essential oils in your life. The first part is to read books, such as this one, so you are well versed in the subject and its implications. Then, start with a few conventional oils in very dilute forms to test how your body reacts to them. With confidence, you can expand your horizons by using more complex oils and blends. This book will be a major reference point throughout the process. The book is, by no means, exhaustive, and you may have to supplement a lot of the information it contains. Nevertheless, it has broadly achieved the objectives with which it started. Here, you have an overview of the origins and basics of essential oils, so you can be inspired to explore the topic further. As for the prospects for the industry, they seem excellent. Many more people are overcoming their traditional prejudices against alternative medicine. They increasingly see it as a way of countering some of the worst impacts of the conventional methods. In practice, that experimental beginning has not meant it is a free fall. Indeed, many governments set out stringent criteria for what is and what is not an essential oil. These rules are there for your safety, as a consumer. That is why this book has emphasized the need for care and precaution when using essential oils. Nevertheless, this is a fun way to develop healthful living habits. If you get it right, you could get rid of some ailments that are not responding to conventional medicine. Try the essential oils today and see what they can do for you.

After reading through this book, you will be aware of many of the uses that essential oils have, as well as how to utilize the oils to accomplish many different health and beauty products.

You have also learned about all the other applications essential oils can have in your life. Remember that many of the essential oils only require a few drops that make it easy to replace many of the products in your home with essential oils, and save yourself a lot of time and money.

The next thing for you to do is decide which recipe you want to try first. Remember you aren't limited to the methods that we have provided here for you. With the information you now have on carriers and essential oils, you have what you need to make whatever you want with your essential oils!

BOOK 11: HERB GARDENING FOR BEGINNERS

Introduction

Growing your own herbs forms a genuine relationship between the plants you use and the medicine you create. It fosters a hearty appreciation for the craft of herbal medicine. There are those who buy herbs from a company and have no idea what the plants actually look like. They only know them by the label on the bag of dried and processed herbs. Creating your own herb garden will help you bridge this relationship gap as you work with these plants from seed to harvest.

When you buy herbs in bulk, you run the risk of buying old herbs that create weak remedies. They often have to be shipped to you in excessively cold or hot conditions, which further works to weaken them. Simply put, the fresher the herbs, the more potent your formulations will be.

You can control the quality of your herbs when you grow them yourself. Certain plants need to be harvested at certain times for maximum potency. You never know when the plants you buy were harvested, so it is nice to be able to control this aspect of herbal medicine-making. Not all bulk herb vendors sell organic herbs. Unless they have the USDA Organic labeling on their package, you have no way of knowing what toxins were sprayed on your herbs. When you grow your own herbs, you don't have to spray them with dangerous pesticides. This means you can grow truly pure, medicinal herbs.

Certain herbs suck toxins out of the soil. You really have no way of knowing if the herbs you buy in bulk have been planted in an area with soil that is high in lead, etc. When you grow your own herbs, you can have your soil tested prior to growing anything, so you know without a doubt that your plants are pure and your remedies are safe.

You will find that when you grow your own herbs, it is a truly gratifying, worthwhile, and fulfilling experience on many levels. You will have a better understanding of the plants you work with, fresher plants, and the highest quality plants possible. This means your herbal remedies will have the potential to be the most potent and highest quality remedies one can make.

Simply Herbs

This is a beginner guide, so let's start from the beginning. The first thing is that you should have a clear idea about why you should consider growing plants. Well, if you are reading this, you probably already know what herbs are, but let's have a little brush-up anyway in case you have any small gaps.

So, what are herbs? In the culinary arts, the term 'herb' refers to any green or leafy part of a plant that can be used for your medical remedies, season your dish or flavor a recipe, and other amazing things such as essential oils, pomades, and so on.

You may be wondering if herbs are used to flavor or season a dish without them being the main ingredient; aren't they the same thing as spices? Well, that's a very valid question, and the truth is that no, they are not the same. Their difference lies in the part of the plant they come from. In fact, spices are made from plant parts such as roots, seeds, twigs, dried bark, and more. For example, cinnamon is the bark of a tree, and cloves are dried flower buds. Notice that spices are often used in dried form, while herbs can be used both dried and fresh.

So, why should you grow herbs at home? as we have already established, growing your garden at home can be physically and mentally beneficial for you. It can turn into a beautiful, healthy hobby that you can teach the people around you to help them improve their lifestyles. It is something on which you can focus your mind on, and it can bring you closer to nature and the many possibilities it offers you. Expert growers assure that herbs are hands down the easiest plants to grow. Also, they simply look beautiful. Don't they? They can turn your garden or your empty home spaces into pieces of work art with their wonderful colors.

In conclusion, herbs are not only an amazing addition to your cooking, but they also have great health benefits that help you live a healthier life, not to mention the great psychological effects an indoor garden, being able to visualize and appreciate the product of your hard work, right at your fingertips. Other members of your family and your friends can see them too, and they can learn from your experience.

We will continue to list the benefits an indoor herb garden can offer you, but as of now, we hope you can see the wonders these little plants can give us beyond their rich flavors and fragrances. So how about starting a new hobby today? One that can help you improve your life, both mentally and physically!

Annual, Biennial, And Perennial Herbs

Plants fall into one of three categories, depending on how long they live when they flower, and when they seed. These are:

- Annual
- Biennial
- Perennial

Annual plants live for a year, meaning they complete an entire growing cycle, i.e., flower and seed, in a single year. Many hot climate plants such as basil and chilies are grown as annuals in temperate zones because they cannot survive the cold winters.

Commonly grown annual herbs include dill, cilantro, and summer savory. Parsley, although a biennial, is usually grown as an annual as the flavor decreases in the second year. You can cut and use annual herbs throughout the growing season, but before they die off for winter, harvest the entire plant. Some annual plants such as dill will self-seed if you let them flower.

Biennial plants, such as parsley, stevia, and sage, live for two years. They will usually grow lots of leaves in the first year, and then flower and seed in the second before dying off.

Perennial plants such as fennel, feverfew, ginger, and chives, live year after year, flowering and seeding each year. Many perennial herbs will die back to ground level and remain dormant over winter until spring comes and they grow back. Winter hardiness of perennial herbs does vary, so you need to check whether the herbs you want to grow will survive the winter where you live. If they will not, then either grow them in containers and move them to a protected location in winter, or grow them as annual plants and re-sow every spring.

Understanding which category each herb falls in helps you to plan your herb garden and know which plants you have to buy or grow again every year. When you read the herb directory, each section will tell you which of these categories each herb falls into. Some may be in more than one as they are grown as annuals in colder areas and their proper category when grown in their native environment.

How To Plant in Your Garden

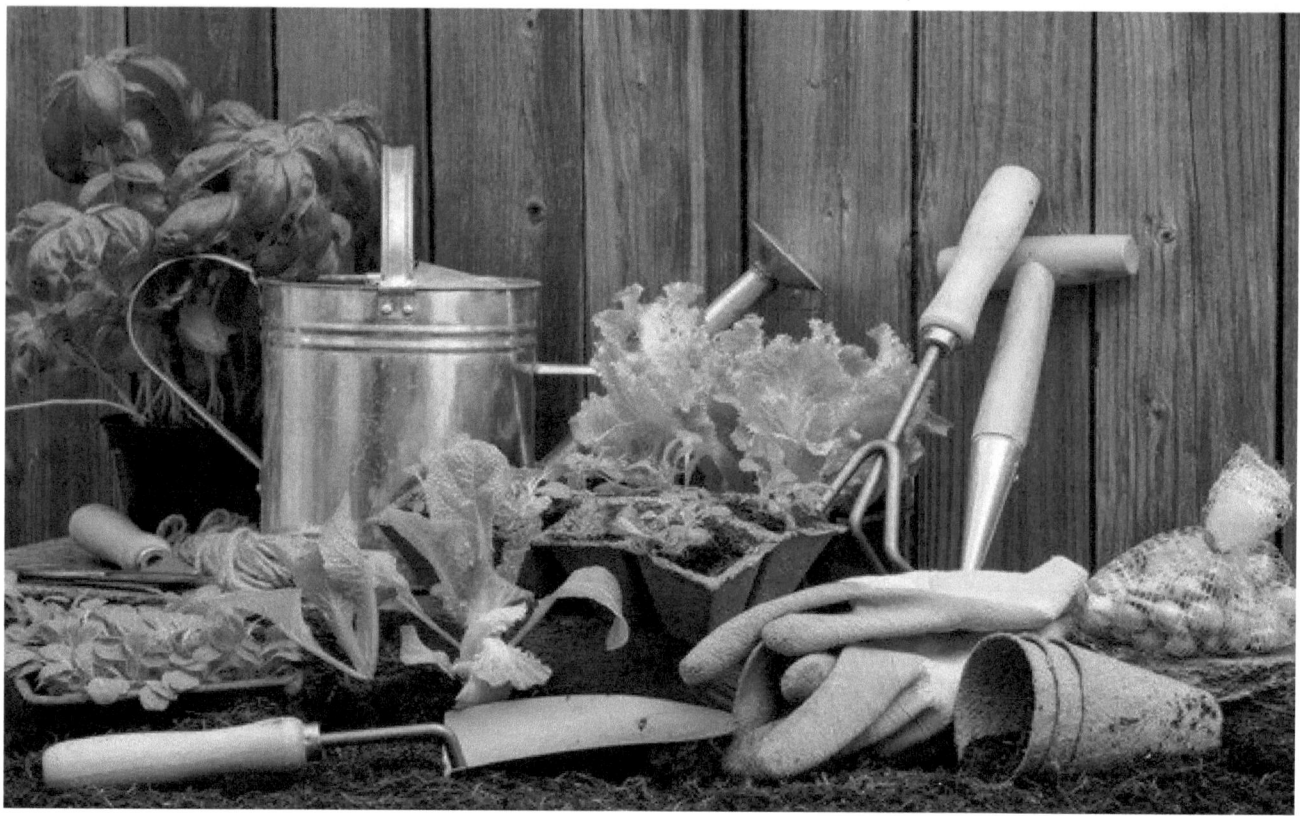

Plant growth refers to the process through which a plant increases in size, height, and breadth, with the process being aided by photosynthesis.

For the plant to grow properly, it would need rich soil, lots of sunlight, and enough water, which aids in initiating the photosynthetic reaction. It also demands a moist soil environment and appropriate temperatures, humidity, and other environmental factors.

A seed must be entirely dry and solid before it is planted in the ground and allowed to germinate. Immediately after planting a seed of this kind, the outer shell of the seed cracks or breaks apart, enabling the growing plant to take root and grow. This is possible if the seed is provided with sufficient water and is exposed to adequate temperatures.

In later stages, the seed absorbs the water, which allows the nodes to sprout and grow properly. The nodes pierce the seed's outer layer, exposing the primary root system of the growing plant under the ground's surface. During the plant's development from seedling to a fully grown plant, a rush of absorbed, well-balanced nutrients fuels the plant's growth as the roots continue their expansion and disseminate across the plant's developing environment. Meanwhile, the plant's roots continue to spread throughout the soil, and the plant's first leaves emerge from the ground, where they can absorb sunlight and begin to create the first photosynthesis, which takes place at this point in the plant's development.

It is for this reason that excavating a large hole while planting is not recommended.

Among other things, nitrogen is a critical component of chlorophyll, the green pigment in plants that allows photosynthesis.

Phosphorus initiates the plant's reproductive cycle, which is the switch from developing leaves to creating buds. Phosphorus is essential for plant reproduction. The plant is preparing to pollinate by developing its reproductive organs.

The first fruits are formed after the flowers have been pollinated. The watering schedule for flowers and fruit should be between ten and fifteen days to utilize all of the nutrients they have previously acquired from the soil throughout their maturation stage. When the fruits are harvested, they contain seeds that will sprout into new plants if planted in the ground.

Essential Tools

To begin with, the essential tools for home gardening have to be at one's beck and call, although it varies in a way due to different locations where the herb might be planted.

- Hand trowel

This looks like a little hand tool with a scoop-shaped blade and a short metal handle at the end. It is a great thigh workout since it requires the user to squat or bend to utilize it correctly and effectively. Even though it is more portable than a spade, this does not imply that it is any less sharp! The hand trowel is essential in the gardening toolbox when transplanting seedlings from a temporary site to a more permanent position.

Because of the scoop-shaped blade, hand trowels may also be used to apply manure. They can also be used for light weeding and mixing the soil and manure, particularly useful in the garden. For others, the desire to begin herbal gardening may be a strong drive that necessitates using a portable container to facilitate the process. After a few days, when the herb is germinating, the curiosity and interest may become so strong that it would need the establishment of a more permanent location.

- Gloves

Gloves are a requirement for any future herbal gardener who doesn't want to get their hands dirty. Some people don't see them as a necessity, but they are, irrespective of the scale of gardening, i.e., greenhouse, portable tins, or patch of land. Dirt can easily slip into the fingers, some plants with thorns can easily scratch your wrist or forearms, and it's not all types of water that a human can tolerate.

My tip when purchasing a pair of gloves is to get water-resistant ones, not surgeon gloves, because they aren't durable enough. Also, the gloves need to be long enough to cover up your wrist and possibly reach your elbows. Moreover, ensure the gloves are not too big for your fingers. They do not need to be a smug fit, but it is better not get gloves that would be falling off your fingers.

Gloves are tricky in a way, but with the right fit, they will last for a long time before they need of replacement.

- Hand fork

Hand forks are useful when turning the soil because it has three or four short flat prongs. It can even dig into denser soil. First, it is easier to lift; it has slightly more flexibility, allowing you to see the depth you require.

Some hand forks have a more extended handle because gardeners want a wide range of longer handle forks. In addition, hand forks can be used for light weeding, ensuring that manure is properly mixed into the soil, and even for breaking muddled ground.

- Hoe

This is a tool with either a round or somewhat rectangular blade. Sometimes, the handle is short, or it could even be longer.

The hoe is a good gardening tool for making ridges and heaps where the stalk or seed of the herbs can be planted. It can be used for weeding as well when large-scale greenhouse gardening is involved. It can also be used in transplanting some particular type of crops, for example

A hoe usually has a wooden handle while the blade is metallic. This allows durability of the hoe and also maximum use.

- Watering wand/ Watering can

A watering can is a metallic and portable container with a handle and a funnel used to water plants and herbs.

Being portable, a gardener can intentionally water the plant base, limiting the growth of weeds to an extent in the garden.

Also, a watering can serves as a container to grow herbs in. Using a watering wand provides a gentle rain-like spray that doesn't blast and pulverize fragile seedlings or tender herbs. Using a long wand allows gardeners to water the roots without bending.

- Garden hose

The garden hose is a good substitute for the regular watering can. It is made of rubber with a metallic nuzzle; ensure that water directly from the source (i.e., tap or a tank) is sprayed all over the crop.

- Rake

A rake is a garden tool that consists of a long wooden handle or a metal handle with a strong metal/wooden head consisting of several prongs that would be used to level the soil's surface.

Rakes vary in length; some are long and can reach a sizeable distance, while some are short and can break soil lumps into finer particles.

Rakes cover vegetable seeds when they are dispersed and gather fallen leaves of herbs in autumn. Raking up leaves ensures that they don't block the soil from receiving what it needs: water, sunlight, and a healthy air flow.

Metal rakes are durable and not as effective as plastic rakes when moving large quantities of leaves. Also, rakes break up the soil and smoothen the ground with lines and drills to plant seeds. They can also be used to draw back the ground to cover seeds.

- Wheelbarrow

This is a small metallic cart with a single wheel at the front, two supporting legs, and two handles at the rear used in carrying tools from the store to where they are needed.

A wheelbarrow can be used to move compost to the garden, mix fertilizer, and even be a good location for gardening itself.

With enough loamy soil, a few micro-organisms that would start the process, and seeds can be a good spot for gardening more than two different types of herbs. The regularity of watering the herb is the most crucial aspect of this, as well as sunlight. The wheelbarrow is a source of transportation in gardening, relatively easy to move, and can bear the weight of tools.

- Secateurs

Secateurs is a scissors-like tool that consists of two short metal blades and two short wooden/metal handles.

This garden tool is used in pruning herbs and plants, removing excess material from the plant to make its growth more effective. As many as five to six stalks can start growing during seeding, but one or two would have to be removed over time to ensure enough nutrients.

Secateurs is also used to trim plants with voluminous growth, i.e., spreading their branches and leaves in a poof pattern. It can also be used during harvesting to cut the flowers from the plant or the leaves from the plants.

Step-By-Step Guide
Choosing Your Herbs

Choosing the herbs, you wish to grow in your garden can be overwhelming. Start by making a list to keep track of what you want and have an idea of how much space you will need. When creating your herb list, start by thinking about what herbs you will be using the most. It can be tempting to purchase herb seeds because they look pretty, but ask yourself whether or not that herb will benefit you. You want to tailor your herb garden to fit your specific needs.

Consider the issues that have the most impact on your life. Those who suffer from indigestion may want to consider adjusting their list to include herbs that help relax the stomach, such as chamomile and fennel, if they do so often. If you are prone to skin problems such as rashes and eczema, consider placing herbs such as calendula and lavender on your shopping list. Continue to add herbs to your list as you come across them for various conditions.

It is essential to include herbs useful for strengthening the immune system and attacking viruses in any herb garden. Consider including plants such as elderberry in your garden for this purpose.

Garden Size

When it comes to selecting how many herbs you will grow, the size of your garden is critical. Once you've compiled a manageable list of herbs, you'll be ready to make your purchase. Get comfortable and examine the size of your garden area in more detail. How much space will you have left when everything has been properly laid out? Fortunately, with pot gardening, even the tiniest of areas may house a large number of plants.

Make a note of the requirements for each of the plants you've discovered, paying close attention to the quantity of sunlight necessary for each plant. On the area you have designated for their cultivation, will all of your herbs access the materials they need to thrive? Along with putting together your herb list, you'll gain a better knowledge of the kind of garden you want: whether it'll be huge and sprawling or small and intimate. You'll also learn if you want a garden that gets primarily the sun, mostly shade, or a little of both.

If you know where your plants should be located, whether they should be near a source of irrigation or not, and how/where to position your plants so that they can flourish in their environment, you will be much more successful. Your master list will be very beneficial to you as you begin your journey on this mission. While you are establishing your garden and even after your plants have begun to grow, you may want to return to it periodically to ensure that you provide the best possible care for them.

Finding the Best Location for Your Plants

Once you have a detailed list of herbs you would like to plant based on your particular needs and information next to each herb detailing their sunlight, soil, and watering needs, you are ready to determine where you will put each plant.

Just make sure you have a realistic plant list that will accommodate the area you choose to plant. Put all the plants that require full shade together. Put all the plants that require partial shade together, etc.

Designing Your Garden

You should create a garden design specifically tailored to the plants you pick while also taking your specific needs into mind. Make certain that the place where you want to start growing plants has a sufficient water supply and is close to a water tap (if outdoors). Rather than running many hoses to bring water to the place in issue, this will save time and effort overall.

Keep in mind where you want to acquire your soil and whether or not you wish to utilize dirt already in your garden area while planning your project. You must submit your soil samples to your local extension office so that they may be properly evaluated. As a result, you'll be able to identify precisely what is lacking in your soil and take steps to rectify the condition. Your soil may need a little amount of lime or fertilizer to enhance its general condition, depending on the findings of the tests.

Fertilizers

It is also a good idea to start thinking about what kind of organic fertilizer you would want to use, if any, in your garden. Fertilizers can help a garden grow. Several gardeners make use of horse manure, while others make use of poultry dung from their chicken coops. Some gardeners utilize manure from cows or turkeys. These fertilizers are frequently superior since they are made from natural ingredients rather than synthetic chemicals. If you already have animals, consider collecting manure for use in your garden. Don't be too aggressive with the manure spreading, or you may end up damaging the plants. Even a little amount here and there might help to keep your soil healthy.

Start with growing some herbs inside for a few weeks before transplanting them into a container or garden bed. This will give them a better start in the long run. Check to see if you have a little area in your house that receives adequate sunshine where you can set up some tiny seed trays for the seeds to germinate. Because many seeds do not need sunshine to germinate if they are not exposed to enough sunlight, they will depend on heat instead. However, for the seedlings to grow, you will need to provide them with sunshine as soon as they emerge. You may want to consider investing in seedling starter lights to aid in the germination of your seedlings. You'll be able to grow them in almost any part of the home this way.

Determining If You Need a Greenhouse

Several gardeners use greenhouses in which they cultivate plants before transplanting them to a different location. Greenhouses are also used for year-round plant cultivation by these individuals. Because they imitate plants' ideal growth environment, greenhouses are useful if you are a serious gardening enthusiast.

Additionally, if you reside in a place with lower temperatures, greenhouses may be beneficial. They make it possible to cultivate plants that would not otherwise be able to grow in that environment. Growing tropical plants such as turmeric and ginger, as well as citrus fruits such as lemon and lime, may be possible in your garden. Many medicinal plants need more tropical temperatures to thrive, and a greenhouse may make it much easier to cultivate these plants successfully. Keep in mind that a greenhouse designed to grow tropical plants in colder areas will need to be equipped with a watering system and a heating system to function properly.

Because of the high cost of timber, it may be quite costly to construct a greenhouse. However, if you decide that you want one, it would most likely be well worth your effort to look into it. To avoid spending the money on a custom-built greenhouse, you can simply purchase pre-built greenhouses or greenhouses made of metal frames and plastic tarping material. These may be more cost-effective, but they seem more unstable and are susceptible to damage during wind storms and other natural disasters.

A greenhouse is not required for gardening, but it is a good idea to investigate whether or not one would be a good match for your requirements before investing in one.

How to Plant Herbs in a Container

Herbs will grow very well in containers outdoors which means you can grow them in an easy to reach location, such as by the kitchen door, or they can be brought indoors or put in a greenhouse to protect them during cold or inclement weather. Containers could be placed on the floor, or there could be hanging baskets or planters attached to walls or fences, to keep herbs away from the prying hands of children and curious household pets.

Although the initial cost of container gardening is much higher than growing direct in the soil, long term maintenance tends to be lower as you are not battling weeds growing through the soil. Containers are a great way to make a herb garden if you have limited space, a balcony, or even a full garden. Some of us are banned by our significant others from growing herbs in the flower beds and must use strategically placed containers!

It is possible to grow different types of herbs in a single container, though you need to make sure that they have similar soil and sun needs. There is no point growing a herb that likes a moist soil with one that likes a dry soil as one or the other will suffer. It is best to use annual herbs when putting multiple plants in a single container as perennial herbs will grow too big and crowd out the smaller herbs. However, if you have rosemary or lavender in a container, you can always grow a trailing herb such as creeping thyme which will hang over the edge of the container and not compete for space with a larger plant.

Seeds can be planted directly into containers or you can plant seedlings or store-bought plants, depending on the size of the container. A good way of extending your growing season is to start your herb seeds off indoors and then transplant them outdoors to containers when they have grown to a reasonable size and the risk of frost has passed.

There are many different types of containers on the market made from anything from stone to plastic to resin or metal. What you buy will depend on your budget, the size container you want and the style container you like for your garden. Porous materials such as clay dry out much faster than those made of plastic or resin due to evaporation, which will influence the amount of watering you need to do.

All containers need drainage holes so that excess water can seep out at the bottom. If there are not sufficient drainage holes, then you need to create some. Most herbs will die if their containers get waterlogged. Self-watering containers are a good idea if you are growing in a greenhouse, but when used outside, they fill up with rainwater and drown your plants.

The key to making your herbs happy in containers is to use a good quality soil mix. Adjust the soil mix based on what the herb you are growing requires, but generally, a mixture of a third each of vermiculite or pearlite, good quality compost and peat moss provides an excellent growing medium. Fill the container with soil and then push it down gently without compacting it as it is easier for the herb to grow in looser soil. Do not use soil from your garden as this will contain pests, weed seeds and potential diseases as well.

Container plants are completely reliant on you for water and food. Once the herbs are established, their leaves will act as an umbrella and direct rainwater away from the container, so you still need to water them when it rains. Water directly onto the soil when required rather than onto the leaves to prevent run-off and mold forming if the leaves get too damp.

Your herbs will need fertilizing regularly too, typically starting two weeks after planting mature plants and four weeks after planting seedlings or after seeds have germinated. After this time, the plants will have depleted the nutrients in the soil, and they will need replenishing. Use a liquid feed such as a tomato feed or a general-purpose vegetable feed. This will have plenty of nitrogen in it that your plants need to grow healthy leaves. Seaweed based feeds are ideal for containers because they are packed with micro-nutrients and plants love these fertilizers. Avoid any fertilizers that are higher in potassium (K) or phosphorus (P) as these will encourage the herbs to form flowers at which point the taste of the leaves can often diminish. Feed once a week during the growing season and no more than once a month during the dormant season.

To encourage leafy growth, cut or pinch off any flower heads that form. This forces the plant to direct its energy on producing more growth so it can produce more flowers. Many herbs produce attractive flowers which will look great and attract beneficial insects to your garden.

Feel free to put some flowers in the containers with your herbs for some extra color and interest. Nasturtiums, marigolds, and pansies all look great in containers plus they have edible parts. These can brighten up a container of otherwise drab green herbs.

What Do I Need for Container Herb Gardening?

Alright, so you have learned a bit about container gardening and what it involves, at least broadly. There is actually good news when it comes to this: the list is not long at all, but it will be quite specific, so make sure to write down a list of all the things you will need when you finally go shopping for your gardening supplies.

Many edible plants can grow in enclosed containers, but herbs are a popular choice for at least two reasons: they don't require much space at all (as compared to, let's say, eggplants, which will require a larger container in which they can develop properly) and their yield is quite rich, considering they are very small in volume. Yet, if you want your efforts to reap benefits, you should always make sure that you place the herb container in a very sunny area in your house–preferably a balcony or a smaller outside area. If not, simply placing them in your most well-lit room, near the windows, will work well (but not as well as those that have the chance to grow outside of your apartment or house).

Herbs do not need much attention.. Fertilizer is not needed and most of the herbs grow naturally and beautifully in the plainest and most ordinary of soils. Yet, while you will not need to add fertilizers, you will need to water the plants when they need it. Most of the herbs grow in dry weather/climate conditions, but some of them will require to be a bit damper to grow healthy.

Many types of herbs can survive even when they are kept outside year-round, as long as the pots are large enough (of at least 5 gallons of soil, for example). Also, if the herbs are good for the climate in which you live and if they have good waste, they stand every chance to survive. However, if you intend to do this, always make sure that you keep them in plastic containers throughout the winter because ceramic and glass can very easily crack and break due to lower temperatures. You can move the plants from their ceramic pots to the plastic containers during the late summer, so that they have enough time to root themselves into their new "home" by the time winter kicks in and so that they resist the harsher weather. If you do not want to bother with this, you can treat your herbs as annuals and completely dispose of them for the winter, but it may not be very advantageous to do this.

You need to make sure that your pot can drain excess water off it. This is extremely important for the well-being of the plant because when there is no space (or not enough space) to allow the water to go out of the pot, the dirt will get excessively wet and it will kill the base of the plant instead of providing it with the necessary nutrients. Of course, you can buy herbs that are already planted in pots, but most of them do not have enough drainage space, so you will either need to enlarge those holes or you will need to buy a separate pot with larger drainage holes. To get an idea of how large the drainage hole should be, you should know that half of one inch is enough for a small or medium pot. Also, one inch is suitable for larger pots.

The terrible news is that numerous herb pots that are sold basically do not have enough seepage. You can regularly expand the drainage that is available to your plant, by penetrating, punching, or cutting greater gaps. In any case, it is simply simpler to purchase a pot that has enough drainage area available for your plant. I would say that the base size for a drainage gap is about half an inch in measurement for small or medium-sized pots. For bigger containers, search for drainage area that is about an inch in measurement to make sure that there is sufficient area for the water to drain.

What about The Soil?

Potting soil is widely available in grocery stores and in specialty shops as well, so you should have no issue with purchasing some for your new garden. Most of the potting soil available for sale does not have any kind of nutritional supplements in it, so you will have to think of purchasing these as well. Also, you may need to add compost as well and mix it with the soil. There are many types of potting soil and compost from which you can choose. You can purchase them from the specialty store or grocery store, or you can use all-natural homemade compost and purchase 100% natural potting soil as well. The choice is up to you. Either way, you will most likely end up with the same range of prices because the difference between the money you pay for different types of soil and compost is quite small.

For instance, some people use fluid compost, while others use fish emulsions, ocean growth mixes. These may not smell very nice, but they are absolutely essential for the good health of the plant. Also, other people use chemical compounds (Miracle Go, for example). While these chemical solutions can be efficient when it comes to the way in which they help the plants grow, they kill the soil's micro=organisms, which are essential for the good growth of the plant. In other words, if you use such chemicals on your plant once, you will always need to use it because it will not be able to re-build its natural stock of micro-organisms.

The Seeds and the Plants

If you have decided to do this, you will also need to purchase seeds and plants. You can check out ranchers and nurseries in your close vicinity if you want to, but if you cannot find what you need there, then you may want to search online. Chives, mint, basil, parsley, rosemary, sage, thyme, and many other herbs are quite easy to find when you want to start your container garden.

Also, keep in mind that no matter what herb in particular you choose, you should make sure that you purchase it in a healthy state and that it is certified by the local authorities in this field. Also, you may have to look around for a bit and see if it would be better to purchase certain plants as seeds or as sprouts. Either way, a bit of research can truly go a long way, so make sure not to rush into anything.

For plants, you ought to check the nearby ranchers' markets or nurseries. Attempt chives, mint, basil, parsley, rosemary, sage, thyme, and that is just the beginning! There are lots to choose from, just make sure that the seeds or plants that you buy are healthy and certified by the place that you buy them from. You may have to look around a bit to figure out whether it's best to buy certain herbs as seeds or as sprouts, but either way, a little bit of time goes a long way and you can find lots of resources to buy your seeds and/or plants from for your container garden.

Generally speaking, herb plants usually go outside, and you can find them in various gardening centers and even order them via mail. However, although you may think it is easier to start with this, it is not necessarily so. If you do order them though, make sure that they will not be delivered before the time when the weather is warm enough as to allow you to plant them.

On the other hand, seeds are much less expensive, and they are much more diverse when it comes to the assortments and flavors. However, in most cases you will have to start with the planting process before the weather is warm enough (1-2 months before). You will most likely have to plant them in a smaller pot and keep them on the inside of the house in a well-lit area and place them on the outside only when there is absolutely no concern about frosting.

Other than these basic things presented here, there is not much to know about container gardening. Once you learn the ropes, everything else should come fairly easy. Even more, you may even come across places that sell container gardening supplies in particular, which means that your job may be even easier than it was described here. Keep your eyes and your ears open and make sure you don't rush into anything–after all, your plants will take their time to grow and you should take your time to grow in the art of gardening as well.

Harvesting

Harvesting herbs can be a rewarding experience. Not only do you get some delicious food, but you also feel like someone who has some serious gardening skills! Harvesting herbs is simple and won't take up too much time or energy; plus, it will make everything you make taste delicious.

Unlike harvesting vegetables, you don't actually have to eat the stuff when you harvest herbs. In fact, many herbs have sharp thorns or prickly leaves that could hurt you when you try to pick them. The best thing to do when picking herbs is to use a pair of sharp shears or garden scissors, which will allow you to safely cut the stems and leaves from the plant without getting hurt in the process.

For some delicate herb plants, such as basil and mint, the best time to harvest them is actually in mid-summer or in September. This way, you can grow new plants from the same seeds and you will not have to replant the cuttings.

Once you have harvested your herbs, consider giving them a drink of water or a little bit of fertilizer to help them resist diseases. Just make sure that the herb flowers are dry before your plant goes into storage, otherwise, it could rot away. Lastly, store your herbs in airtight containers with paper towels or coffee filters on top to keep mold at bay. This way, they will stay moist until you are ready to use them again.

How to Harvest

Many people around the world eat herbs and vegetables, but they probably don't know how to harvest them. The process is not difficult, though it does require patience and time. This will tell you everything you need to know about harvesting herbs such as thyme, parsley, sage, chives, and more!

Before we get started on this guide on how to harvest herbs, we're going to give a brief introduction to the subject. Herbs are plants that grow in temperate zones like Europe and North America that can be used for both culinary purposes and medicinal purposes. Healing herbal remedies like tea or soup made from these plants has been used for centuries because of their strong medicinal properties.

Herbs are harvested by cutting the plants with pruning shears or scissors. The plants should be picked while they are still in their growing season, so it's best to go out and pick them the morning after the plants have flowered. If you don't trim your plants right away, they will regrow and it will take quite some time until you harvest them again.

Ways to Harvest Herbs

There are many ways to harvest herbs, but here are just a few of them:

• Pulling the Oldest Leaves: this method is very practical because you can use it anytime if you want to use just a handful of leaves at a time. Simply pull the oldest leaves on the plant and hang them upside down in bunches. This will give you a beautiful display of herbs.

- Harvesting Whole Plants: this method is important if you want to collect large amounts of herbs at once because you can use them directly without trimming or drying. Simply cut the stems off of the plants with shears (preferably pruning shears) and place them all in some kind of containers like a bucket or an old jar so they can start to dry out till they get used up. Trim them again when they get too big for your container.
- Small Potted Plants: this is a rather minor way to harvest herbs because you only need a few at a time. All you have to do is cut your plants with pruning shears or scissors and place them in some kind of pot, preferably one that the herbs can be moved around in.
- Herbal Recipes: these can be used to make herbal soups, tea, or any other type of herbal product depending on the herb. To make a soup, for example, you will want to finely chop the leaves and put them in some water (1 cup of water per 5 leaves). Allow the plant to soak for 10 minutes, then boil it in some water until it softens (about 15 minutes). Some herbs will have a stronger effect, so you might want to boil them longer. Once it's finished, strain the herbs out. You can follow the same process with the leaves of other herbs as well.

You can also use fresh herbs for tea instead of dried ones. However, only fresh ones will have enough potency especially if you're using very strong herbs like sage or rosemary, which are prone to lose potency over time because they contain essential oils that evaporate after drying.

How Much to Harvest and When to Harvest

When the time comes to harvest herbs, gardeners know that timing is key—but exactly how much harvesting should take place? How long are the different herb plants in their prime? And what are some general guidelines for when to harvest each type of plant?

There are many factors that go into deciding how to harvest an herb. Obviously, the greatest factor is the type of herb you are harvesting. But if you are harvesting for personal use, there is no need to harvest a huge quantity of an herb at one time. In most cases, it will be more efficient to make several small harvests rather than one big harvest.

For example, if you were harvesting rosemary for cooking purposes, it would not be practical to try and harvest a large number of rosemary plants all at once. The best way would be to wait until you need some for a specific recipe or meal and then harvest a small amount from one or two plants. If you need rosemary in the future, you can harvest it in the same manner.

One of the reasons you may want to wait until you need herbs for cooking is that if they are left to dry on their own, they will lose their flavor. For example, after harvesting basil, it is best to dry basil quickly by hanging it upside down in a cool dark location or in a paper bag lined with newspaper or paper towels. This way, it will retain its flavor until you are ready to use it. When drying herbs for storage purposes only, they can be placed on paper plates in a cool dark location and allowed to dry naturally without losing any flavor.

Some herbs are best harvested right after harvest time. These are usually the herbs that dry well. Examples of this are basil, coriander, chives, cilantro, marjoram, parsley, sage, and tarragon. Many herbs such as mint and spearmint do not dry as well as those listed above and it is best to harvest them right before use.

Some herbs such as cilantro and mint may be susceptible to powdery mildew if they are not harvested soon after picking. This means that you do not want to wait too long to harvest them or they will be ruined and uncluttered and must be thrown away (not composted!).

Some herbs are best left for several weeks to several months before they are harvested. This is especially true of the ones that do not dry well. If you want to harvest these herbs before they are ready, you should harvest the leaves and not the tops of the plants. The tops of these types of herbs usually need to be pulled up in their entirety.

If you want to harvest an herb that needs time to mature, then wait until just before or just after flowering time before harvesting it. This applies to herbs such as chamomile, lemon balm, peppermint, rosemary, lavender, sage, thyme, and more.

Some herbs do have a specific harvest time, however. These herbs include anise hyssop, borage, calendula, chamomile, chervil, fennel, lemon balm, and sweet cicely. If you are not sure when the best time to harvest these herbs is, then it is best to wait until you have a specific recipe that requires them in order to know exactly when they should be harvested.

Another factor in harvesting is the amount of lighting that the plants receive. If you are harvesting indoors, then you will want to harvest the herbs in the late afternoon or early evening when there is less sunlight. This will help to prevent wilting and help maintain freshness.

If your plants are grown outdoors, it is better to harvest them when it is slightly cloudy rather than in direct sunlight. When they are harvested in direct sunlight, they may be more susceptible to wilting and color fading.

The most essential thing to remember about harvesting herbs is that you do not need a large quantity of each herb for your own personal use. It is most efficient and economical to harvest only what you need at that specific time. If you are harvesting for commercial purposes, though, it may be necessary to harvest a larger number of each herb at one time.

<u>Tools Needed</u>

If you're a cook who likes to use fresh herbs in your daily cooking, then harvesting and stocking up for the winter months is going to be an important job! You can do this whole process with a few simple tools, which we will cover in more detail below.

Herbs need very little maintenance, but it's still worth having the right equipment on hand. For instance, if you are running out to harvest your herbs in the middle of fall, then you are going to want to have the right tools ready.

In general, there are three basic tools that you will need when harvesting fresh herbs from your garden: a pair of garden clippers, a pair of scissors, and a good knife.

- The first is the garden clippers. A good set of shears or clippers can be essential in making sure that every bit of herb is harvested without damage to the plant.
- The second piece of equipment, the scissors, will be used to prune the plant gently. If your herb is growing too high or too close to a wall, then clippers won't be able to reach it. The shears will do the job perfectly!
- The third and final piece of equipment is a good knife. You can use this for a variety of tasks, from pruning stems and making cuts to trimming off a few leaves here and there before you put them in a container.

While these are the basic tools that you will need, there are also other things that you will want to keep in mind. You can find more details below!

Methods in Harvesting Herbs

There are two methods used for harvesting herbs: cutting your plants with scissors or taking out small sections with shears. You will find these methods equally effective in getting all of the leaves without damaging the plant.

Garden clippers and shears will both work well for harvesting herbs. However, garden clippers are better for larger plants and certain herbs while shears are better for smaller plants and some more delicate herbs.

To make sure that you avoid damage to the plant, it is important to prune your plants exactly as you want them. This can be done by cutting off any branches that are too close to the ground or hitting the stem on a wall or fence.

Once your plants have been pruned, use your scissors or shears to take out all the leaves in the space where you plan on putting them in a container.

7 Herbs to Grow At Home

Although there are plenty of plants you can grow in your garden, we will not review all them. These herbs are tolerant and do not require much attention. Most importantly, they are potent with healing compounds and can treat almost all diseases that affect humanity. Here are the top plants to consider for your backyard herbal garden.

Rosemary

Rosemary is one of the most potent herbal plants to grow in your garden. Officially known as Salvia Rosmarinus, the plant is a woody perennial with fragrant evergreen leaves. It blooms with white, pink, blue, and purple flowers. The flower is native to Mediterranean regions and treats various diseases, including indigestion, vomiting, and nausea, among others. The herb thrives in climate zones 5 to 8, but it is only perennial in climate zones 6 and 7.

Basil

Basil is another of the most common herbs that are grown in backyard gardens. Basil thrives in pots and containers as opposed to planting directly in the soil. This herb is known for its culinary and medicinal benefits. It is native to Asia and central Africa. Still, it can also be grown in the US and other parts of North America. The herb thrives in soil with a pH of 5.1 to 5.8 and can do well in climate zones 2 - 11. However, it is only perennial in climate zones 10 and 11.

Ginger

Ginger is one of the most useful plants you can grow in your garden, and it is easy to see why. This sweet and spicy herb is a rhizome and not a root, as many people believe. The herb is an excellent additive to tea and fermented foods and acts as a spice in recipes.

Ginger can be grown in some parts of the US and takes about ten months to mature. The stem and leaves are dark green and will remain green throughout until it's time to harvest. Ginger does not thrive in every zone but does well in zone 7.

Ginger is used in treating various conditions, including colds, nausea, arthritis, migraines, and hypertension. The herb is also anti-inflammatory and increases the flow of blood in the body. The herb also helps in reducing flatulence and stomach issues such as diarrhea and nausea.

Garlic

Garlic is another of the best all-around medicinal herbs with plenty of uses. Garlic can be grown in most zones and soil types and is tolerant to pests. With that said, if you wish to grow garlic in your garden, you have to get the timing right. In hardiness zones, 3-5, garlic should be planted during September and October. Plant your garlic between early September and October so that they are out of the ground by December. In climate zones 5 - 7, you should plant the garlic in late October. In climate zones 7-9, you can plant from October to November. In zones 9 to 10, you should plant in late October to November. If you do not get the timing right, you may mess with the plant's growth.

Garlic is used to treat respiratory ailments such as colds and coughs. It is also used to boost the immune system, treat asthma, and manage heart disease. Some people also use garlic to manage pain caused by arthritis or toothaches.

Thyme

Thyme is one of the herbs that every gardener must grow. Thyme is beautiful and has a sweet scent that attracts bees and butterflies. It is also tolerant of most soil types hence easy to cultivate even for beginners. Although it can grow in the US and other parts of North America, it does not fare well in cold winters. The herb will thrive in hardiness zone 5 but can be grown through to zone 10. However, in higher zones such as 10 and 9, more care should be taken. Due to its sweet scent, thyme is used as a relaxant. It is also used to treat coughs and other upper respiratory conditions. Some studies have suggested that it can be used to treat bronchitis.

Peppermint

Peppermint is one of the fast-spreading perennial herbs. It usually takes over the garden and may end up overpowering other crops in the garden. However, it can be contained with proper management. This herb is known for its spicy, aromatic scent and can be recognized from a distance. Peppermint is grown within climate zones 3 to 8 and is perennial in most regions. This herb is used to treat flatulence, menstrual pains, diarrhea, nausea, and anxiety.

Oregano

Oregano is another herb that can be planted within your garden. The beauty of this herb is that once it is planted in soil, it thrives and develops quickly. The plant originates from Southern and Easter Eurasia and belongs to the mint family. Oregano is used as a spice in most Mexican, Spanish and Italian dishes. It is a hardy perennial plant that can grow in most backyard gardens. Although it can grow in most climate zones in the US and Canada, it mainly thrives in hardiness zones 5 to 10.

Oregano herbs have plenty of health and dietary benefits, including fighting bacterial infections, reducing viral infections, and decreasing inflammation, among other uses.

Benefits Of Self-Cultivation Of Medicinal Plants

As of now, you must have already understood that Native American herbs are considered as the basic necessities for human beings to live healthy lives. For several ages, the plants have been integrated with tradition and culture to make you aware of future generations. In the past centuries, it was quite easy for Native Americans to locate the herbs they needed for treating a certain health condition. But currently, it is quite hard for people to find or source herbs organically for themselves. It means that they cannot just walk around in the wild and get the herbs anymore. It is because the big herbal retail stores and the supplement manufacturers are taking the lands of herbs into their possessions. As a result, the commoners have to buy the herbs from them in order to avail their medicinal benefits.

This shouldn't be the case! Therefore, the idea of growing medicinal plants at home boomed among the common people across the globe. Growing such Native American plants in your garden is not just going to help you with healthy functional outcomes but will also help you out with greenery and beauty around the space. Before ending the book, it is important to give you a subtle explanation of the fact that you did the right thing by walking on the path of growing herbs in your garden. Here are some benefits of the same, to support your initiative:

4. Enhances Mental Clarity and Focus

Beginners who intend to take the job of planting indoor and outdoor herb plants for adapting the herbal remedies in the long run for health concerns will also improving their mental clarity and focus in the process. You are studying this book with utmost focus and clarity in order to learn the steps on how to plant herbs in your garden. This is one kind of prime focus that you are developing by giving your time, effort, and patience to this subject. This might not be in direct relation to the medicinal benefits of the herbs, but this development still counts! It is because you can use the same amount of focus and mental clarity to learn anything and everything in life, which you desire to master!

5. Eradicate the Air Pollutants

The prime reason behind planting the herbs is to reap their health benefits! But beyond that, these plants also have the capability of filtering the air from pollutants and improving their quality. The more plants you add to your indoor or outdoor gardens, the fresher the air will be around the space. As a result, you will be breathing fresh air directly being filtered by the medicinal plants. Hence, this itself will work upon enhancing your physical, mental, and heart health. Some of the specific Native American plants do have the reputed potential of improving the quality of air and making it free from irritants to breathe healthily.

6. They are Economical

One of the most common reasons why people turn to growing Native American herbs in their garden rather than buying them from the stores is the cost. The amount you spend on buying bulk herbs can be utilized in planting the same seeds or plants in the garden. The plus point is that the plant will keep on giving you its herbal limbs and parts throughout the year and more till the time you shower care upon it. And this won't be the case with single-use packages. If you are want to try out the herbs and their efficacies first before planting them, then you can surely go for the packaged herbs from such stores. But if you are a herbal enthusiast and your health depends upon such plants and their herbal extracts, you cannot buy them all the time! Therefore, grow them in your garden to have unlimited accessibility over time.

7. Healthy Engagement with Mind and Body

The plants will need care and pampering throughout their growing period just like any other living being would need! Therefore, you will feel engaged throughout your free time, as you will be spending more time with the plants. Hence, this gives you an opportunity to build compassion within yourself, and you will develop a connecting mind to socialize with others on a better note. Living around plants is always credited for rejuvenating the mood of a person.

These are the four major benefits that prove the efficacy of growing medicinal plants in your home. This totally explains what nature has to offer to the people till eternity. The Native Americans have passed on their knowledge and expertise of herbs to their offspring through positive word of mouth and practical applications. Modern-day scientists have tried extreme ways in order to derive the maximum potential of the Native American herbs. And the commoners are keeping their best foot forward by growing the plants in their private gardens.

Conclusion

Herbs have a whole host of uses in your garden from attracting pollinating insects, to culinary, health, and beauty uses, and let's not forget, a lot of them look fantastic!

In general, herbs are easy to grow, and for those that are hard to germinate, you can usually buy the part-grown plants from a local nursery or plant store. Many supermarkets now stock living herbs and sell them very cheaply, and these can usually be planted outdoors after they have been hardened off and adjusted to sunlight.

Every gardener should be growing some herbs. Fresh herbs are great in the kitchen, and as you start to experiment with the healing and beauty properties of herbs, you realize how incredibly useful they are. Today, a lot of the traditional uses of herbs have been backed up by scientific research, showing that they are effective treatments for many conditions. Of course, for any serious complaints, you should not self-medicate but must seek professional medical advice.

If you are on any prescribed medication, be careful taking herbs as many of them can interact with these medicines and change their effect or render them useless. If you have been prescribed any medication, no matter what it is, then talk to your doctor before taking herbs medicinally as they could negatively interact with your medication. Some herbs boost estrogen production and can stop the birth control pill from working, whereas others stop anti-depressants from working or allow drugs like lithium to build up in your system to potentially harmful levels.

Growing herbs is incredibly rewarding. You have learned a lot about herbs in this book, from what they are to how to use them and now you can start planning out your herb garden. Think about the herbs that you regularly buy from the supermarket to use in your kitchen and start by planting them. As you gain more experience, start growing new herbs to use in your cooking. Then try making some tea as a change from coffee or black tea. Many herbal teas have a delicious flavor, and you can combine different herbs to make a tea specifically for you.

Remember when planting herbs together, ensure they have the right soil conditions. The biggest problem people have when growing herbs is planting herbs with very different environmental requirements together. Planting an herb that loves dry soil in the same container with one that likes moist soil is a recipe for disaster as one of the herbs, if not both, will die off.

Whether you grow herbs indoors or outdoors, in large quantities or small ones, is entirely up to you. Herbs are wonderful plants and you have had an introduction to some of the most popular and commonly used culinary and healing herbs. There are many more herbs out there plus many of those listed here have a wide variety of cultivars that may not have healing properties or be edible, but look fantastic! There is no reason why an herb garden should be drab and boring. In fact, many herb gardens are alive with insects and abundant in color from the purple flowers of chives to the blue of borage and the orange of calendula.

Your herbs can be frozen or dried to store, so you can enjoy your herbs all year round. Literally, nothing needs to go to waste.

Growing your own herbs is very beneficial for you because you are reducing your environmental footprint by not buying herbs that have been transported to supermarkets. You recycle glass jars for storage, reducing the garbage from your home. Your home-grown herbs will also be free from pesticides and chemicals, and you will know exactly what has gone into the herbs.

BOOK 12: FORAGING WILD EDIBLE PLANTS

Introduction

Have you ever wondered whether a plant you saw was edible? Have you ever plucked fresh fruit from a tree or gathered berries from stray bushes? Have you ever looked at beautiful berries and fruit in the outdoors and wondered whether they were edible or not? Have you met people in the woods looking for valued mushrooms? Have you considered foraging? If yes, this is the book for you.

Agriculture was not developed until a few thousand years ago. Agriculture is so important in today's society that we can't envision a future without it. So, what did our forefathers do before the first agricultural seeds were planted? They had to rely on nature for their food. Hunting and gathering were the sole means of survival for the bulk of human existence. However, fire wasn't always accessible, and meat wasn't always available. In such situations, our forefathers' sole option for survival was to harvest natural edibles. Natural foods discovered in the outdoors were utilized to both feed and treat their bodies. All of this was accomplished by foraging.

Foraging is used as a form of sustenance only by a few societies these days. However, the act of foraging itself is neither lost nor unsatisfying. Even in modern society and the concrete jungle most of us live in, foraging is still possible. From herbs and edible flowers to mushrooms, plants, and other natural elements, there's plenty available from nature. All you need to do is look. Foraging has several benefits. It is not only a relaxing activity, but is a means to unplug from the hectic lifestyles most of us lead these days. It's also a great way to bond with your family and teach young ones about nature. Apart from that, foraging helps build a better relationship with nature.

So, what is foraging? Foraging is the simple act of identifying, gathering, and harvesting edible plants, weeds, flowers, and mushrooms in the wild. Before the advent of agriculture, foraging was a significant source of sustenance for humans. Now, it is time that we went back to our roots and reconnected with nature. Chances are, you may have foraged in the past but did not know it was called foraging. For instance, if you have ever plucked fresh fruit from trees or gathered wild berries, this is foraging. Once you learn about it, you will see how beneficial it truly is. When it comes to foraging, the most important aspect is learning about different plants to know their value as edible plants. Unless you do this, you cannot effectively differentiate between edible and poisonous varieties.

Wild edible plants will be identified and used. Also covered are the benefits of foraging, becoming an ethical forager, safety tips, and equipment. Start foraging right now if you want to learn a new hobby, reconnect with nature, or save money on groceries.

And the greatest part? Foraging improves with practice. You'll learn to identify edible and inedible plants. The more edible plants you forage, the better. So, are you keen to discover more? If yeah, let's go!

Foraging

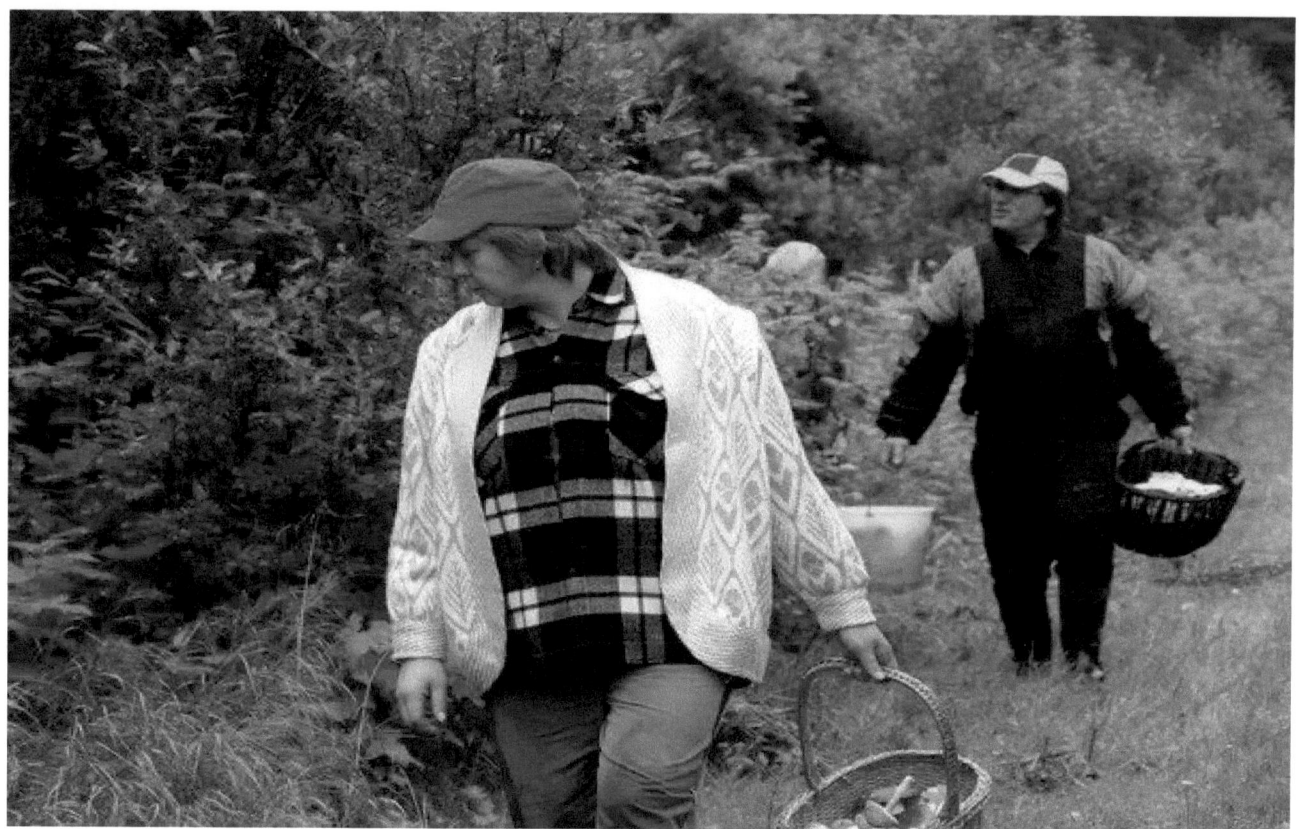

Searching for, locating, and gathering food in the outdoors is called foraging. Plants, mushrooms, herbs, and fruits of all kinds may be found growing wild around us.

It's safe to say that almost everyone has eaten an apple or a blackberry that they picked from a tree themselves. Foraging has been a part of existence for centuries. It was common practice for people to eat what they could find in their own backyard.

After that, urbanization altered our way of life, and people's appetites for wild foods waned. Nowadays, almost everything can be obtained at a grocery store, so most people never get the opportunity to learn about the growing and harvesting processes or the origins of their food.

The food industry's recent crises have increased public awareness of environmental concerns and the carbon impact. Foraging may have a significant influence on our health, and many individuals are rediscovering the advantages of reconnecting with nature.

Any mushroom or plant that has not been cultivated to maximize its yield might be considered a wild food. This includes seaweed, mollusks, fish, and game on occasion. In addition, wild food does not include any plastic packaging, does not use any artificial fertilizers, and may be harvested right in front of your eyes.

What Is A Forager?

By foraging for wild foods in our own backyard, we are able to maintain a meaningful connection to the earth. We get acquainted with nature's sights and sounds, as well as the geography and history of our area.

A forager observes the yearly changes in the terrain and provides an alternative to our present globalized food system, which allows us to purchase anything at any time of year.

Getting food from your area during a period when it naturally grows may create a genuine feeling of connectivity to the landscape.

In addition to providing essential nutrients, foraging helps us better comprehend the world around us.

What are Wild Edibles?

Foraging for edible plants is a terrific way to connect with our primitive nature and the natural environment. This may be a healthier option than the pre-packaged items we get at the supermarket. Foraging is not only a great way to get some exercise, but it's also a great source of vitamins and minerals. To do this, you'll need to do both trekking and gardening. In order to guarantee that foraging is safe and sustainable, it is a good idea to be familiar with a few fundamental standards.

Do not eat endangered creatures - Some locations may include species that are on the verge of extinction. Do not feed on these animals. Over-harvesting is the most common cause, although climate patterns or even other alterations in the ecosystem may also play a role. This might result in the extermination of that species in the region if you choose the final one.

Even though a plant is listed as edible, it doesn't indicate that all components of it may be consumed. For example, although the bark, stems, and roots of elderberries, when ripe and cooked, are safe to consume, the berries themselves are deadly. Additionally, certain plants may only be eaten at particular seasons of the year, so it's vital to keep this in mind. Stinging nettle, for example, should not be used after flowering.

Avoid Overharvesting Plants - There is a limit to every population. Even in areas with high concentrations of wild edible plants, the colony should always be respected. Ten percent should be your goal. Then, don't accumulate more than you can utilize.

In general, it's a good idea to just take a third or so of the leaves, roots, and fruits that are accessible. There will be enough leftover over for the following forager and adequate for the plant to keep multiplying if everyone who finds the identical bramble bush picks this quantity.

Prickly bushes and spiky plants may be uncomfortable and difficult to harvest if you don't have the correct protective clothing on. You'll want to pack some essential gear and apparel to make the trip enjoyable.

Don't Eat Dangerous Plants - If you have even the least uncertainty about whether or not a plant is poisonous, don't eat it. Also, if you're having trouble identifying a plant or animal, collaborating with other local foragers or joining a foraging group can provide you with additional resources to narrow your search.

Know the few harmful species in your region before traveling into the outdoors to forage. Learn about them. You'll be more confident exploring edible plants if you understand what harmful plants you may find.

Foraging requires permission, so ask ahead of time. Not adhering to property rights and rules in this area might result in negative repercussions, even if it isn't visible. As an added bonus, it's just good manners.

What Methods Do Foragers Use To Gather Resources?

Wild garlic foraging in the woods, blackberry picking in the hedgerows, or picking crab apples in your local park are all examples of foraging.

Foragers who have honed their craft know exactly where to go at any time of year to acquire whatever ingredient they want. We feel it's crucial to get to know the place and get to know the seasons in the area.

Because humans and the other creatures that live in the region rely on the resources in the terrain, it is always handled with care.

The Fundamentals of Foraging

Gathering wild plants and fungus is a way to eat well and connect with nature at the same time. In return for the food, you choose, however, you must treat it with care and respect! When you learn the fundamentals of foraging and wildcrafting, you'll begin to perceive weeds and wild creatures in a whole new way.

Plants (fungi) and other organisms that give food may be found via foraging. If an animal's capacity to live and reproduce is dependent on its ability to forage, then its fitness will be affected. In fact, it seems that human beings may live and reproduce even if they do not hunt for food across uncultivated areas. This ancient technique has a good effect on physical, mental, and emotional wellbeing!

Ethical Foraging

Foragers are often attracted by the promise of "free food." Our hyper-commodified civilization certainly welcomes direct access to the Earth's abundance. Foraging for wild food does not imply that it is worthless or available for the taking because of the absence of a price tag. You should learn about the plants you choose, their histories, migratory routes, cultural settings, and wonderful attributes since the significance of such knowledge can't be understated. Always thank the plant you've just harvested. For the sake of your own existence, another living creature is willing to give its life.

In addition, harvesting must be done in a manner that does not harm the ecology. Only abundant plants, such as invasive species, should be harvested. It also entails leaving a beautiful and well-cared-for environment rather than digging up a lot of trash and walking away. Make sure you know everything about the plant's life cycle and demands before harvesting or using it. Your crop will be more sustainable if you use this method.

Safe Forage

Some plants and fungi may be harmful to people, according to a recent study. You might become ill or possibly die if you consume a deadly plant or fungus. Your family and friends might be put at risk by your consumption of dangerous plants or fungus.

Learn how to identify plants before you go out in search of wild food. We've included a collection of helpful ID resources below.

In addition, harmful pesticides may be sprayed on a large number of so-called "wastelands," as well as the banks of streams and highways toward the outer reaches of civilization. A potentially poisonous region should not be the source of any food you want to consume.

Beginner Foragers' Guide to Basic Rules

- Keep an eye out for dangers

Before handling or ingesting any plant, be sure you know exactly what it is. Attend plant walks with an expert, learn basic botany, cross-reference several guidebooks, or use websites like gobotany.nativeplanttrust.org to improve your abilities.

- Know where you're going

Investigate the region where you want to go foraging. Is there an abundance of delicacies and toxic plants in this area? Stay away from regions near industries, golf courses and highways, as well as areas where water and soil may be polluted.

- Responsible harvesting

Limits and limitations on harvesting might be found in local land management rules. Do not congregate outside of allowed places or in excessive quantities. You should only take what you require, leaving adequate space for animals and regeneration in your wake. Take care not to disturb delicate ecosystems, such as marshes, tundra, or the desert. Beginners may start out in areas that are often disturbed, such as trailside, grazing fields, and campgrounds, since their influence will be minor.

- Feed on the weeds

Seek weedy areas with a high concentration of edible plants. Weeds are plants that are undesired and grow quickly and aggressively, particularly in disturbed areas. As long as you don't deplete them by eating too much, dandelion and other weeds may be enjoyed in plenty.

- Walk lightly

In the quest for flora, be aware of your influence. Travel over logs and rocks and be aware of trampling other plants as you make your way through the wilderness. Leave no trace. Principles should be followed at all times.

- Recognize the toxins

Being able to tell which plants you might eat and which ones you can't is just as vital as being able to tell which ones you can't. Poisonous plants may cause a rash or even death, depending on how toxic they are. Toxic species, particularly those that resemble edible or therapeutic plants, should be easy to spot if you do your research.

Foraging Tips

- With experience, your taste, smell, and sight senses will become more adept at assisting you in the identifying process.
- Avoid spreading invasive seeds or diseases to new regions by thoroughly cleaning your instruments and clothing between harvests.
- Allow the plants to continue to grow by snipping off leaves and other plant components with a sharp knife.
- Suffocating your crop in plastic containers will result in mildew growth. A permeable cotton bag, basket, or even your shirt may be used to collect plants.

Tools For Foraging

Similar to any endeavor, coming up with the right tools and techniques greatly enhances your chances of being successful. In foraging, other than knowledge and your senses, a good set of tools can assist you in picking not only the right herbs but the best ones too. To get started, here's a quick list of the tools you need to prepare in foraging.

Picking Tools

Although your hands can be enough to pick herbs and plants, it's still a good idea to use the right picking tools particularly if you are harvesting an herb that might potentially cause an injury. Gardening gloves can help prevent irritation and offer protection if you want to pick herbs using your hands. Using plastic mitts is also a good idea particularly if you're targeting a prickly herb.

However, for plants that need to be cut at the lower stem and you don't want to spend a lot of time yanking the needed part off, using a good pair of scissors can really be helpful. If you're aiming high, using a long stick can greatly lengthen your reach. In case you are digging for roots, using a shorter stick or even a trowel can make your work less laborious than using your hands. For larger areas, you might want to keep a spare shovel in your car just in case.

Knives

Knives or shears are important tools in foraging. Aside from harvesting, a knife is also a helpful tool in cutting branches and vines that hinder your path. You can also use it as a grasping tool and in marking your trail in the woods.

Storage Containers

Another thing you need to prepare beforehand is your transport containers. You may not need any special type of containers when it comes to foraging. Typically, you only need a few covered containers, big plastic shopping bags, or even freezer bags will do.

First Aid Kits

Because you are in the wild and accidents are always possible, it's a wise idea to be ready in case something happens while you are foraging. In setting up your first aid kit, you can add the following:

• Tweezers and even needles are essential first aid tools in cases of splinters and thorns.
• Antiseptic solutions can come in handy while you are foraging. While slips and bruises are fairly common when you are in the wild, bringing an antiseptic solution even if it's just alcohol or povidone iodine can help ward off infections.
• Keep a fresh set of plantain leaves in your first aid kit. It can help you manage insect bites and even poison ivy rashes.

Water and Rags

Walking under the sun for a certain period of time can cause your body a certain degree of dehydration. If you're going to forage, make sure to bring a few bottles of water with you for hydration. You'll also need water to clean up your hands and your tools. A spare rag can also help you clean up berries, plant parts and even your fingers.

Illustrated Books

Bringing a few illustrated books is necessary in making sure you identify plants and herbs correctly. It's not necessary to take all books with you while you walk because they carry a certain weight. Instead, you can just take one and leave the others in your car for easier cross checking when you've collected all needed herbs.

Sun Protection

Being exposed in the sun is never healthy and safe. However, as foraging makes sun exposure inevitable, it's wise if you can bring a hat or a good sunscreen with you. You may need to frequently reapply the product particularly if you'll be spending a good couple of hours walking outside the shade of trees. Aside from sunscreen, you may also want to bring a good bottle of bug spray just to keep insects away.

Magnifying Glass

You may not always need it but bring a magnifying glass in your foraging. It can help make sure you get your hands on the right herbs. The glass can allow you to visually inspect small herbs and plants for any discernable features that can set them apart from the rest of their family and specie. A difference in hair or even tiny holes in the stem can be all you need to properly identify an herb. As the eyes are limited in terms of what it can see, a good magnifying glass can make the job a lot easier.

Proper Clothing

While there aren't any strict guides on what you can and can't wear while foraging, the idea is to use something that's both protective and comfortable. Clothes that have long sleeves as well as long pants are good choices because they can help prevent insects from biting you and thorny shrubs from irritating your skin. It's also a good idea to wear a scarf for added protection against the sun. For your feet, it's best if you can stick with a pair of socks and boots.

Snacks

You don't need to bring a lot of food particularly if you'll be spending most of your hours looking for herbs and plants. However, because the activity can be tedious and laborious, it's wise to bring a few snacks with you while you forage.

Wild Edibles

Best Wild Edibles and How to Gather Them in WINTER

Big Leaf Maple

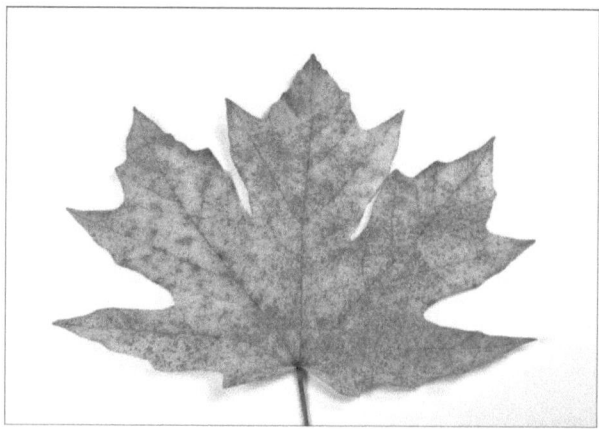

The maple family is most well-known for its syrup. The sugar maple produces the very best syrup, but the big leaf maple can produce earthy-sweet syrup, too!

How to Gather

The most popular part of the big leaf maple to gather is the flowers. These flowers contain deliciously sweet nectar. They grow in bunches in the spring and are the focus of our recipe for this tree.

This maple can also be tapped for syrup. It takes some hardware but making syrup is a great way to forage, and you can come back to those same trees year after year.

Bittercress

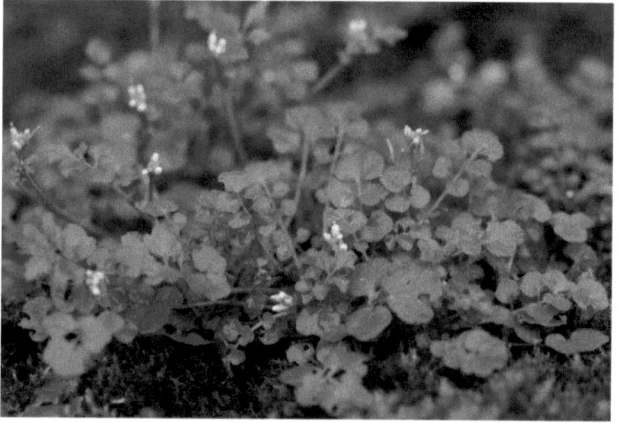

Also known as hairy bittercress, this wild edible got the short end of the stick on the name, but it has a big flavor and is part of a family of mustards filled with character, nutrition, and flavor.

How to Gather

When it comes to harvesting this wild edible, use the forager's shears. They are going to become very handy when trimming the stems of bittercress.

Crab Apples

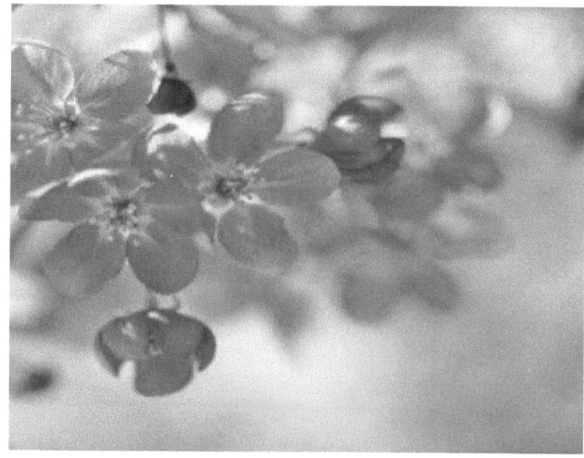

These smaller apples are very prolific and easy to identify. They lend themselves less to raw eating and more to cooked preparations. This is because they have a very tart flavor.

How to Gather

Gathering crab apples is a great opportunity to bring out the tubtrugs. You can fill large baskets or other containers with these ripe crab apples.

Grab the fruit and twist. The stem will separate from the tree, and you will have your first crabapple. For taller trees, you are going to need a fruit picker basket to extend into the trees.

Peppergrass

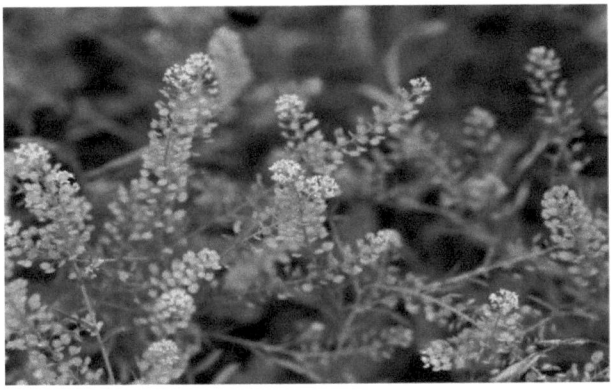

Wild peppergrass or poor man's pepper is a well-documented wild edible used by the Incas and written about by the Roman author Pliny, the Elder. We have been harvesting wild peppergrass for a very long time.

How to Gather

The wonderful thing about gathering peppergrass is that the entire plant is edible. All parts can be consumed, and they can all be consumed raw. It would be a great plant harvest in the same trip as chickweed; they would likely be near one another, too!

Your shears are going to be very useful for harvesting peppergrass.

Siberian Miner's Lettuce

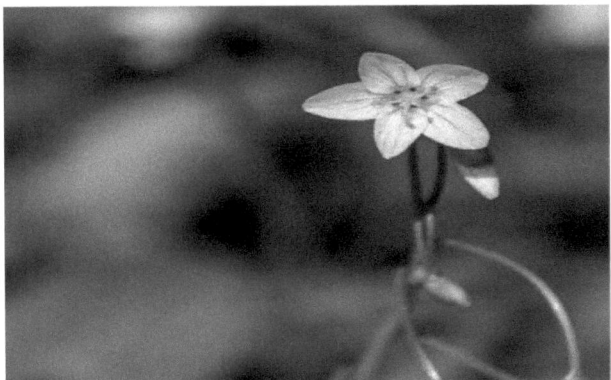

Siberian Miner's Lettuce is easy to find, full of nutrition, and goes by many names: Indian lettuce and clasp leaf miners lettuce.

How to Gather

Siberian Miner's Lettuce is edible in all its forms. Everything from the stems to the roots is edible. It's an easy plant to gather because of that. If you are not interested in gathering roots along with your lettuces, then bring some shears to deal with that.

Best Wild Edibles and How to Gather Them In SPRING

Asparagus

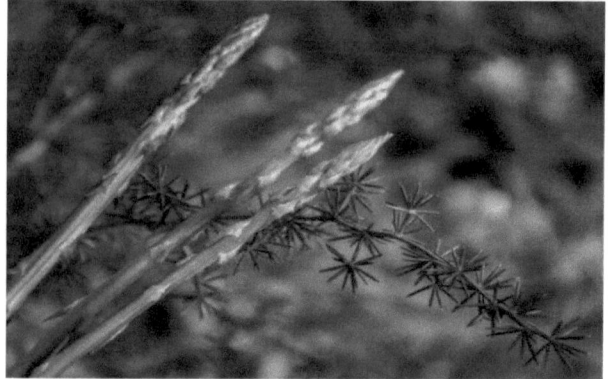

Wild asparagus is a must forage in the spring. There is something magical about finding those pencil-thin stalks popping up from the ground.

How to Gather

Wild asparagus should be treated much like fresh cut flowers. Your sharp knife is the best tool for cutting stalks close to the woody base. When you get them home, store the cut stalks so that water touches the cut parts.

You can keep going back to it when you find a patch of wild asparagus. New stalks will sprout.

Blue Camas

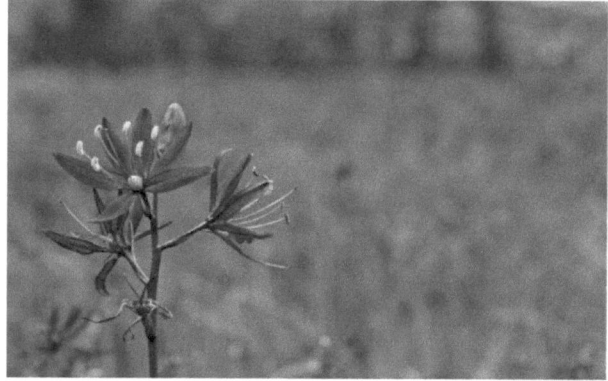

This perennial wild herb grows nearly 2 feet tall in the wild and has a beautiful blue flower.

How to Gather

You are after the bulbs to get the most bang for your buck. These can easily be had using your hori hori to harvest them. Dig around the bulbs, or roots, just underground and pry them loose.

They are sturdy and can be piled atop one another when carrying them.

Catnip

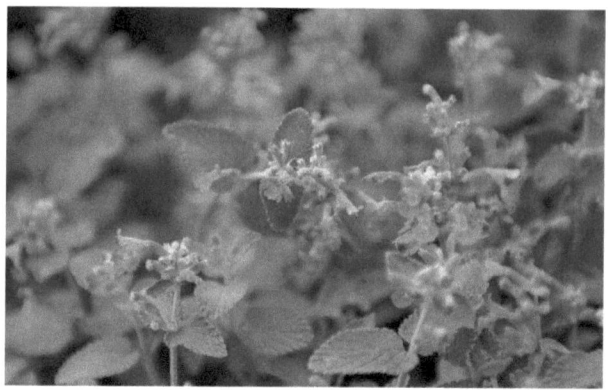

Catnip is a wild herb that is not just for cats. Many parts of the plant are edible and can be used in herbal remedies.

How to Gather

The best tool for gathering catnip will be the forager's shears. They will give you the ability to cut these plants off at the base and gather them.

You could bring your small shovel or hori hori as many people forage wild catnip and then bring it home, root and all. This plant is great to cultivate and grow on your property.

Common Plantain

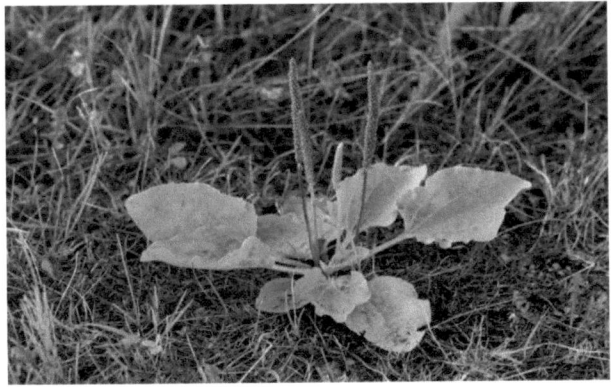

Common plantain is probably the first wild edible you can find as a new forager. There is a good chance you can walk 100 feet from where you are sitting and look down in the grass to find some common plantain.

How to Gather

The trusty shears are going to be your best tool for trimming the leaves of the common plantain. If you find a field that is full of them, you can actually snip some leaves from several plants and never endanger any one plant by taking all its leaves.

Mustard

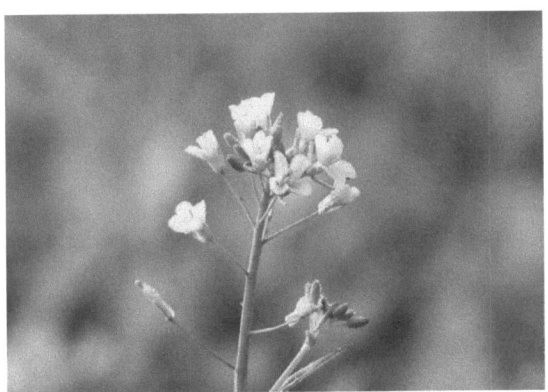

The mustards are a highly opportunistic plant that likes hanging near humans and are packed with nutrition. They are in the brassica family with broccoli and cauliflower.

How to Gather

All parts of this plant are edible. The best time to eat mustard is before the plant bolts or starts to flower. After the flowering begins, mustard can get very bitter.

Your forager's shears are the perfect tool for this wild edible, and some baskets to pile with mustard are great, too.

Sheep Sorrel

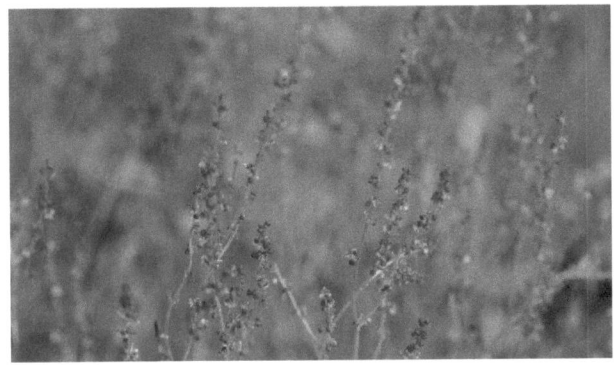

This tangy wild edible is very common and could be growing in your garden this spring!

How to Gather

This is an easy plant to gather, and your forager's shears will make quick work of the arrow-shaped leaves. The small seed pods can just be picked by hand.

Wild Ginger

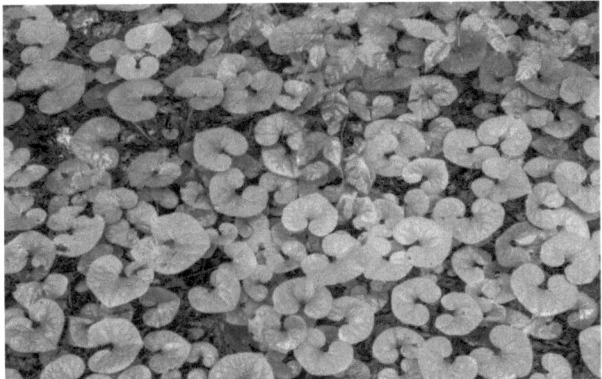

Ginger has been an ingredient and medicine all the way back to the days of Ancient China.

How to Gather

You can gather the flowers and rootstocks. Your hori hori will be great for digging out the roots, and your shears will take the flowers easily.

Wild Strawberry

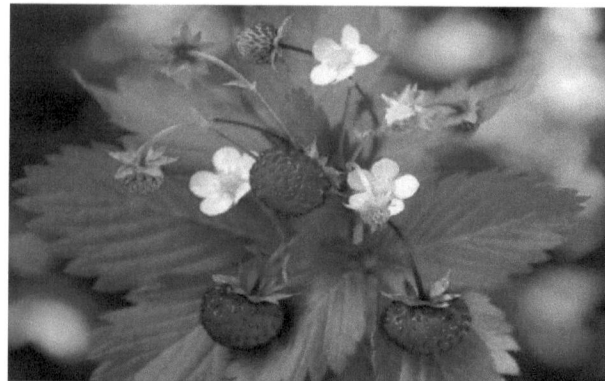

We have all happened to come across these little small wild strawberries snaking through yards and fields in spring.

How to Gather

You can gather the fruit of the wild strawberry, but the flowers and leaves are also nice to have.

Wild strawberry is a delicate plant, so your forager's shears should do the job just fine.

Yarrow

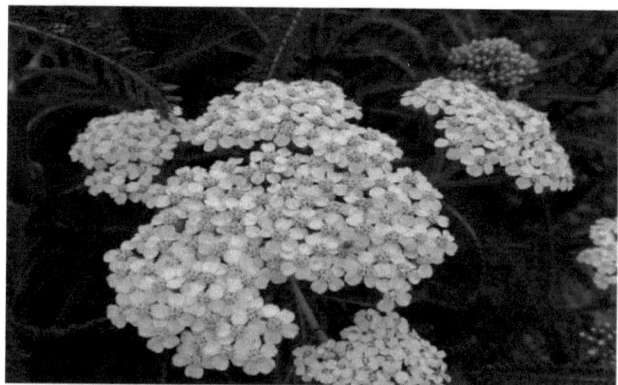

Yarrow is a wild edible with a special power. It can help stop bleeding.

How to Gather

All parts of the yarrow plant are edible. The root is a big part of foraging it so bring the hori hori or even a small shovel to help harvest this rhizomatous plant.

Best Wild Edibles and How To Gather Them In AUTUMN

Arrowhead

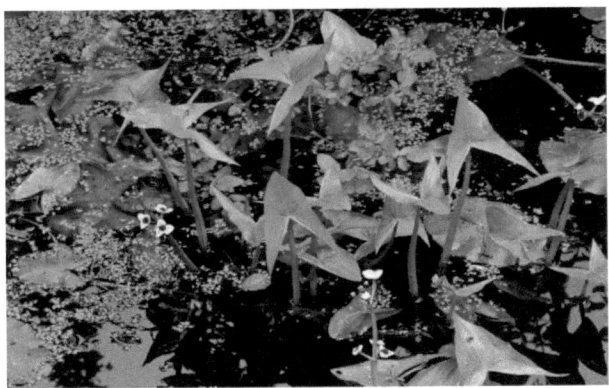

Arrowhead has a very funny nickname. It is also known as duck potato.

How to Gather

If you eat the stalks and leaves, then you should focus on harvesting younger plants. The tubers can be harvested at all times, and they are a good source of carbohydrates.

Black Hawthorn

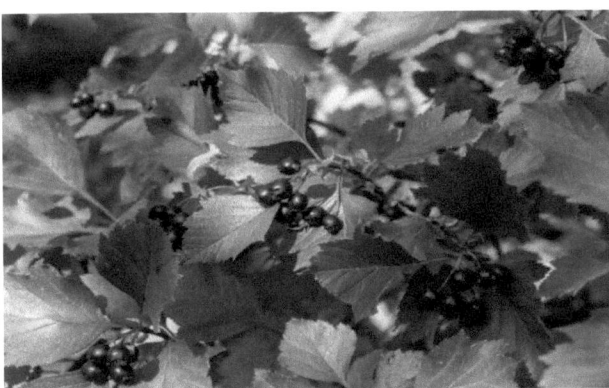

Black hawthorn puts off long and strong spines that can be used as needles or hooks in wilderness survival.

How to Gather

The shoots and bark of this plant have medicinal properties and are worth gathering. Wear strong gloves to deal with the spines.

The berries are delicious and should be gathered at any opportunity.

Bog Cranberry

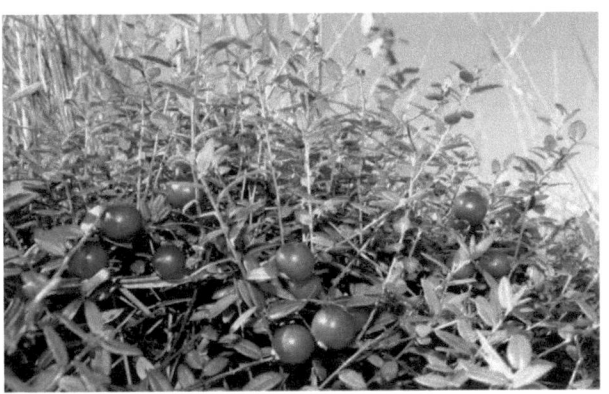

The bog cranberry is also known as the small cranberry or the swamp cranberry.

How to Gather

The cranberries can be gathered by hand, but because of the nature of their habitat, you will want some waterproof boots to keep your feet and legs dry.

Evergreen Huckleberry

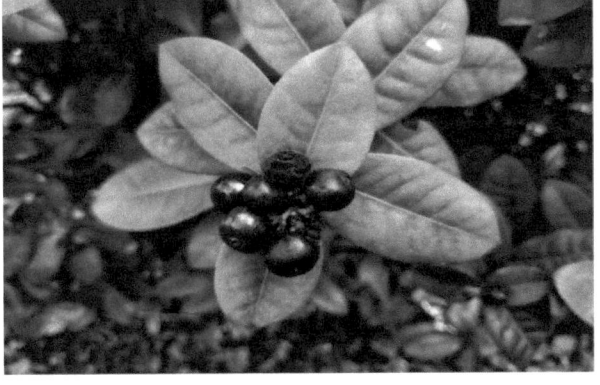

This evergreen species is found in the wild but is also very popular in native landscaping in the Pacific Northwest.

How to Gather

Huckleberries are easy to gather by hand in the late summer and early fall. Just bring gloves as the berries can stain your fingers.

Hazelnut

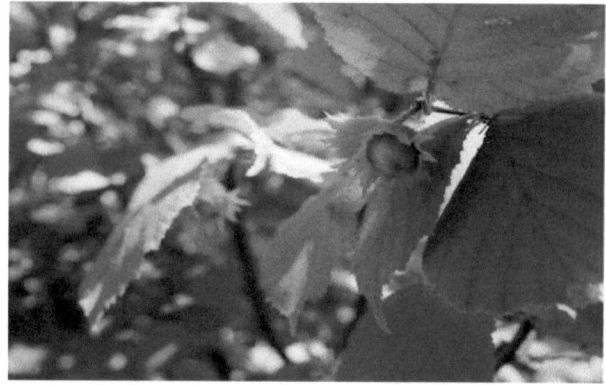

The hazelnut is a luxurious wild edible and is the main flavoring in Nutella.

How to Gather

The nuts are the only edible part of this shrub, so you are just grabbing nuts and gathering them. Bring a bag with you for storage and carrying.

Jerusalem Artichoke

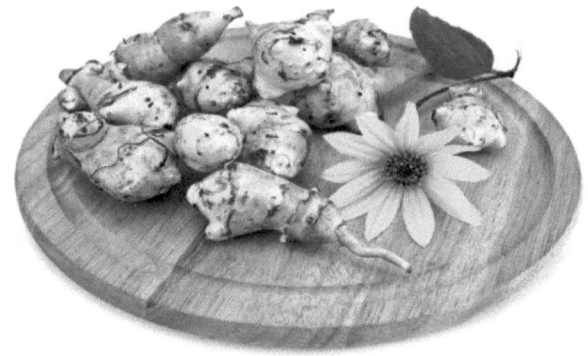

This tuber is also called a sunchoke.

How to Gather

You are after the potato-like tuber that has an outer skin. The hori hori is great for digging these tubers.

Juniper

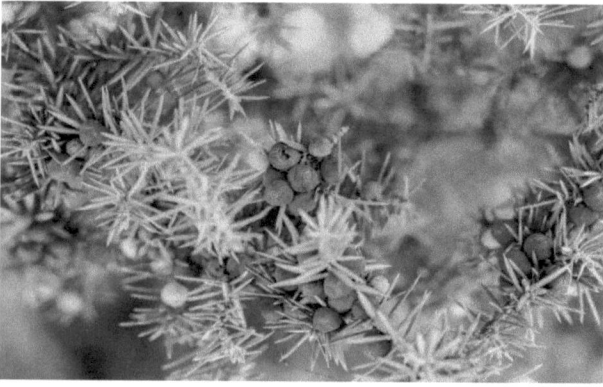

The juniper can live up to 200 years!

How to Gather

The berries are the true edible part of this plant. They are most often used as a flavoring and are the main flavoring ingredient in gin. The berries can be gathered by hand.

Oregon Grape

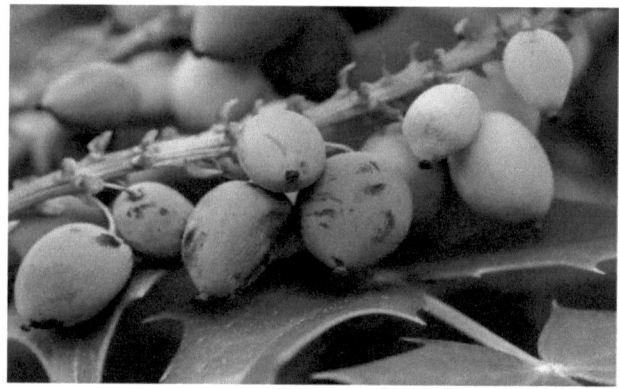

The flower of the Oregon grape is Oregon's state flower.

How to Gather

The grapes themselves are easy to harvest and can be done with some simple gloves and a basket. Pick the whole cluster of berries to be quicker. You can separate them at home.

Silverweed

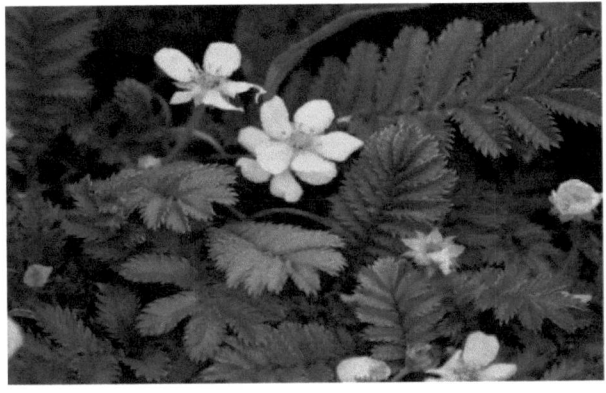

The best part of silverweed is in the roots, which taste similar to sweet potatoes when roasted!

How to Gather

The leaves and the roots of this plant are edible. Gather them with your shears. The roots should be harvested in Autumn and can be dug up using the hori hori.

Springbank Clover

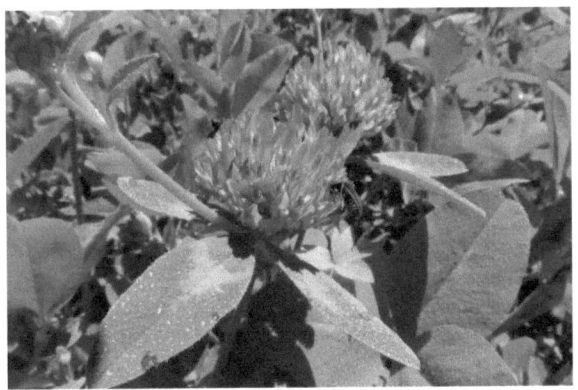

This wild edible is also known as cow's clover, sand clover, and seaside clover.

How to Gather

Unlike red clover, this edible is known for its tender white tuber. They share a similar taste with Chinese bean sprouts. The flowers are also edible.

Milk Thistle

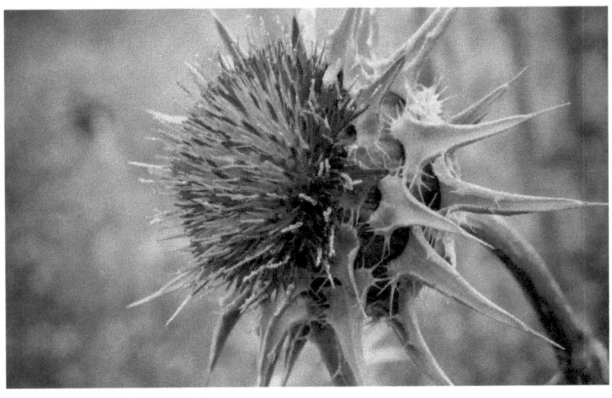

This plant has been in the human diet for over 2,000 years!

How to Gather

You can gather all parts of the milk thistle as it all can be eaten. The leaves are great if you remove the spines. The stems are a great asparagus substitute. Even the seeds can be roasted as a coffee substitute.

Wild Licorice

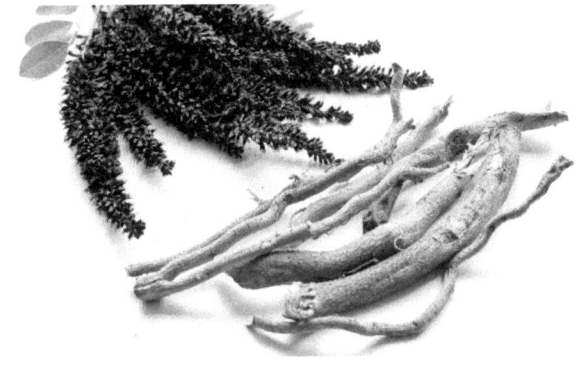

The roots of licorice are very fibrous and can be used as a substitute for a toothbrush.

How to Gather

The roots can be gathered using your hori hori. These have a strong licorice taste and many uses.

Best Wild Edibles and How To Gather Them In SUMMER

Chokecherry

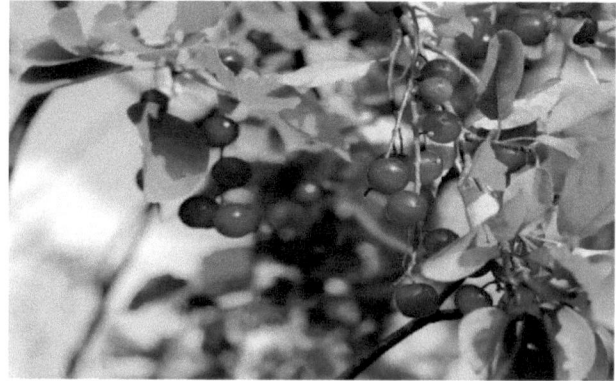

With a name like this, you might not think it's edible, but the chokecherry is delicious.

How to Gather

The chokecherries can be gathered when they are ripe and stacked in baskets or satchels. They are tasty and unique. However, you cannot eat the pit of the fruit as it contains hydrocyanic acid, and this is toxic to humans.

Cloudberry

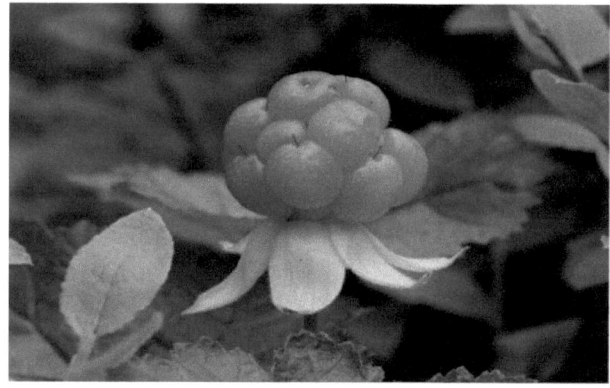

The cloudberry looks like something from a video game or another planet. It's a beautiful orange-yellow berry.

How to Gather

Gathering cloudberries is very simple. You just pluck the berry off the stem and move on to the next one.

Coastal Black Gooseberry

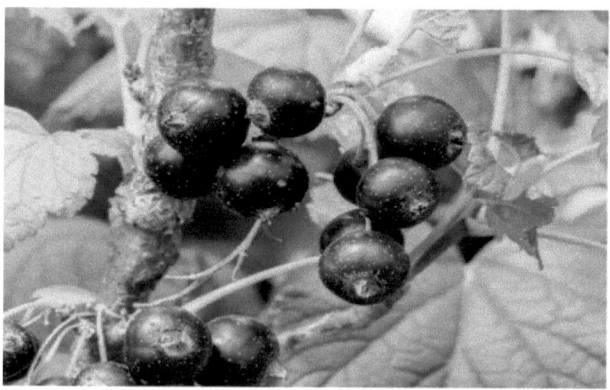

This is the tastiest variety of gooseberry in North America.

How to Gather

The gooseberries can be gathered by hand and plucked. Be sure you wear gloves because the spines hurt!

Oval Leaf Blueberry

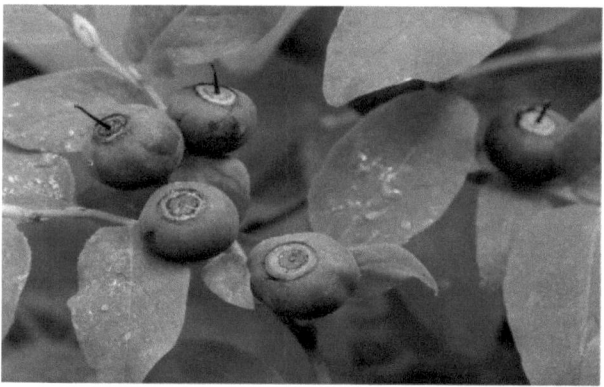

There are many forms of blueberry in the nation, and all of them are edible.

How to Gather

Blueberries can be plucked by hand, but you might want to wear gloves to protect your fingers from staining.

Pearly Everlasting

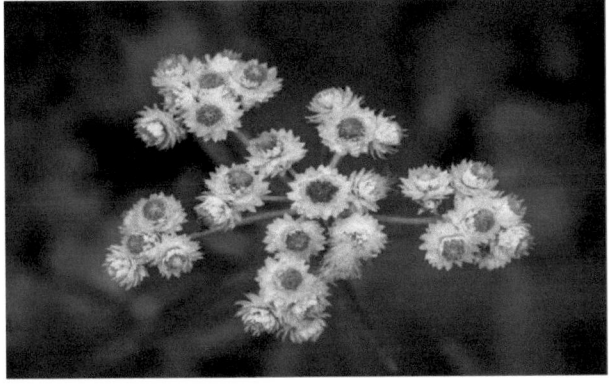

This is a powerful healing plant that has been used to treat many ailments.

How to Gather

If you wish to eat this plant, then you are going to eat the young leaves of the plant. They can be trimmed with shears. Gather the flowers for medicinal uses.

Pipsissewa

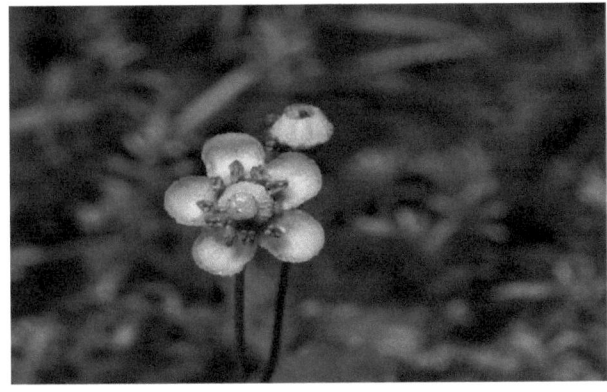

A Native American medicine and flavoring herb.

How to Gather

The plant's leaves can be harvested with shears and used to make medicinal tea or to flavor things like root beer and candy.

Red Currant

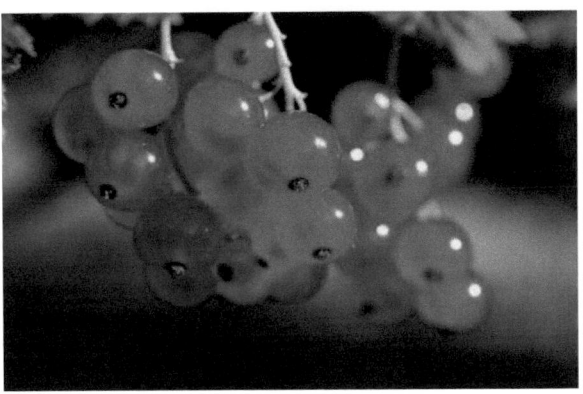

This is one of the tastiest members of the gooseberry family.

How to Gather

The ripe red currant berries can be gathered by hand, and they are easy to pick.

Salmonberry

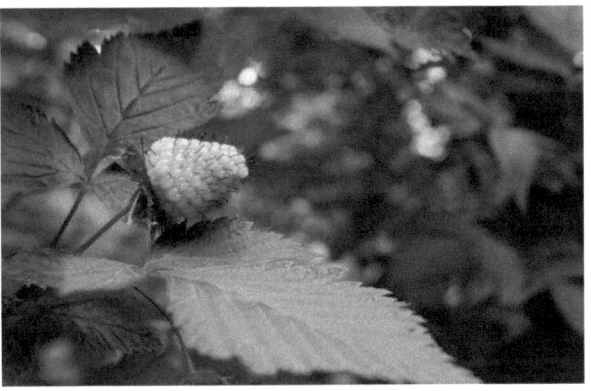

These berries are in the same family as raspberries and blackberries.

How to Gather

These berries are easy to gather and can be done so by hand. Just make sure you have plenty of storage because they are often plentiful. They are delicate, too.

Yerba Buena

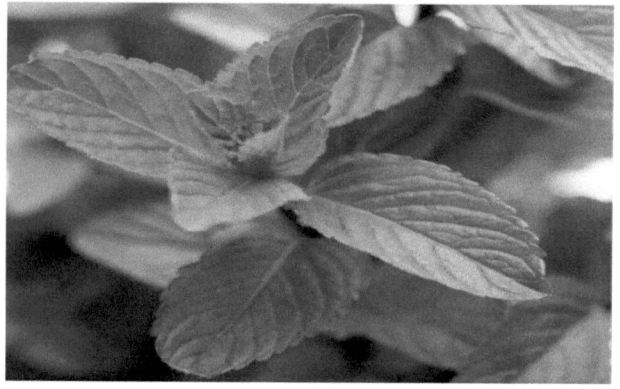

This is one of the best wild edibles for stomach aches and digestive issues.

How to Gather

Using your forager's shears, trim the plant at the bottom and take the stalks with leaves and flowers.

Conclusion

Foragers that are new to the field may be interested in learning how to identify different types of plants in the wild. That is why we have put together this book for you. It has been a joy going through the basics of what to expect when out in the field, as well as a method of identifying one of your favorite plants with you. Because there are so many edible plants to pick from in the wild, and each one has its specific identifying characteristics, you'll want to practice with and get familiar with some of the most common edible plants in the area.

Thank you for taking the time to read our book on wild edibles; we hope you enjoyed it. It is possible to find fantastic edible food in a variety of locations across the world. This book contains a list of wild plants that can be discovered and used as food in the area. This information has been created with the hope that you will find it helpful and that you will be thrilled about discovering edible wild nutrition in your backyard!

BOOK 13: ROSEMARY BASIL AND THYME BEST RECIPES

Introduction

Rosemary

Rosemary is a Mediterranean herb that grows wild. Rosemary was thought to help with memory and brain function by the Greeks. This plant was once used as incense at wedding parties throughout Europe, and it was also known as a symbol of fidelity. Judges in Europe likewise burnt rosemary to protect themselves from the ailments that the inmates had exposed them to.

Uses:

Rosemary is used for enhancing memory, indigestion, arthritis-related joint discomfort, hair loss, and other ailments, but there is no acceptable experimental proof to support most of these applications. The effectiveness of rosemary includes treatment of eczema, myalgia, toothaches, as well as for improving menstrual flow in ladies.

In cooking, rosemary is used as flavoring. The leaf and oil are used in cooking, and oil is used in drinks. In production, rosemary oil is used as an aromatic ingredient in perfumes and soaps!

It can be used to Improve Memory: Taking rosemary by mouth may moderately enhance memory in young grown-ups. Using rosemary aromatherapy appears to raise some measure of memory. Rosemary aromatherapy also seems to boost sharpness.

Growing:

Rosemary grown in the ground rarely requires supplemental irrigation. Potted rosemary should be monitored occasionally to ensure the soil doesn't dry out completely.

Basil

The mint family, Lamiaceae, has a genus of annual herbs known as basil (sweet basil). Basil, a popular culinary herb, is said to have originated in India. It is used to flavor meats, seafood, salads, and sauces while basil tea is an aphrodisiac; and the leaves may be used fresh or dried. Its glossy, oval-shaped leaves have smooth or slightly serrated margins that cup slightly; the leaves are placed in opposing directions on the square stems. Clusters of white to magenta-colored blooms are seen at the top of the plant. Frost-sensitive, the plant thrives in warmer areas. The Fusarium wilt, blight, and downy mildew are all problems that may plague basil plants when they are planted in humid environments.

Uses

For stomach cramps, lack of appetite and intestinal gas, renal disorders, and fluid retention, as well as head colds and wart and worm infections, basil is a good remedy. Insect and snake bites were also treated with it. Basil is a common pre-and post-partum remedy for increasing blood flow and kicking-starting the production of breast milk.

Growing

To initiate the growing season, many home gardeners start their basil plants from the seed inside. Four to eight weeks before the final day of frost, basil seeds start inside. Basil can thrive in a broad range of environments, making it an excellent choice for beginners. As long as your growth circumstances are the same, you can grow basil in a decorative pot inside just as effectively as you can outside. I like to start my basil inside rather than directly plant it in the garden once the spring frost danger has passed.

Thyme

Thyme has a distinct fragrance that makes it simple to recognize. During the spring and summer, tiny oval leaves cling to thin, woody stalks, and small pink flowers bloom. There are approximately 350 different varieties of this plant, each with minor differences in appearance but comparable therapeutic properties.

Uses

Thyme is a mainstay in many kitchens across the globe because of its ability to give a deliciously savory taste to dishes. This beautiful tiny herb is a great all-around cold treatment that soothes sore throats, clears chest congestion, reduces coughing spasms, and helps you sleep comfortably.

Growing

Thyme is easy to cultivate, especially if you buy established plants and move them to a sunny location. If not maintained in a container, this plant likes well-drained soil but will creep. After the first spring frost, you may start picking the plant tops, and you should finish cutting about a month before the first autumn frost. Harvesting your thyme plants on a regular basis will prevent them from getting too woody and encourage them to keep producing delicate new leaves for you to appreciate.

10 Rosemary Recipes

Best Recipes as A Medicine

Rosemary Oil

Preparation Time: 30 minutes

Cooking Time: 1 hour

Ingredients:

- 3-4 sprigs of Dried rosemary
- 2-3 cups of olive oil

Directions:

- Wash the rosemary to remove the dust and debris.
- Take the oil in a saucepan and heat it.
- Add chopped rosemary to it and cook for 20 minutes at least.
- Drain the oil and let it cool.
- Store the rosemary oil in a glass jar.

Rosemary Tincture

Preparation Time: 20 minutes

Cooking Time: 25 minutes

Ingredients:

- 4-6 sprigs of chopped rosemary
- ¾ cup of vodka

Directions:

- Bruise the rosemary with the help of a fist.
- Take the alcohol in a glass bottle.
- Add the bruised rosemary to it.
- Cover the glass bottle.
- Shake it for 60 seconds.
- Place the bottle in a dark and cool place for 5-8 weeks.
- Now strain the tincture.
- Store in a cool place.

Rosemary Tea

Preparation Time: 1 minute

Cooking Time: 5 minutes

Ingredients:

- 2 cups boiling water
- 2-3 tsp. rosemary leaves

Directions:

- Put the rosemary in boiling water.
- Set it aside for five minutes.
- Strain the rosemary leaves.

Enjoy!

Rosemary Salve

Preparation Time: 60 minutes

Cooking Time: 3-4 days

Ingredients:

- 8 oz. Of almond oil or olive oil
- 8 oz. Of dried rosemary herb
- Mason jar
- stockpot or crockpot

Directions:

- Chop the dried rosemary herb and put it in a mason jar.
- Cover with the oil and gently shake the herb in it.
- Place the jar in the water bath.
- Now heat the oil and water for 3-5 days and keep the oil temperature around 11 degrees.
- After 4-5 days, remove the jar from heat and let it cool.
- Strain the oil.
- Store in an airtight jar and put it in a dark place.

Orange Rosemary Salt Scrub

Preparation Time: 20 minutes

Cooking Time: 1-2 hours

Ingredients:

- 1 cup of salt
- orange zest
- 1 Tsp of rosemary leaves
- 1/3 cup of olive oil

Directions:

- Take rosemary, orange zest, and salt in a food processor.
- Pulse it until a homogenous mixture is obtained.
- Now add the olive oil and again pulse 3-4 times.
- Sore in a jar.
- To use it, take some scrub and lightly rub it on the skin.

Best Recipes for the Home

Rosemary Shampoo Bar

Preparation Time: 20 minutes

Cooking Time: 1 hour

Ingredients:

- 1 lb. Of glycerin of goat milk
- 1 Tsp. of mango butter
- 2 Tsp. of castor oil
- 16 drops of rosemary oil
- 16 drops of cedar wood oil
- 1 tbsp. rosemary, chopped
- Boiler
- 1 soap mold
- 1 spray bottle

Directions:

- Melt the soap base over low heat.
- Add mango butter to it. Let the mango butter melt.
- Remove it from the heat and add castor oil.
- Mix well.
- Now mix the rosemary and cedar wood oil in it.
- Add the chopped rosemary to it.
- pour the mixture in the mold. To avoid air bubbles, spray some rubbing alcohol.
- Let it cool for 3-4 hours.

Now remove it from mold and store it in a container.

Rosemary Pest Deterrent

Preparation Time: 10 minutes

Cooking Time: 25-30 minutes

Ingredients:

- 1 cup of dried rosemary
- Quarter of water

Directions:

- Take the rosemary leaves and water in a pot and boil for 5-10 minutes.
- Strain the rosemary water in a container and pour the blend in the squirt bottles to spray the water directly on the skins and pits.
- It can also be stored in the refrigerator.

Rosemary Tooth Paste

Preparation Time: 20 minutes

Cooking Time: 1 hour

Ingredients:

- 3 tbsp. of coconut oil
- 16-18 drops of rosemary oil
- 2 tbsp. of baking soda
- ¼ Tsp of stevia powder

Directions:

- Take a small bowl and mix the baking soda and coconut oil in it.
- Add the essential oils in it along with the stevia powder.
- Mix well until everything is combined well.
- Store the paste in a container.

Rosemary Conditioner

Preparation Time: 5 minutes

Cooking Time: minutes

Ingredients:

- 2 C. natural, unscented herbal conditioner like Stonybrook Botanicals
- 55 drops of rosemary essential oil

Tools Needed:

- Large bowl; plastic bottle
- Whisk or fork

Directions:

- Get a big bowl, mix the conditioner with the essential oil, and use a fork or whisk to mix it. Transfer the mixture into a Biphenyl-free plastic bottle with a very tight lid. Alternatively, you can use a glass jar with a tight lid.
- After applying shampoo, add a small amount of conditioner to the scalp and wait for 3–5 minutes before rinsing with cool water.

Rosemary Toner

Preparation Time: 3 minutes

Cooking Time: 0 minutes

Ingredients:

- 1 ½ C. witch hazel
- 2 ½ tbsps. rosemary tincture

Tools Needed:

- Glass bottle
- Cotton

Directions:

- Combine all the ingredients into a dark-colored bottle and shake gently to mix well.
- Using the cotton cosmetic pad, apply ¼ tsp. of the mixture on your face 2 to 3 times daily.

10 Basil Recipes

Best Recipes as a Medicine

Fresh Basil Steam For Congestion

Preparation Time: 5 minutes

Cooking Time: 5 minutes

Ingredients:

- 2 quarts water
- Basil leaves

Directions:

- Take a pot and pour water into it
- Boil water over medium heat.
- Add basil leaves in water and soak for 5 minutes.
- Now make a tent with a towel over your head.
- Inhale the steam for five to ten minutes.

Basil Essential Oil

Preparation Time: 5 minutes

Cooking Time: 0 minutes

Ingredients:

- 2 oz. basil
- 12 oz. olive oil

Directions:

- From the stem, discard the basil leaves.
- Put the oil in the jar and fill basil into it with a shut top.
- Place the jar in sunlight for one day.
- Strain the oil and, with a spoon, mash it.
- Remove the basil leaves and move them to another jar.
- Freeze it for one week.

Basil and Honey Tea For Digestion

Preparation Time: 5 minutes

Cooking Time: 2 minutes

Ingredients:

- 1-quart water
- 3 leaves mint
- 1 tbsp. honey
- 1 tsp. lemon juice
- 1 tsp. cumin
- 1 tsp. lime zest
- 1 tsp. ginger

Directions:

- Place the pot over medium heat.
- Put in water and boil.
- Shake in lime juice, cumin, honey, lime zest, mint, and ginger.
- To infuse the flavor, shake well and cook for two minutes.

Simple Basil Tea For Cough

Preparation Time: 5 minutes

Cooking Time: 0 minutes

Ingredients:

- 1 black tea bag
- ½ lemon slice
- 6 basil leaves

Directions:

- Boil the water into the pot.
- Mix lemon and basil leaves well in the glass.
- Now put the teabag in the cup and pour the boiled water into it.
- Soak it for 5 minutes to infuse the flavor.
- Drink and enjoy.

Basil Vinegar For Warm Bath

Preparation Time: 10 minutes

Cooking Time: 0 minutes

Ingredients:

- 1 cup basil
- 1/8 tsp. pepper
- ½ cup olive oil
- ½ cup shallot
- 3 tbsp. red wine vinegar
- ½ tsp. salt

Directions:

- Put all the ingredients in a blender.
- Bled well for 1 minute until mixture is completely mixed.

Best Recipes for The Home

Basil Hair Oil

Preparation Time: 5 minutes

Cooking Time: 10 minutes

Ingredients:

- 30-gram basil leaves
- ¾ cup olive oil

Directions:

- Take a pot and boil the water over medium heat.
- Put in the basil leaves and boil.
- Strain the water and discard the basil leaves.
- Now dry basil leaves with a towel.
- Take a blender and put in the olive oil and leaves.
- Blend the mixture completely until the mixture is smooth.
- Now move the oil to cover the top container.
- Place the oil in the refrigerator.
- Use oil within two to four days.

Basil Perfume

Preparation Time: 6 weeks

Cooking Time: 0 minutes

Ingredients:

- 1 lemon zest
- 8 oz. vodka
- 1 grapefruit zest
- Basil oil

Directions:

- Take a glass and mix citrus zest in it.
- Put in vodka and stir until liquid appears above the zest.
- Cover it tightly and stir well 1 or more than one time every day.
- Strain the mixture after 6 weeks and discard the peel from the cologne.
- Transfer the cologne to a decorated bottle with a diffuse top.
- Now put in few drops of basil oil in it.
- Increase the quantity of oil to want the strong cologne.

Basil Based Insect Repellent

Preparation Time: 4 hours

Cooking Time: 0 minutes

Ingredients:

- Basil leaves
- ¼ tsp. basil oil
- ½ cup boiling water
- ½ cup vodka

Directions:

- Take a cup and pour water into it. Soak the basil leaves in it for two to four hours.
- Take the liquid from the leaves by compressing the leaves.

- Take a spray bottle and put it in the infused liquid.
- To increase the potency, put in basil oil.
- Shake in the vodka to mix all the content completely.
- Spray on the skin to repel the mosquitoes.

Unclogging Steam Bath

Preparation Time: 10 minutes

Cooking Time: 0 minutes

Ingredients:

- 8 oz. pine needles
- 4 oz. dried sage
- 4 oz. dried thyme
- 4 Garlic minced cloves
- 32 oz. water

Directions:

- Combine the herbs. Bring the water to a boil, remove from heat and place the pot on your kitchen table (be sure to use a trivet).
- Put ½ cup of the mixture and the garlic in the hot water and use a towel to make a tent with your head at the apex.
- Steam your face for 10 to 20 minutes max.

Basil Salt

Preparation time: 10 minutes

Cooking time: 30 minutes

Ingredients:

- 1 cup rock salt /sea salt, coarse
- 1/3 cup (fresh) basil, packed

Directions:

- Getting the Basil Salt Ready
- Weigh out your fresh basil, then slice it into little pieces so the blender can mix it with the salt more easily.
- Place the basil in a blender or a large mixing basin if using an immersion blender.
- After that, pulse for a few seconds till the basil is totally broken up and combined with the salt. During this procedure, you may need to pause and combine the salt using a rubber spatula. It has a habit of sticking to the base of the blender. The salt will have a fine texture after you're done. When drying basil salt, use the following method:
- Preheat the oven at 220 degrees Fahrenheit and place the baking sheet inside.
- Bake for 30 minutes, stirring halfway through, or till the salt has no moister. The basil salt should be green after drying, but it should be a lighter tint than when you started. With a spoon or fork, break up any clumps in the finished salt and keep it in a sealed jar in your pantry. Use within 3 months for the best taste.
-
- Air-Dried Method (Slower, but without the need for heat):
- Use parchment paper to cover a big surface, such as a chopping board or baking sheet.
- On the parchment paper, distribute the salted basil mixture in a thinly single layer.
- With your fingers, break up any big clumps and cover carefully with a towel.
- Put it somewhere cold and dark. Allow the sea salt to remain for 12 to 24 hours, or till it has absorbed all of the basil's moisture and is totally dry. The basil salt should be green, but it should be a lighter hue than before.
- To get the finest flavor, put it in a jar with a tight cover and use it within three months.

10 Thyme Recipes

Best Recipes as A Medicine

Thyme Essential Oil

Preparation Time: 10 minutes

Cooking Time: 3 hours

Ingredients:

- 50 g thyme
- 1 L vegetable oil

Directions:

- Place the thyme and oil in a vacuum sealer.
- Cook sous vide at 131 Fahrenheit for three hours.
- Transfer it to an ice bath. Allow it to cool.
- Strain the oil and remove thyme.

Thyme, Ginger, Garlic, and Mint Tea for Tonsillitis

Preparation Time: 2 minutes

Cooking Time: 5 minutes

Ingredients:

- One glass water
- Two branches of fresh mint
- One piece of fresh ginger
- Five sprigs of thyme
- Two garlic cloves

Directions:

- Take a pan and fill it with water.
- Take ginger chunks and put them in the pan. Boil for five minutes.
- Rinse the herbs.
- Chop garlic cloves. Add the garlic along with herbs to the pan.
- Let it steep for eight minutes.
- Serve with honey.

Thyme Tea

Preparation Time: 1 minute

Cooking Time: 5 minutes

Ingredients:

- 1 ½ cup boiling water
- Three sprigs of fresh thyme

Directions:

- Take a teacup. Put thyme sprigs in it.
- Add boiling water into the cup and cover it.
- Set it aside for five minutes.
- Uncover it and remove the sprigs. Enjoy!

Honey Thyme Cough Syrup

Preparation Time: 5 minutes

Cooking Time: 10 minutes

Ingredients:

- 1 cup organic raw honey
- 2 cups water
- 3 tbsp. organic fresh thyme

Directions:

- Take a saucepan. Add water into a saucepan and let it boil.
- Remove the pan and add thyme to it.
- Cover the pan and set it aside for ten minutes.
- Strain it and mix honey in it.
- Put the mixture in the refrigerator.
- Take 1 or 2 tsp. whenever needed.

Thyme Tincture

Preparation Time: 15 minutes

Cooking Time: 0 minutes

Ingredients:

- 300 ml vodka
- One hand dried thyme

Directions:

- Take a glass jar. Add herbs to it.
- Put vodka in it.
- Set the jar aside after covering. Don't expose it to direct sunlight.
- Set the jar aside for forty days. Shake it from time to time.
- Drain the mixture after forty days.
- The tincture is ready; now, just store it in a jar in a dark place.

Best Recipes for The Home

Thyme Based Repellent for Mosquitoes

Preparation Time: 5 minutes

Cooking Time: 0 minutes

Ingredients:

- 10-15 drops citronella essential oil
- 1 tbsp. extra virgin olive oil
- 1 tbsp. dried thyme
- 2 tbsp. neem seed oil
- 1 tbsp. coconut oil

Directions:

- Start by melting the coconut oil.
- Take a jar and mix all the ingredients in it.
- The jar should contain an eyedropper.
- The repellent is ready to use.

Thyme Based Mouthwash

Preparation Time: 30 minutes

Cooking Time: 0 minutes

Ingredients:

- One drop of lemon essential oil
- 4 drops thyme essential oil
- 1 tbsp. sodium bicarbonate
- 3 drops peppermint essential oil
- 1 tsp. salt
- 250 ml distilled water

Directions:

- Take a glass jar. Add sodium bicarbonate and distilled water in it. Mix well.
- Put all the ingredients in the jar as well.
- Mix well by shaking the jar.
- Put the mixture in the refrigerator for one week.
- Mouthwash is ready to use.

Thyme Disinfectant

Preparation Time: 5 minutes

Cooking Time: 20 minutes

Ingredients:

- 5 drops tea tree oil
- 1 tsp. lemon essential oil
- 1 tsp. baking soda
- 1 tbsp. thyme extract
- A bunch of garden-fresh thyme
- 2 cups water
- ¼ tsp. thyme essential oils
- 2 tsp. castile soap
- 2 tsp. borax
- 2 cups lemon verbena hydrosol
- One lemon

Directions:

- Take a small pot, put thyme, lemon, and water in it. Allow it to simmer over medium heat.
- Turn off the heat and set it aside for one hour.
- Strain the mixture.

- To the strained liquid, add borax and baking soda and mix well.
- Add other ingredients as well.
- Transfer the mixture to a spray bottle.
- Don't forget to label the bottle.

Homemade Thyme Insect Repellant

Preparation Time: 5 minutes

Cooking Time: 0 minutes

Ingredients:

- 2 tablespoons of either olive, jojoba or almond oil (known as carrier oils)
- 10 drops of thyme essential oil

Directions:

- Mix the carrier oil with the thyme essential oil.
- Apply to areas of exposed skin or clothing before heading outdoors.
- Alternatively, you can put the repellent in a misting bottle and spray it on as needed.
- If you need to make more, add 5 drops of essential oil for every tablespoon of carrier oil. You may experiment with mixing essential oils to create an insect repellent that also smells nice.

Frozen Thyme Cubes

Preparation time: 5 minutes

Cooking time: 10 minutes

- Ingredients:
- Thyme herbs
- Olive oil (Gustare Vita) /Hy-Vee (unsalted) butter

Directions:

- Remove and discard the stems; cut the herbs as required.
- Fill the ice cube tray's wells with herbs about 2/3 full. You may combine the herbs if you choose; for example, you might freeze sage, rosemary, and thyme together and use them to roast entire chickens, sweet potatoes, or root vegetables.
- Over the herbs, drizzle olive oil or butter.
- Freeze overnight, loosely wrapped in plastic wrap. Take the frozen cubes out of the freezer and place them in tiny bags.
- Make a note of the kind of oil and herb in each bottle or bag. The frozen cubes may be thrown into your favorite spaghetti sauce, used to sauté veggies, poultry, or pork, or used as a basis for soups while sautéing onions.

Conclusion

This book was such a fun journey to take. We enjoyed telling you all about recipes you can make with different plants.

Now, it is not much different with herbs; they are green leaves, so they are great to add to your recipes.

Think about it. If you have a garden, you will enjoy smelling around different smells of each herb and pick out just exactly the one you need. Also, if you need more than anticipated, it is as easy as walking back in the yard and getting more!

Herbs have been used for many years for their medicinal properties, just as much as some spices do. Before refrigeration, herbs and spices were used to help food stay fresh longer.

Herbs are just extraordinary to use as a medicine or for home use.

This book has come to an end, but we hope or know you will keep making recipes with herbs.

Printed by Libri Plureos GmbH in Hamburg,
Germany